Malignant Tumors of the Thyroid

Rhoda H. Cobin David King Sirota
Editors

Malignant Tumors of the Thyroid

Clinical Concepts and Controversies

With 83 Illustrations

With Foreword by Terry F. Davies

Springer-Verlag
New York Berlin Heidelberg London Paris
Tokyo Hong Kong Barcelona Budapest

Rhoda H. Cobin, M.D.
Division of Endocrinology
Mount Sinai Medical Center
New York, NY, USA

David King Sirota, M.D.
Division of Endocrinology
Mount Sinai Medical Center
New York, NY, USA

Library of Congress Cataloging-in-Publication Data

Malignant tumors of the thyroid: clinical concepts and controversies
Rhoda H. Cobin, David King Sirota, editors.
p. cm.
Includes bibliographical references and index.
ISBN 0-387-97570-5 (alk. paper).—ISBN 3-540-97570-5 (alk. paper)
1. Thyroid gland—Cancer. I. Cobin, Rhoda H. II. Sirota, David King.
[DNLM: 1. Thyroid Neoplasms—pathology. 2. Thyroid Neoplasms—therapy. WK 270 M251]
RC280.T6M35 1992
616.99'444—dc20
DNLM/DLC
for Library of Congress

91-5201

Printed on acid-free paper.

Production managed by Christin R. Ciresi; Manufacturing supervised by Jacqui Ashri.
Typeset by Asco Trade Typesetting Ltd., Hong Kong.
Printed and bound by Edwards Brothers, Inc., Ann Arbor, MI.
Printed in the United States of America.

9 8 7 6 5 4 3 2 1

ISBN 0-387-97570-5 Springer-Verlag New York Berlin Heidelberg
ISBN 3-540-97570-5 Springer-Verlag Berlin Heidelberg New York

To David, Jonathan, Jeremy, and Jessica

and

To Teddy, Miriam, Eliot, and Ida

Foreword

Thyroid carcinoma is an uncommon malignancy. In the vast majority of patients, if treated appropriately, it is associated with a benign clinical course. Why then does it hold a continuing fascination for so many physicians?

The answer is probably directly dependent on the very benign nature of most thyroid malignancies. While there are terrible exceptions, the follicular and papillary thyroid cancers behave in a way quite alien to "common" neoplasia, since they grow and metastasize slowly. We believe that if only we could understand such a transformed state, we would be able to learn a great deal about the normal and abnormal regulation of the cell cycle and improve our understanding of cancer.

However, recent advances in the biology of normal cell division in general, and malignant cells in particular, have to date shed only dim light on our understanding of the human thyroid cell. There are clear and important reasons for this. First, the human thyroid cell has proven a difficult in vitro model and immortalized, fully differentiated thyroid cell lines are still not available (although they are under development in a number of laboratories). Second, only a few cell biologists have attempted to utilize the thyroid cell, including the available non-human lines, as models for cell cycle studies and oncogene/anti-oncogene regulation, because they are unaware of the often fundamental dichotomy between thyroid malignancy and prognosis. Third, the very nature of the benign clinical course has suggested to the major health research funding agencies that thyroid cancer is not worthy of study in a time of scarce resources.

Nothing could be further from the truth. This gratifying clinical course is the very reason why the study of human thyroid cancer has the potential for contributing further to our fundamental understanding of malignancy and, perhaps more importantly, the mechanisms by which the human body can resist neoplastic cells. In this regard, my colleagues are to be congratulated on putting together a timely review of the clinical nature and treatment of thyroid cancer. They have dealt with the common and the rare, the benign and the deadly, and have tried to bring clarity to an often "polluted" literature. Let this book be widely read in order that these diseases may become better understood within the general scientific community as well as by the many physicians and surgeons who will so obviously benefit from reading this book.

Terry F. Davies, MD, FRCP
New York, NY

Preface

Malignancies of the thyroid gland account for only a small fraction of all neoplasms, occurring in about 10,000 patients per year in the United States, or 40 per 1 million people.

Most of these tumors are well-differentiated and have a good prognosis; nonetheless, significant morbidity and mortality do occur. Appropriate management is essential to achieving optimal therapeutic success; however, there is considerable variability in current approaches to many aspects of the management of these tumors.

The purpose of this volume is to review analytically the major topics relating to malignant tumors of the thyroid gland. The contributors have presented an extensive overview of all areas of tumor biology—etiology, pathogenesis, pathophysiology, biochemistry, and genetics. As practicing clinical thyroidologists, they emphasize clinical presentation and therapy. In each chapter, recommendations for management are suggested by members of the division of endocrinology of the Mount Sinai Medical Center.

The Mount Sinai Medical Center has been a major center for the study and treatment of thyroid disorders for over a century. The contributors to this volume, current members of the faculty and staff, have benefited from the teaching and clinical expertise of such pioneers as Sergei Feitelberg, Solomon Silver, Louis J. Soffer, J. Lester Gabrilove, Solomon Berson, and our current division chief, Terry F. Davies.

An important aspect of division activities has always been the teaching of students, house staff, and endocrine fellows. This volume evolved from a series of seminars presented at our Thursday afternoon conferences to highlight new developments and controversies in the management of thyroid cancer.

It is our hope that the combined efforts of our contributors will provide the reader with information that is both up to date and comprehensive, as well as providing them with our guidelines for the care of patients with thyroid malignancy.

Contents

Contributors

Steven D. Averbuch, M.D. — Assistant Clinical Professor of Neoplastic Diseases, Mt. Sinai School of Medicine, New York, N.Y.; Associate Director, Clinical Research, Merck, Sharp, and Dohme Research Laboratories, Rahway, N.J.

Rhoda H. Cobin, M.D. — Associate Clinical Professor of Medicine and Endocrinology, Mt. Sinai School of Medicine; Associate Attending Physician, Mt. Sinai Hospital, New York, N.Y.

Terry F. Davies, M.B.B.S., MRCP, M.D. — Professor of Medicine and Endocrinology, Chief, Division of Endocrinology, Mt. Sinai School of Medicine; Attending Physician, Mt. Sinai Hospital, New York, N.Y.

Robert P. Fiedler, M.D. — Assistant Clinical Professor of Medicine and Endocrinology, Mt. Sinai School of Medicine; Assistant Attending Physician, Mt. Sinai Hospital, New York, N.Y.

Eugene W. Friedman, M.D. — Professor of Surgical Oncology, Chief Division of Head and Neck Surgery, Mt. Sinai School of Medicine; Attending Surgeon, Mt. Sinai Hospital, New York, N.Y.

Jeffrey I. Mechanick, M.D. — Assistant Clinical Professor of Medicine and Endocrinology, Mt. Sinai School of Medicine; Assistant Attending Physician, Mt. Sinai Hospital, New York, N.Y.

Edward Merker, M.D. — Assistant Clinical Professor of Medicine and Endocrinology, Mt. Sinai School of Medicine; Assistant Attending Physician, Mt. Sinai Hospital; Associate Physician, Lenox Hill Hospital, New York, N.Y.

Arthur F. Schwartz, M.D. Associate Clinical Professor of Surgery, Mt. Sinai School of Medicine; Associate Attending Surgeon, Mt. Sinai Hospital, New York, N.Y.

Robert L. Segal, M.D. Associate Professor of Medicine and Endocrinology, Mt. Sinai School of Medicine; Associate Attending Physician, Mt. Sinai Hospital, New York, N.Y.

Marvin W. Sinkoff, M.D. Senior Clinical Instructor in Medicine and Endocrinology, Mt. Sinai School of Medicine; Assistant Attending Physician, Mt. Sinai Hospital; Attending Physician, Beth Israel Hospital, New York, N.Y.

David K. Sirota, M.D. Associate Clinical Professor of Medicine and Endocrinology, Mt. Sinai School of Medicine; Associate Attending Physician, Mt. Sinai Hospital; Attending Endocrinologist, Jewish Home and Hospital for Aged, New York, N.Y.

Alex Stagnaro-Green, M.D. Assistant Professor of Medicine and Endocrinology, Mt. Sinai School of Medicine; Assistant Attending Physician, Mt. Sinai Hospital, New York, N.Y.

Andrew J. Werner, M.D. Assistant Clinical Professor of Medicine and Endocrinology, Mt. Sinai School of Medicine; Associate Attending Physician, Mt. Sinai Hospital, New York, N.Y.; Consultant Physician in Endocrinology-Metabolism and Internal Medicine, Hospital for Joint Diseases-Orthopedic Institute, New York, N.Y.

Li-Teh Wu, M.D. Instructor of Neoplastic Diseases, Mt. Sinai School of Medicine; Assistant Attending Physician, Mt. Sinai Hospital, New York, N.Y.

1

Papillary Thyroid Carcinoma

ALEX STAGNARO-GREEN

Thyroid cancer is the most common form of endocrine malignancy; papillary cancer accounts for more than 50% of all thyroid carcinoma. Despite over fifty years of research on papillary carcinoma and hundreds of published articles, many questions remain unanswered.[1] In particular, the actual mortality rate from papillary cancer and the optimal therapeutic approach remain unknown. Furthermore, although prognostic indicators at diagnosis are known and predictive models have been formulated, the constellation of signs and symptoms yielding the best and worst prognosis needs further refinement. Confusion in the literature is caused by the following problems: (1) the lack of prospective studies comparing various treatment regimens or predictive models, (2) inconsistencies in the literature in regard to the pathologic definition of papillary cancer, (3) the failure of many articles to evaluate papillary cancer separately from follicular cancer, and (4) the need for a 20- to 30-year follow-up—papillary carcinoma is often deadly decades after initial diagnosis.

Pathology

The pathology of papillary carcinoma is marked by tremendous microscopic variability. Nevertheless, the constellation of findings present on examination by light microscopy typically makes diagnosis easy.[2] In this section we will discuss not only the gross pathology of papillary cancer but also the findings obtained by light microscopy, as well as by electron microscopy. Special attention will be given to distinctive features of the nucleus, specifically the "Orphan Annie Eyes," as well as to nuclear folding. Furthermore, the origin and significance of psammoma bodies in papillary cancer will be reviewed. This section will conclude with a discussion of the rationale for the present system of calling a cancer papillary carcinoma in spite of the fact that the majority of the tumor may be follicullar.

On gross examination the majority of papillary cancer are tan in color. In cases in which hemorrhage has occurred or in which fibrosis is prevalent the tumor may have areas of either red or gray.[3] On palpation the tumor is firm.[4] Nevertheless, in 47% of the cases in one series small cysts are present and are filled with a "thin brown fluid".[3] Encapsulation of the tumor is seen on examination in 22% of the cases[3] and is more commonly seen in predominately cystic lesions as compared with solid tumors.[2]

In 1971 Woolner described papillary cancer seen by light microscopy: "The typical histologic picture is a mixture of papillary excrescenses and neoplastic follicles containing varying degrees of colloid"[5] (Fig. 1.1). The percentage of papillary versus follicular elements in papillary cancer is quite varied.[6] The papillae have a central fibrovascular area that is composed of a vascular network with interspersed connective tissue.[7] Lining the fibrovascular core is an epithelium of cells, typically a monolayer, that is cuboidal in shape although it sometimes approaches a columnar morphol-

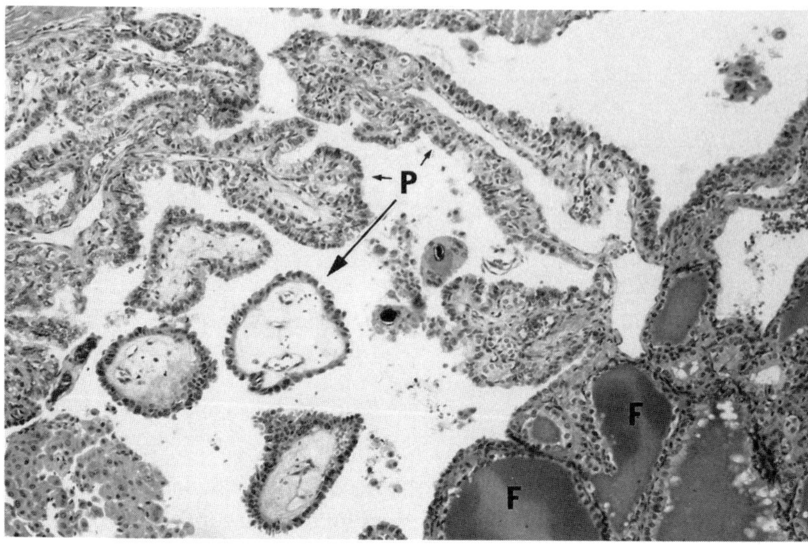

Figure 1.1. 100x original magnification hematoxylin-eosin stain of papillary thyroid carcinoma with papillae (P) and follicular differentiation (F).

ogy.[3] The cytoplasm is typically described as amphophilic; it has an abundance of both mitochondria and cytoplasmic filaments as documented by electron microscopy.[4]

The most intensely studied aspect of papillary cancer pathology is the nucleus. The appearance of the nucleus under a light microscope reveals a round or oval nucleus that is somewhat enlarged (Fig. 1.2). The nucleus is hypodense with large areas that appear empty and are apparently devoid of chromatin.[4,8,9] Consequently, the nuclei appear opaque and have been given many names including "clear," "pale," "watery," or—the most imaginative—"Orphan Annie Eyes" (Fig. 1.2). Furthermore, a nuclear groove, which at times seems to almost divide the nucleus in half, is frequently found (Fig. 1.2). Electron microscopic evaluation of the nucleus reveals chromatin that is very dispersed, as well as a high degree of nuclear folding.[4,7] Furthermore, there are frequent and deep invagations of the cytoplasm into the nucleus. Some authors believe that the nuclear groove is a reflection of the cytoplasmic intrusions into the nucleus.[10]

The etiology of the "Orphan Annie Eyes" nucleus has been the subject of much debate. Some authors believe it is simply an artifact since the phenomenon is not present in frozen sections.[7] On the other hand, other researchers argue that because it is so reproducible it must reflect a fundamental abnormality.[4] Still others believe that the dispersed nature of the chromatin as shown by electron microscopy is demonstrated in light microscopy by the presence of a clear nucleus.[11] Nevertheless, the empty nucleus is one of the most consistent findings in papillary cancer. Hapke and Dehner found the Orphan Annie Eye in 83% of thyroid cancer but in only two nonmalignant thyroid lesions (2%).[12] They concluded that "clear nuclei when present as a diffuse change in a thyroid tumor are a reliable sign of papillary carcinoma but are not pathognomonic."

Two studies have evaluated the sensitivity and specificity of the nuclear groove as a means of diagnosis of papillary cancer. Chan and Saw found the nuclear groove to be present in 89 consecutive cases of papillary cancer but present in only 2 thyroid specimens that were non-malignant.[10] Shurbaji et al. evaluated 124 consecutive thyroid aspirates for the presence of a nuclear groove.[13] They found grooved nuclei in all 11 cases of papillary cancer but in only 2 out of the 113 cases that were not papil-

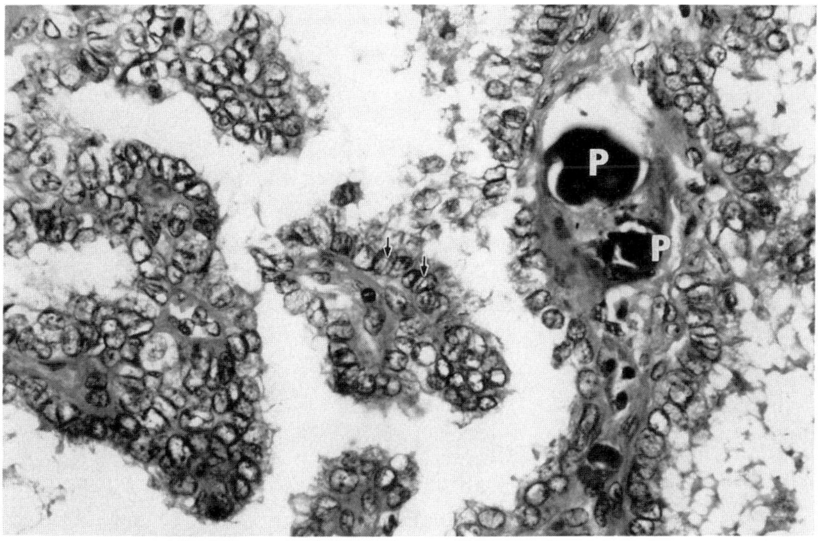

Figure 1.2. 100x original magnification hematoxylin-eosin stain of papillary thyroid carcinoma with papillae lined by uniform cells containing "Orphan Annie Nuclei," nuclear grooves (arrow), and psammoma bodies (P).

lary cancer. Consequently, the nuclear groove may be the most sensitive indicator of papillary cancer, with a specificity that approaches, but does not reach, 100%.

Consequently, the diagnosis of papillary cancer via pathology is not based on any single criteria, but on a constellation of findings. In particular, papillae projecting into open spaces, as well as clear nuclei with prominent nuclear grooves, are all important features of the diagnosis. Another important indicator of the presence of papillary carcinoma is psammoma bodies (Fig. 1.2). Psammoma bodies (Greek *psammoma* is "sand") are calcific areas that are laminated.[3] Their rate of incidence in papillary cancer is 50% in most series.[7,9,14] Although their etiology is still unclear, in general they are believed to represent the remains of dead papillae.[2] Psammoma bodies are quite specific for papillary cancer and are rarely seen in other thyroid lesions.[9] They can be found some distance from malignant cells; therefore they serve as a signal for the physician to search thoroughly for papillary cancer.[2]

A source of much confusion in the classification of thyroid cancer has been the dilemma of how to classify a lesion which has papillary elements intermixed with follicular components (Fig. 1.1). Early studies based the diagnosis on that histologic type that predominated. However, over the years it has become apparent that tumors that possess papillary tissue, regardless of the amount, behave in a manner similar to a lesion that is completely papillary in nature (Crile and Hazard).[15] In 1973 Franssila evaluated the course of 230 cases of thyroid cancer that ware recorded in the Finnish Cancer Registry.[16] He found that a comparison of tumors that were mainly papillary with tumors that were a mixture of papillary and follicular components demonstrated a similar prognosis. The survival curve for patients with these tumors differed markedly however from the group of patients with follicular cancer. These results confirm the findings of Crile and Hazard in addition to presenting strong evidence for the classification of tumors as papillary even if follicular elements predominate.

Discussion of the clinical characteristics of papillary carcinoma of the thyroid is divided into tumors greater than 1.5 cm and tumors that are less than or equal to 1.5 cm (occult papillary carcinoma of the thyroid). This reflects the exceedingly benign course that occult papillary cancer has compared with papillary tumors that exceed 1.5 cm

Table 1.1. Papillary cancer of the thyroid greater than 1.5 cm

	Years of study	Follow-up (years)	No. patients	Age (years)	Sex	Mortality (%)	Death due to local recurrence (%)	Death due to distant metastase (%)	Age associated with increased mortality (years)	Recurrence (%)
Frazell & Foote (1958)[17]	1930–1954		393	—	111M/280F	12	50	50	>40	—
Underwood et al. (1958)[18]	1924–1955		62	—	12M/50F	5	—	—	—	—
Beahrs et al. (1959)[19]	1938–1947		136	42	—	5	—	—	—	—
Hirabayashi et al. (1961)[20]	1920–1959		286	—	—	11	—	—	>40	—
Tollefsen et al. (1963)[21]	1930–1957	11	282	—	—	7	—	—	—	—
Noguchi et al. (1970)[22]	1967–1968		71	—	—	—	—	—	—	—
Crile (1971)[23]	1937–1964	10	307	—	—	5	—	—	—	—
Franssila (1973)[16]	1958–1962	12	100	49	1M/3.3F	21	56	44	—	—
Beaugie et al. (1976)[24]	1945–1972		81	—	1M/2.5F	20	63	37	>50	—
Mazzaferri & Young (1981)[25]	1962–1977	10	576	32	221M/355F	1	—	—	>40	14.6
Samman et al. (1983)[26]	1951–1975		574	—	—	9	—	—	—	18
Rossi et al. (1985)[27]	1931–1970	15	554	—	—	11	—	—	>50	24
Carcangiu et al. (1985)[7]		6.3	241	41	67M/174F	6	—	—	>40	—
McConahey et al. (1986)[29]	1946–1970	18	859	44	276M/583F	7	36	61	>50	—
DeGroot et al. (1990)[30]	1968–1988	12	269	—	88M/181F	8	—	—	>45	25
Total			4791			8				

Papillary Cancer Larger Than 1.5 cm

A review of 15 series of papillary cancer is presented in Table 1.1.[16–30] All series that had a confirmed pathologic diagnosis of papillary cancer and had follow-up data are included. Some of the studies include tumors less than 1.5 cm in their analysis; however, for purposes of completeness these will be included. Excluded from review were studies that did not have the diagnosis proven by pathology or in which subsequent studies published by the same group either clarified the earlier data or repeated large sections of the data. Areas left blank in the table reflect data that were not available. Mortality data included reflect death directly due to papillary cancer. The data reviewed represents a total of 4791 cases of papillary carcinoma of the thyroid.

The series reviewed includes studies with as few as 62 cases of papillary cancer and as many as 859 cases. Six of the studies were part of a larger review of all types of thyroid carcinoma. In these studies papillary cancer of the thyroid comprised 44% to 81% of the total cases of thyroid cancer. Only in the papers by Franssila[16] (Finland) and Beaugie et al.[24] (England) did papillary cancer comprise less than 50% of the total. It appears that papillary cancer is clearly the predominant form of thyroid cancer.

Table 1.1 shows that women are prone to develop papillary cancer. Every study that included the sex of the patient demonstrated that women had a greater tendency to develop papillary cancer than men did. Analysis of all the available data reveals a female-to-male ratio of 2.1:1 (1623:775). Although well documented, the reason that women have a tendency to develop papillary carcinoma of the thyroid is not yet understood.

McConahey et al. found in the Mayo Clinic series that the two most common presenting symptoms of papillary cancer were a mass in the neck and cervical adenopathy, which were reported, respectively, by 64% and 22% of their patients.[30] In their series of 859 patients, examination of the neck revealed a solitary nodule in 56% of the patients and two or more nodules in 21%. Of the 158 patients who had a nuclear medicine scan performed, 84 revealed a cold nodule, 3 had a hot nodule, 6 demonstrated "patchy uptake," and 65 had scans that revealed "no focal uptake."

Papillary cancer consistently affects a younger age group than follicular, medullary, or anaplastic cancer. In those studies where the mean age at the time of initial presentation was available it ranged from 32 to 49 years. It should be noted that there appears to be a direct correlation between mortality and mean age at presentation. Consequently, the study that included patients with the lowest mean age at presentation had the lowest mortality rate.

The mean size of the cancer in studies where this data was available was 2.4 to 2.5 cm. Length of follow-up in the studies varied from 6.3 to 18 years. An extended period of follow-up is needed because papillary carcinoma has been shown to be the cause of death as long as 39 years following the initial diagnosis of the cancer. It should be noted that despite the existence of this wide range, the majority of deaths occur within the first five years.

The extent of spread of papillary cancer at the time of diagnosis has been an area of great interest. In particular, the degree of multicentricity of papillary cancer has been utilized by many to advocate subtotal thyroidectomies as opposed to more conservative surgical procedures. A true estimate of multicentricity is difficult to obtain because an accurate determination requires that all patients have cervical neck dissections and that serial sections be performed by the pathologist. The literature shows an incidence of multicentricity ranging from 11% to 46%. The majority of studies reveal an incidence of approximately 20%. This correlates well with a 1960 study by Black et al. who concluded that the incidence of multicentricity of papillary cancer is at least 20%.[31] Degroot et al., in the most recent study published on papillary cancer of the thyroid, found multifocality in 46% of all cases.[30] The high percentage found in their study probably reflects the extensive nature of the surgery performed in their series (65.8% had total or near total thyroidectomies). It can be concluded that multiple foci of papillary cancer are present in a minimum of 20% of all cases but that the actual incidence is probably closer to the 46% found by Black et al.

The extent that papillary cancer spreads through the thyroid capsule to surrounding local structures at the time of initial diagnosis has been reported by only a few authors. This lack of information probably reflects the retrospective nature of all of these studies, as well as the fact that many of the studies that were reviewed combined all differentiated thyroid cancers into one group. Although the range of local extrathyroidal spread in the literature was quite marked (5% to 33%), extrathyroidal spread of papillary cancer at the time of diagnosis was associated with an increased mortality rate in every study. In these patients death was secondary to obstructive symptoms caused by the tumor growth as well as to invasion into local structures. Furthermore, Mazzaferri and Young reported that the recurrence rate was adversely affected by the presence of extrathyroidal spread at the time of diagnosis.[25]

Cervical node metastases present at the time of diagnosis have been found to be present in as few as 11% of the cases and in as many as 72% of all patients. Comparison of the various results is again difficult because the surgical procedure performed, as well as the diligence of the pathologist, has a direct effect on the results obtained. Nevertheless, a compilation of all the results shows that 45% (1412/3196) of the reported cases had documentation of cervical nodal metastasis. The effect that the nodes have on mortality is, however, intriguing. Unlike most cancers, in which the presence of adenopathy is an indicator of a poor prognosis, no study has shown an increased mortality rate associated with the presence of spread of this cancer to cervical nodes. In fact, early literature in this area hypothesized that cervical nodes are somehow protective and decrease mortality; indeed, two studies show an inverse relationship between cervical metastases and mortality. However, the majority of the studies show no relationship between cervical node involvement and survival. The lack of increased mortality in individuals with cervical metastases remains baffling. It appears to be related to the fact that the presence of cervical nodes is much more frequent in younger patients and, as discussed previously, mortality is directly related to age. Nevertheless, the explanation of the benign behavior of nodal metastasis in papillary cancer remains an unanswered question.

Six studies presented data on the presence of distant metastases at the time of initial diagnosis. The incidence of these metastases was always under 10%, ranging from 0.75% to 8.7%. The average rate of distant metastasis was 4.2% (109/2624); pulmonary metastases were the most common, followed by metastases to bone sites.

The rate of recurrence of papillary cancer of the thyroid was relatively consistent among the various studies, ranging from 14.6% to 25.3%. In most studies recurrence was defined as the reappearance of thyroid cancer, diagnosed by either pathology or radioiodine uptake, following a disease-free interval. The frequency of recurrence appeared to be highest in the cervical nodes, followed by distant metastasis and local extrathyroidal recurrence.

The mortality data presented in Table 1.1 reflects deaths that were directly due to papillary cancer. The range from the various studies was 1% to 21% with an overall average mortality of 8% from all studies combined. Analysis of the studies with the lowest and highest mortality rates may yield insights into the results obtained. Mazzaferri and Young's study revealed the lowest mortality rate (1%).[25] However, of all the studies their patient population was the youngest (32 years). Furthermore, the 21% mortality discovered by Franssila was found in a population with the oldest mean age (49 years).[16] Consequently, the low and high mortality rates found in these studies is probably a reflection of the mean age of the population sampled, as almost every study has shown a direct correlation between age and mortality. Deaths were evenly divided between those caused by local spread and those due to the effects of distant metastasis (mainly pulmonary).

It can be concluded therefore that the overall mortality of 8% is accurate in general, but for any individual it is affected by a variety of factors. In particular, the following variables were found to typically correlate with a poor prognosis: (1) increased age (above either 40 or 50 years), (2) increased size of the tumor (typically above 4 cm), (3) the presence of extrathyroidal spread at the time of diagnosis, and (4) the presence of distant metastasis at initial diagnosis. Two of the studies reviewed found that males had a higher mortality rate compared to females, but three other studies found no such relationship.

Two studies are noteworthy because they reviewed the characteristics of a large number of deaths due to papillary cancer that occurred in a single medical center. Tollefsen et al. reported on 70 fatal cases evaluated at Memorial Hospital for Cancer and Allied Diseases[32] and Smith et al. discussed 56 fatal cases from the Mayo Clinic and Medical Center.[33] Due to the uniqueness of these studies, they will be discussed separately.

Tollenfsen et al. reviewed 70 deaths caused by papillary cancer from 1930 to 1962. They found 64% of the deaths occurred in women, as opposed to 36% in men. Furthermore, the mean age at diagnosis was 52 years. These results were compared to a control group of survivors (n = 262) whose mean age was 39 years and was 28% male. At diagnosis, 20% of the patients who eventually expired had recurrent laryngeal nerve paralysis, versus only 3% of the controls. Furthermore, at the time of diagnosis 29% had tumors greater than 5 cm, in contrast to 9.5% of the controls. The median survival time for all 70 patients was 5 years; however, those individuals (n = 28) whose initial surgery was not curative survived only 14 months. The cause of death was due to local recurrence in the neck (40%), pulmonary dissemination (31%), brain metastasis (10%), and bone involvement (10%).

Smith et al. performed a case-control study matching (for age and sex) 56 patients who died from papillary cancer with 56 survivors selected from a total of 803 survivors of papillary cancer. The mean age for the fatal cases was 59 years versus 42.4 years ($p < .05$) for the survivors as a whole. Interestingly, the fatal cases had a male-to-female ratio of 1.0:0.93 compared to 1.0:2.25 in the group of survivors. The group in which the cancer proved lethal showed a significant increase in hoarseness, vocal cord paralysis, and extrathyroidal invasion as well as larger tumor size (4.3 cm vs. 1.9 cm) compared with the control group. Furthermore, local tumor recurrence was seen in 41% of the fatal cases and in 0% of the cases in which patients survived ($p < .001$), and distant spread was seen in 80% of those who died and in 0% of the survivors ($p < .0001$). The mean survival time for the 56 individuals who died was 8.5 years (range: 1 month to 31 years) with 14% of the deaths occurring after 20 years. The most frequent cause of death was pulmonary involvement (37%), followed by local extension (36%) and neurologic involvement (21%).

These two studies confirmed some indicators of poor progosis and shed new light on another. Confirmed are the associations of increasing age, size of the primary tumor, and extrathyroidal invasion with an increased mortality rate. The studies also provide further support for the widely held belief that death due to papillary thyroid cancer needs to be monitored over decades, as opposed to a limited 5 year follow-up. On the other hand, these studies support the notion that, although papillary thyroid cancer has a higher incidence in women, it is more often lethal in men. This was found to be particularly true in the study by Smith et al. in which the male-to-female mortality ratio was greater than unity.

Occult Papillary Carcinoma of the Thyroid

The concept of occult papillary carcinoma of the thyroid is one that has evolved over time. In 1942 Frantz et al. described thyroid tissue that was normal but displaced laterally in the neck and coined the term "lateral aberrant thyroid."[34] What was not appreciated was that these were, in actuality, metastasis from small foci of primary neoplasm within the thyroid gland. In 1948 Wozencraft et al. clarified their true nature as being a thyroid metastasis from a small, nonpalpable focus within the thyroid.[35] The first series published on this topic came from Memorial Hospital in 1948, in which three cases were described.[35] That paper strongly advocated careful pathologic review of the thyroid to try to locate a primary lesion, arguing that it is never normal to find thyroid tissue lateral to the carotid sheath.

The definition of occult carcinoma is a thyroid cancer the longest axis of which is equal to, or less than, 1.5 cm.[16,24,25,28,29,36–45] There is disagreement in the literature regarding whether or not to include primary tumors that are palpable. For the purposes of this discussion we will define occult carcinoma as being tumors that are equal to or less than 1.5 cm, regardless of whether or not they are palpable. This definition is consistent with the majority of the published literature. What will become apparent in this review is the benign course individuals have with this disease despite the frequent presence of cervical metastasis. A total of 1579 cases of papillary cancer less than or equal to 1.5 cm were reviewed (see Table 1.2). Five studies were performed in America, four in Japan, and data are included from eight other countries. It should be noted that five of the studies were autopsy studies, whereas the rest of the studies were retrospective analysis of patients who underwent thyroid surgery. In the following discussion, comparison will be made between the autopsy and retrospective studies of occult papillary cancer. Furthermore, both groups will be compared to these studies reviewed earlier which included patients whose primary thyroid tumor was greater than 1.5 cm.

Review of the retrospective studies reveals that occult cancer comprises 14% to 46% of all papillary carcinoma. In particular, all the studies done in the United States show an incidence of 25% or greater. The percentages of occult papillary cancer of the thyroid detected at autopsy in a given population are even more revealing. Although the overall range is 5% to 28%, there is a clear dichotomy between indi-

Table 1.2. Occult papillary carcinoma of the thyroid

	Years of study	Follow-up (years)	No. patients	% of patients with occult	Sex	Definition of papillary carcinoma (cm)	Autopsy study	Cervical metastases (%)	Country	Age (years)	Mortality (%)	Multicentricity (%)
Hazard (1960)[36]	1926–1953		56	25	9M/47F	≤1.5	N	23	US		1.8	36
Sampson et al. (1969, 1970, 1970)[37–39]	1951–1968		525	17	251M/274F	≤1.5	Y	27	Japan		0.2	33
Sampson et al. (1974)[40]	1969–1970		8	6	—	<1.5	Y	—	US		—	38
Franssila (1973)[16]	1958–1962	12	19	19	—	—	N	—	Finland		—	—
Fukunaga & Yatani (1975)[41]						<1.5	Y	2			0	—
			6	6	3M/3F				Canada			
			29	28	16M/13F				Japan			
			10	9	2M/8F				Poland			
			33	5	23M/11F				Columbia			
			60	24	29M/31F				Hawaii			
Beaugie et al. (1976)[24]	1945–1972		13	16	—	—	N	38	England		7.7	—
Sobrinho-Simoes et al. (1979)[42]	1972–1977		39	6.5	9M/30F	—	Y	5	Portugal	61	—	31
Hubert et al. (1980)[43]		25	137	25	1M:3F	≤1.5	N	40	US	41	1	—
Mazzaferri & Young (1981)[25]	1962–1977	10	153	34	—	<1.5	N	—	US		0	—
Bondeson & Ljungberg (1981)[44]			32	6.4	14M/18F	<1.0	Y	—	Sweden		0	—
Schroder et al. (1984)[45]	—	7.7	32	18	1M:3F	≤1.5	N	56	Germany	45	0	—
Carcangiu et al. (1985)[7]	—	6.3	31	14	—	≤1.0	N	65	Italy		0	—
McConahey et al. (1986)[29]	1946–1970	18	396	46	—	≤1.5	N		US		0.3	—
Total			1579									

viduals of a Japanese background and those of other nationalities. The studies that were either performed in Japan or include Japanese living in Hawaii reveal an incidence of occult cancer of 17% to 28%. In contrast, the range for the rest of the studies is 5% to 9%. In contrast to the increased rate of occult papillary cancer seen in the Japanese population, their incidence of clinically apparent papillary cancer of the thyroid is similar to that of other populations. This has led some authors to speculate that although more thyroid carcinogens are present in Japan there is a relative paucity of promoting factors.[41,46]

Of the eight retrospective studies, three presented data regarding the sex distribution of individuals with occult papillary cancer. The three confirmed the marked tendency for women to develop cancer found in the earlier review of papillary cancer. In contrast, the autopsy studies do not show this tendency. An analysis of all the autopsy data reveals a male–female ratio of 10:11 (347:388). Consequently, occult papillary cancer of the thyroid diagnosed at autopsy lacks the distribution by sex seen in papillary cancer, even in occult papillary cancer that had come to surgical excision. The reasons for this discrepancy are not known.

Cervical nodes involved with tumor were present in 23% to 65% of the retrospective studies—an average of 41% (111/269). Surprisingly, this is only somewhat decreased from the 45% found in papillary tumors larger than 1.5 cm. The percentage of involved cervical nodal metastasis in the autopsy studies was considerably lower, ranging from 1.5% to 27%. It is impossible to tell if this reflects a true difference or if it is instead secondary to differences in the extent of cervical neck dissection and/or pathlogic review performed in the various studies.

Mortality data reveal five deaths attributable to occult papillary cancer in the 1579 patients reviewed. Review of the literature reveals one other case of death due to occult papillary cancer.[47] Consequently, the mortality rate is

0.38% (6/1580). This confirms the benign course of this tumor; an outcome suggested by Woolner et al. in 1960[48] and confirmed in every subsequent study. Clinical information on the cause of death in five of the six patients was available. All five of these individuals had distant spread of the tumor; one patient also exhibited local recurrence. In the three instances where sex and age were available all three individuals were men with a mean age of 61 years. Although these data are obviously limited, there is a suggestion of an increased mortality in older men, with occult papillary cancer with distant spread (most frequently pulmonary) being the cause of death.

In conclusion, occult papillary carcinoma of the thyroid, although frequent, is rarely deadly. Consequently, once the diagnosis is made it portends an excellent prognosis. One caveat to this is that older men may have a slightly worse prognosis than the group of occult papillary cancer patients as a whole.

Nuclear DNA Content

The challenge in treating patients with papillary cancer is to identify those individuals who have the worst prognosis. Clearly, certain characteristics such as advanced age, larger tumor size, and extrathyroidal and distant metastasis are associated with increased mortality. Nevertheless, the majority of individuals with these risk factors do not die from papillary cancer. Consequently, a novel marker is needed to identify more precisely those individuals with a poor prognosis. Research in the past decade has focused on the cellular DNA content of individuals with papillary cancer. The assumption is that patients with nondiploid nuclear DNA, be it aneuploid or tetraploid, would have a worse prognosis. To be of use, this predictor would need to serve as an indicator independent of other known prognostic indicators, as analyzed by multivariate analysis. This section will review eight studies that attempt to answer this question.

Johannessen et al. (1983) reported a case of a 70-year-old woman with papillary cancer who in a 9-year period had tumor spread to the thoracic wall, groin, and thigh before she died from an unrelated disease.[49] Flow cytometry of the DNA revealed that although diploid cells were present, the majority of the cells were tetraploid. They postulated that the aberrant nature of the cellular content was responsible for the tumor's invasive behavior. They noted that DNA cellular analysis of papillary cancer had in no prior case revealed a tumor with tetraploid cells.

In 1986 Joensuu evaluated the DNA content of 125 patients with differentiated thyroid cancer, 82 of whom had papillary cancer.[50] Flow cytometry revealed that 75% ($n = 62$) of the papillary group had diploid cells, whereas 24% ($n = 20$) had aneuploid cells. Analysis of the 10-year survival rate for the two groups revealed a 95.7% survival rate in patients with diploid DNA versus 75.4% in individuals with aneuploidy. For the entire 125 patients of the study, aneuploidy was associated with increased mortality ($p < .0001$) as well as with an older age group ($p < .002$). However, utilizing Cox's stepwise proportional hazard model, the age of the patient, pathology, and tumor size were independent prognosticators of survival, but aneuploidy was not. They postulate that the poor prognosis seen in older patients with papillary cancer is due in part to an increase in aneuploidy with age.

Further data on the role of nuclear DNA content in papillary cancer appeared in an article in the *World Journal of Surgery* in 1984 by Cohn et al.[51] Ten individuals who died from papillary cancer were compared to a control group of 80 survivors. Analysis of the DNA content revealed that all 10 nonsurvivors had in excess of 70% aneuploid cells, whereas all of the survivors had less than 60% aneuploid cells at analysis. They conclude that DNA analysis may offer important prognostic information. However their study did not perform multiple regression analysis to determine if DNA cellular analysis is an independent prognostic variable.

In 1986 Bachdahl et al. extended the work of Cohn et al. by performing the requisite statistical tests.[52] They compared the 10 patients who died of papillary cancer to the 80 survivors and performed multiple linear regression analysis. They found that for papillary cancer the nuclear DNA cell content was a better prognostic indicator than all known indicators combined. Furthermore, regression analysis revealed that DNA content added further prognostic information when compared to the other known indicators. They concluded that nuclear DNA measurement should be performed on all patients with papillary cancer.

Smith et al. performed a retrospective case-control study of 56 lethal cases of papillary cancer and compared it to a control group of 56 survivors matched for age and sex.[33] They performed flow cytometry to assess nuclear DNA content in 20 lethal cases and in 20 matched controls. They found that 25% (n = 5) of the lethal group exhibited aneuploidy as compared with 0% of the survivors ($p < .05$). They concluded that DNA ploidy is a prognosticator in papillary cancer; however, they did not perform a multiple regression analysis.

In 1989 Ekman et al. performed nuclear DNA measurement on 32 cases of papillary cancer diagnosed at age 20 or younger.[53] They found that 81% (n = 26) exhibited a diploid pattern and 19% (n = 6) revealed aneuploidy. Despite a median follow-up of 22 years (range: 10 to 35 years) there were no deaths in their series. Furthermore, the 2 patients who presented with lung metastasis and the 5 patients with local recurrence all had diploid nuclei. They concluded that nuclear DNA analysis does not yield prognostic information in young patients. They also demonstrated that a significant proportion of patients under 20 years exhibit aneuploidy.

Another study evaluating the impact of nuclear ploidy in papillary thyroid carcinoma was published in 1990 in the *International Journal of Cancer*. Schelfhout et al. performed flow cytometry on 168 patients whose cases were followed for 9.5 years, 71 of whom had papillary cancer.[54] They found that the cellular DNA was aneuploid in 23% of the cases of papillary cancer and that aneuploidy was more common in individuals with moderately differentiated malignancies than in well-differentiated malignancies ($p < .001$). Furthermore, the 10-year survival rate was lower in those individuals with moderately differentiated tumors. Nevertheless, due to the presence of benign adenomas in their study that were aneuploid, as well as near-diploid undifferentiated carcinoma, they concluded that the relationship between survival and cellular DNA content was nuclear.

The most recent study addressing this topic was published in 1990 and was included in a book on thyroid carcinoma in the *Endocrinology and Metabolism Clinics of North America* series. Hay reported on 209 patients with papillary carcinoma who had had DNA analysis performed.[55] Median follow-up time for the group was 15.5 years. He found that DNA aneuploidy was associated with the highest mortality rate and that diploid tumors had the lowest mortality; patients who were polyploid had a mortality rate between the two extremes ($p < 0.0001$). Furthermore, DNA content was found to be an indepent prognosticator when analyzed by both the EORTC (European Organization for Research on Treatment of Thyroid Cancer) and AGES [A (patient age), G (tumor grade), E (extent of local invasion and distant metastes), S (size of the tumor)] classification schemas. Hay concluded that nuclear DNA analysis yielded important prognostic information and stated that " . . . we at the Mayo clinic plan to offer DNA ploidy as a routine laboratory test. . . ."[55]

Thus two studies have demonstrated that, when subjected to multiple regression analysis, cellular DNA content is found to be an independent prognostic indicator. However, certain caveats remain. Ekman et al. have demonstrated that aneuploidy is common in young patients without adverse effects. Schelfout et al. have shown that benign adenomas may be aneuploid and that deadly undifferentiated thyroid cancer may be diploid. Therefore, the role of flow cytometry still requires further study. Prospective studies controlling for the type of surgery and medical therapy are needed to further clarify the role of nuclear DNA as a prognosticator for those individuals with the worst prognosis.

Predictive Models

Due to the lack of precision in predicting which patients with papillary cancer will have the worst prognosis, three predictive models have been proposed. All three models utilize standard clinical criteria in a multivariate analysis in order to predict which patients have the greatest likelihood of death secondary to thyroid cancer. The models are the European Organization for Research on Treatment of Thyroid Cancer (EORTC, published in 1979),[56] the AGES model (proposed in 1987),[57] and the AMES model (published in 1988).[58] All three models will be reviewed below. However, it is important to note that none of the models have been evaluated prospectively.

From 1966 to 1977 The European Thyroid Cancer Co-operative Group gathered data on 1183 thyroid cancer patients from 23 European Hospitals.[56] Their study included individuals with all types of thyroid cancer and was not limited to patients with papillary cancer. Follow-up data was available on 507 individuals (median follow-up: 54 months). Utilizing multivariate analysis (Weibull survival model) they developed a mathematical model to predict prognosis in patients with thyroid cancer. Specifically, age at the time of presentation, sex, pathologic diagnosis, presence of an anaplastic component, extension of the primary tumor, and presence of one or more distant metastases are each assigned a numerical score, and are then tallied for each patient. Utilizing an actuarial table the patient's score can then be used to predict the expected five-year survival rate.

Three retrospective studies published from 1980 to 1987 evaluated the utility of the EORTC prognostic index for thyroid carcinoma. Hannequin et al. used the EORTC criteria to evaluate 480 French patients with thyroid cancer.[59] They found that although the majority of the EORTC criteria were validated, their own classification system yielded better prognostic information. They concluded that for each population studied, a separate prognostic schema would need to be established using multifactorial analysis. However, Kerr et al. found that the EORTC index was applicable to their 441 patients in England with thyroid carcinoma.[60] They found the EORTC index was predictive of survival in their group and concluded by recommending " . . . the adoption of their (EORTC) prognostic index as an aid to prediction of survival. . . ." Tennvall et al. applied the EORTC prognostic index to 226 cases of differentiated thyroid carcinoma.[61] They found that only three of the EORTC criteria were significantly associated with survival in their study population. They questioned the validity of the EORTC index for patients with differentiated thyroid carcinoma, concluding that separate prognostic indexes should be formed for each of the histologic variants of thyroid carcinoma.

In 1987 Hay et al. published a prognostic scoring system designed specifically for papillary cancer. Hay et al. performed a retrospective analysis of 860 patients with papillary carcinoma of the thyroid who were treated at the Mayo Clinic from 1946 to 1970.[57] Median follow-up was 18.3 years in the group of patients who survived. Fourteen prognostic variable were subjected to a step-up multiple regression analysis. Patient's age (A), the tumor grade (G), the presence of local invasion and distant metastases—the extent (E), and size (S) of the tumor were shown to be independent prognostic variables utilizing their model (AGES). Patients were then evaluated using these four criteria, after which a numerical score was derived that yielded prognostic information.

Cady and Rossi published a prognostic scale based on experience with 821 patients at the Lahey Clinic Foundation.[58] Their scale included patients with both papillary and follicular carcinoma and, similarly to the scales previously reviewed, it was retrospective in nature. Their scale is based solely on clinical criteria and included the following four variables: patient age (A), distant metastases (M), the extent of the thyroid carcinoma (E), and finally, the size of the primary lesion (S). The authors concluded that their AMES scale can be applied to both papillary and follicular carcinoma of the thyroid with equal accuracy.

Hay recently reviewed the experience at the Mayo Clinic treating papillary cancer of the thyroid over a 40-year period (1945 to 1985).[55] A total of 1500 patients were included in this retrospective analysis with a median follow-up of 15.5 years. He compared the EORTC,

AGES, and AMES prognostic indexes in relation to this cohort of patients. The results revealed that all three models yielded important prognostic information. He concluded that "It does, therefore, appear that for patients with papillary thyroid carcinoma it should be possible at the time of initial operation to make an accurate prediction with regard to likely postoperative outcome."

It can therefore be demonstrated through the use of multivariate analysis that models predictive of ultimate outcome in patients with papillary cancers can be formulated. The present models, however, need to be evaluated in prospective studies in which treatment modalities are standardized. Furthermore, analysis of the utility of the DNA content of the nucleus as an independent prognosticator needs to be a component of any such trial.

Treatment

The hallmark of management of papillary cancer of the thyroid is thyroid surgery, regardless of the size of the presenting lesion (see Chapter 5). Following surgical intervention, radioiodine (discussed in Chapter 7) and thyroid hormone suppression therapy are often advocated as adjunctive therapy. Analysis of the utility of thyroid hormone in the treatment of papillary cancer must balance the benefits of decreasing the recurrence and mortality rate of papillary cancer against the deleterious effects on bone density known to occur with suppressive doses of thyroid hormone.

Treatment of papillary cancer of the thyroid following surgery with suppressive doses of thyroid medication has become standard adjunctive therapy. However, no study has prospectively evaluated the efficacy of thyroid hormone treatment. In fact, all the studies that address this issue are retrospective nonrandomized studies. The first series that evaluated the effect of therapy with thyroid hormone on the recurrence and mortality rates from papillary cancer was published by Dr. George Crile in 1957.[62] He reported on 16 patients treated at the Cleveland Clinic for papillary cancer with thyroid therapy following surgical intervention. He concluded that hormonal therapy was definitely beneficial in 10 of the cases and possibly beneficial in the remaining 6. Although it is unclear if he thought that thyroid hormone actually arrested the growth of papillary cancer or if it simply retarded its progression, he concluded by stating, "All patients operated on for thyroid cancer should be given dessicated thyroid to prevent recurrences."

In 1959 Crile, McNamara, and Hazard reviewed 107 cases of papillary cancer followed at the Cleveland Clinic.[63] Patients operated on prior to 1953 were not placed on dessicated thyroid postoperatively, whereas patient operated on after 1953 were routinely treated with 2 to 3 grains of dessicated thyroid daily. The group not placed on dessicated thyroid had a recurrence rate of papillary cancer in the cervical nodes of 24% (15/58), compared to 16% (2/15) in the group treated with hormonal therapy. They concluded: "The routine feeding of 2 or preferably 3 grains of dessicated thyroid daily after all operations for papillary cancer appears to have decreased the incidence of recurrence."

Further evidence for the beneficial effect of thyroid hormonal treatment of papillary cancer was published by Crile in 1966.[64] Nineteen patients with surgically incurable papillary cancer were placed on dessicated thyroid. He found that 12 of the 19 patients had either regression of the tumor or stabilization of the tumor mass, while 7 patients did not respond to dessicated thyroid and eventually died from extension of the cancer. It should be noted that the patients under 40 years old were more responsive to dessicated thyroid than the older age group. This may reflect, of course, the more benign course that papillary cancer patients under 40 years old experience, and may be totally independent of the effect of hormonal therapy.

Crile summarized his experience at the Cleveland Clinic in a 1971 article which reviewed 307 cases of papillary cancer treated at the Cleveland Clinic from 1937–1964.[65] He concluded that the mortality rate for papillary cancer following 1954 (when dessicated thyroid began to be routinely administrated postoperatively) was appreciably lower than the years preceeding 1953. Thus the experience at the Cleveland Clinic, although retrospective, revealed a beneficial effect of thyroid hormone replacement. However, not all studies have found thyroid hormone administration beneficial in the treatment of papillary cancer of the thyroid. Cady et al. published a retrospective series of 761 patients treated at the Lahey Clinic between 1931 to 1970 for differentiated thyroid cancer.[66] Seventy-one percent of the patients had papillary cancer and the median follow-up period was 18 years. Patients treated prior to 1960 were not routinely placed on thyroid hormone postoperatively; their survival curve was compared to individuals operated on after 1960, all of whom received thyroid replacement therapy. No significant difference was found in survival rates between the two groups. They concluded that "these data suggest that the administration of thyroid hormone as an adjunct to operation for differentiated thyroid cancer to suppress TSH does not improve survival times."[66]

The most recent study evaluating the role of thyroid hormone as adjunctive therapy for papillary cancer was conducted by Mazzaferri and Young in 1981.[25] Their study consisted of 576 patients with papillary cancer diagnosed between 1962 to 1972. The mean age for the entire population studied was 32.4 years and the median follow-up period was greater than 10 years. They found a decrease in recurrence rates, as well as an increase in survival rates in patients treated with thyroid hormone. They concluded that thyroid carcinoma greater than 1.5 cm should be treated with a variety of modalities including "life-long thyroid hormone suppression of endogenous thyroid stimulating hormone. . . ."

Clearly, the majority of the studies conclude that thyroid administration should be a standard part of the adjunctive medical treatment of papillary cancer. However, this conclusion is not universally accepted. Furthermore, the studies cited are all retrospective analyses that often compare survival rates in different decades and do not control for the different surgical procedures performed. Furthermore, none of the studies utilized a sensitive thyroid-stimulating hormone (TSH) assay that was able to detect suppressed TSH. Consequently, it is unclear if the group of patients on thyroid hormone was receiving suppressive doses. How effective thyroid administration is as adjunct therapy in the treatment of papillary cancer remains unanswered. However, given that the vast majority of the data reveal a beneficial effect of thyroid suppressive therapy (despite the limitations of the studies already discussed) this treatment should be considered standard medical practice until proved otherwise. Hopefully, a prospective, randomized, double-blind study assessing the role of thyroid hormone in papillary cancer will be performed. In particular, it has not been shown that patients who are at low risk for recurrence or mortality from papillary cancer (which comprise the majority of the patients) benefit from suppressive therapy. Further study of this question has become increasingly important because the benefits of treatment must be compared with the osteoporotic effect of suppressive doses of thyroid hormone.

Summary

In conclusion, papillary carcinoma, although one of the more indolent cancers, still has an 8% mortality rate. We have identified certain variables that are indicative of a good prognosis, the best of which is the presence of occult papillary cancer. The examination of nuclear DNA, although still under investigation, will probably be helpful in prognosticating, but is, at best, only part of the answer. The challenge for the future is to enhance our ability to select those individuals with the worst prognoses. At that point intervention trials can be designed so as to further refine our treatments, thus decreasing the present mortality rate of 8% to 0%.

Acknowledgments. I would like to thank Dr Steven Dikman for review of the manuscript and for supplying the photomicrographs.

References

1. Mazzaferri EL. Controversies in the management of differentiated thyroid carcinoma. Endocrine Society. 42nd Annual Postgraduate Assembly 1990. Bethesda, MD.
2. Oertel JE, LiVolsi VA. Pathology of thyroid diseases. In: Ingbar SH, Braverman LE, eds. Werner's The

Thyroid: A fundamental and clinical text. 5th ed. Philadelphia: J.B. Lippincott Company, 1986:667–672.
3. Meissner WA, Adler A. Papillary carcinoma of the thyroid: A study of the pathology of two hundred twenty-six cases. Arch Pathol 1958;66:518–525.
4. LiVolsi VA. Papillary lesions of the thyroid. In: Bennington JL, ed. Surgical pathology of the thyroid. Vol 22. Philadelphia: W.B. Saunders Company, 1990:136–172.
5. Woolner LB. Thyroid carcinoma: Pathologic classification with data on prognosis. Seminars in Nuclear Medicine 1971;1:481–502.
6. Woolner LB, Beahrs OH, Black BM, McConahey WM, Keating FR. Classification and prognosis of thyroid carcinoma: A study of 885 cases observed in a thirty year period. Am J Surg 1961;102:354–387.
7. Carcangiu ML, Zampi G, Rosai J. Papillary thyroid carcinoma: A study of its many morphologic expressions and clinical correlates. Pathol Annu 1985;20:1–44.
8. Gray A, Doniach I. Morphology of the nuclei of papillary carcinoma of the thyroid. Br J Cancer 1969;23:49–51.
9. Hawk WA, Hazard JB. The many appearances of papillary carcinoma of the thyroid. Cleveland Clinic Quarterly 1976;43:207–216.
10. Chan JKC, Saw D. The grooved nucleus: A useful diagnostic criterion of papillary carcinoma of the thyroid. Am J Surg Pathol 1986;10:672–679.
11. Albores-Saavedra J, Altamirano-Dimas M, Alcorta-Anguizola B, Smith M. Fine structure of human papillary thyroid carcinoma. Cancer 1971;28:763–774.
12. Hapke MR, Dehner LP. The optically clear nucleus: A reliable sign of papillary carcinoma of the thyroid? Am J Surg Pathol 1979;3:31–38.
13. Shurbaji MS, Gupta PK, Frost JK. Nuclear grooves: A useful criterion in the cytopathologic diagnosis of papillary thyroid carcinoma. Diagnostic Cytopathology 1988;4:91–94.
14. Klinck, GH, Winship T. Psammona bodies and thyroid cancer. Cancer 1959;12:656–662.
15. Crile G, Hazard JB. Relationship of the age of the patient to the natural history and prognosis of carcinoma of the thyroid. Ann Surg 1953;138:33–38.
16. Franssila KO. Is the differentiation between papillary and follicular carcinoma valid? Cancer 1973;32:853–864.
17. Frazell EL, Foote FW. Papillary cancer of the thyroid: A review of 25 years of experience. Cancer 1958;11:895–922.
18. Underwood CR, Ackerman LV, Kckert C. Papillary Carcinoma of the thyroid: An evaluation of surgical therapy. Surgery 1958;43:610–621.
19. Beahrs OH, Woolner LB. The treatment of papillary carcinoma of the thyroid gland. Surg Gynecol Obstet 1959;108:43–48.
20. Hirabayashi RN, Lindsay S. Carcinoma of the thyroid gland: A statistical study of 390 patients. J Clin Endocrinol Metab 1961;21:1596–1610.
21. Tollefsen HR, DeCosse JJ. Papillary carcinoma of the thyroid: Recurrence in the thyroid gland after initial surgical treatment. Am J Surg 1963;106:728–734.
22. Noguchi S, Noguchi A, Murakami N. Papillary carcinoma of the thyroid: Developing patterns of metastases. Cancer 1970;26:1053–1060.
23. Crile G. Changing end results in patients with papillary carcinoma of the thyroid. Surg Gynecol Obstet 1971;132:460–468.
24. Beaugie JM, Brown CL, Doniach I, Richardson JE. Primary malignant tumours of the thyroid: The relationship between histological classification and clinical behaviour. Br J Surg 1976;63:173–181.
25. Mazzaferri EL, Young RL. Papillary thyroid carcinoma: A 10 year follow-up report of the impact of therapy in 576 patients. Am J Med 1981;70;511–517.
26. Samaan NA, Maheshwari YK, Nader S, et al. Impact of therapy for differentiated carcinoma of the thyroid: An analysis of 706 cases. J Clin Endocrinol Metab 1983;56:1131–1138.
27. Rossi RL, Nieroda C, Cady B, Wool MS. Malignancies of the thyroid gland: the Lahey Clinic experience. Surg Clin North Am 1985;65:211–230.
28. Carcangiu ML, Zampi G, Pupi A, Castgnoli A, Rosai J. Papillary carcinoma of the thyroid: A clinicopathologic study of 241 cases treated at the University of Florence, Italy. Cancer 1985;55:805–828.
29. McConahey WM, Hay ID, Woolner LB, Van Heerden JA, Taylor WF. Papillary thyroid cancer treated at the Mayo Clinic, 1946 through 1970: Initial Manifestations, pathologic findings, therapy, and outcome. Mayo Clin Proc 1986;61:978–996.
30. DeGroot LJ, Kaplan EL, McCormick M, Straus FH. Natural history, treatment, and course of papillary thyroid carcinoma. J Clin Endocrinol Metab 1990;71:414–424.
31. Black BM, Kirk TA, Woolner LB. Multicentricity of papillary adenocarcinoma of the thyroid: Influence on treatment. J Clin Endocrinol Metab 1960;20:130–135.
32. Tollefsen HR, DeCosse JJ, Hutter RVP. Papillary carcinoma of the thyroid: A clinical and pathological study of 70 fatal cases. Cancer 1964;17:1035–1044.
33. Smith SA, Hay ID, Goellner JR, Ryan JJ, McConahey WM. Mortality from papillary thyroid carcinoma. A case-control study of 56 lethal cases. Cancer 1988;62:1381–1388.
34. Frantz VK, Forsythe R, Hanford JM, Rogers WM. Lateral Aberrant thyroids. Ann Surg 1942;115:161–183.
35. Wozencraft P, Foote FW, Frazell EL. Occult carcinoma of the thyroid: Their bearing on the concept of lateral aberrant thyroid cancer. Cancer 1948;1:574–583.
36. Hazard JB. Small papillary carcinoma of the thyroid: A study with special reference to so-called nonencapsulated sclerosing tumor. Laboratory Investigation 1960;9:86–97.
37. Sampson RJ, Key CR, Buncher CR, Iijima S. Thyroid carcinoma in Hiroshima and Nagasaki. Prevalence of thyroid carcinoma at autopsy. JAMA 1969;209:65–70.
38. Sampson RJ, Key CR, Buncher CR, Oka H, Iijima S.

Papillary carcinoma of the thyroid gland: Sizes of 525 tumors found at autopsy in Hiroshima and Nagasaki. Cancer 1970;25:1391–1393.
39. Sampson RJ, Oka H, Key CR, Buncher CR, Iijima S. Metastases from occult thyroid carcinoma: An autopsy study from Hiroshima and Nagasaki Japan. Cancer 1970;25:803–811.
40. Sampson RJ, Woolner LB, Bahn RC, Kurland LT. Occult thyroid carcinoma in Olmstead County Minnesota: Prevalence at autopsy compared with that in Hiroshima and Nagasaki Japan. Cancer 1974;34:2072–2076.
41. Fukunaga FH, Yatani R. Geographic pathology of occult thyroid carcinomas. Cancer 1975;36:1095–1099.
42. Sobrinho-Simoes MA, Sambade MC, Goncalves V. Latent thyroid carcinoma at autopsy: A study from Oporto, Portugal. Cancer 1979;43:1702–1706.
43. Hubert JP, Kiernan PD, Beahrs OH, McConahey WM, Woolner LB. Occult papillary carcinoma of the thyroid. Arch Surg 1980;115:394–398.
44. Bondeson L, Ljungberg O. Occult thyroid carcinoma at autopsy in Malmo, Sweden. Cancer 1981;47:319–323.
45. Schroder S, Pfannschmidt N, Bocker W, Muller HW, deHeer K. Histopathologic types and clinical behavior of occult papillary carcinoma of the thyroid. Path Res Pract 1984;179:81–87.
46. Sampson RJ, Key CR, Buncher CR, Iijima S. Smallest forms of papillary carcinoma of the thyroid. Arch Path 1971;91:334–339.
47. Silliphant WM, Klinck GH, Levitin MS. Thyroid carcinoma and death: A clinicopathological study of 193 autopsies. Cancer 1964;17:513–525.
48. Woolner LB, Lemmon ML, Beahrs OH, Black BM, Keating FR. Occult papillary carcinoma of the thyroid gland: A study of 140 cases observed in a 30 year period. J Clin Endocrinol Metab 1960;20:89–105.
49. Johannessen JV, Sobrinho-Simoes M, Lindmo T, Tangen KO, Kaalhus O, Brennhovd IO. Anomalous papillary carcinoma of the thyroid. Cancer 1983;51:1462–1467.
50. Joensuu H, Kleimi P, Eerola E, Tuominen J. Influence of cellular DNA content on survival in differentiated thyroid cancer. Cancer 1986;58:2462–2467.
51. Cohn K, Backdahl M, Forsslund G et al. Prognostic value of nuclear DNA content in papillary thyroid carcinoma. World J Surg 1984;8:474–480.
52. Bachdahl M, Carstensen J, Aver G, Tallroth E. Statistical evaluation of the prognostic value of nuclear DNA content in papillary, follicular, and medullary thyroid tumors. World J. Surg 1986;10:974–980.
53. Ekman ET, Backdahl M, Lowhagen T, Auer G. Nuclear DNA measurements on thyroid carcinoma in young patients. Acta Oncologica 1989;28:475–479.
54. Schelfhout L, Cornelisse CJ, Goslings BM et al. Frequency and duration of aneuploidy in benign and malignant thyroid neoplasms. Int J Cancer 1990;45:16–20.
55. Hay ID. Papillary thyroid carcinoma. In: Kaplan MM, ed. Endocrinology and Metabolism Clinics of North America: Thyroid Carcinoma. Vol. 19. W.B. Saunders 1990:545–576.
56. Byar DP, Green SB, Dor P. A prognostic index for thyroid carcinoma. A study of the E.O.R.T.C. thyroid cancer cooperative group. Eur J Cancer 1979;15:1033–1041.
57. Hay ID, Grant CS, Taylor WF, McConahey WM. Ipsilateral lobectomy versus bilateral lobar resection in papillary thyroid carcinoma: A retrospective analysis of surgical outcome using a novel prognostic scoring system. Surgery 1987;102:1088–1095.
58. Cady B, Rossi R. An expanded view of risk group definition in differentiated thyroid carcinoma. Surgery 1988;104:947–953.
59. Hannequin P, Liehn JC, Delisle MJ. Multifactorial analysis of survival in thyroid cancer: Pitfalls of applying the results of published studies to another population. Cancer 1986;58:1749–1755.
60. Kerr DJ, Burt AD, Boyle P, MacFarlane GJ, Storer AM, Brewin TB. Prognostic factors in thyroid tumors. Br J Cancer 1986;54:475–482.
61. Tennvall J, Biorklund A, Moller T, Ranstam J, Akerman M. Is the EORTC prognostic index of thyroid cancer valid in differentiated thyroid carcinoma? Retrospective multivariate analysis of differentiated thyroid carcinoma with long follow-up. Cancer 1986;57:1405–1414.
62. Crile G. The endocrine dependency of certain thyroid cancers and the danger that hypothyroidism may stimulate their growth. Cancer 1957;10:1119–1137.
63. Crile G, McNamara JM, Hazard JB. Results of treatment of papillary carcinoma of the thyroid. Surgery, Gynecology, and Obstetrics 1959;109:315–320.
64. Crile G. Endocrine dependency of papillary carcinoma of the thyroid. JAMA 1966;195:101–104.
65. Crile G. Changing and results in patients with papillary carcinoma of the thyroid. Surg Gynecol Obstet 1971;132:460–468.
66. Cady B, Cohn K, Rossi RL, et al. The effects of thyroid hormone administration upon survival in patients with differentiated thyroid carcinoma. Surgery 1983;94:978–983.

2

Follicular Carcinoma of the Thyroid

ROBERT P. FIEDLER

Introduction

Follicular carcinoma of the thyroid is one of the subgroups of differentiated thyroid carcinoma. This group also includes papillary carcinoma and the follicular variant of papillary carcinoma. Hürthle cell (oxyphil cell, Askanazy cell) carcinoma is now considered a subgroup of follicular carcinoma. Although these tumors are all generally slow growing, late to metastasize, and often associated with a normal life span, there are significant differences among them. This has produced much confusion in the literature, where authors have lumped them all together as "well-differentiated carcinoma" and have reported results of treatment in large series without regard for separating patients in terms of risk factors. Finally, there is great variability in length of follow up in a relatively slow growing lesion. In attempting to understand follicular carcinoma it is important to remember that its etiology, epidemiology, pathology, clinical features, pattern of growth and spread, prognosis, and response to various treatment modalities are different from other tumors in this group.

Epidemiology

The incidence of follicular carcinoma of the thyroid varies with the level of iodine intake. In areas of adequate iodine ingestion follicular carcinoma accounts for approximately 5% of thyroid cancer. In iodine deficient areas there is an increase to 25 to 40%.[1,2] It accounts for approximately 15% of thyroid cancer seen in the United States.[3] In 1981 Woolner reported that in a series of 885 patients with well differentiated thyroid cancer collected over 30 years, 17.7% of the thyroid malignancies were follicular.[4] The female-to-male ratio was 2.6:1 and the mean age was 50 years. This correlated well with Young and Mazzaferri's series of 214 patients with follicular carcinoma selected from the group of 1500 patients described in tumor registry of the Armed Forces—an incidence of 14%.[5] These statistics are not stable with respect to time, nor are they the same in other areas of the world. This variability is best correlated with the incidence of endemic goiter and with the relationship of iodine intake to goiter.

The effect of iodine intake on endemic goiter was seen in 1924 in Michigan by Olin who noted an inverse relationship between the iodine content of drinking water and the incidence of goiter.[6] He suggested the use of iodized salt. After iodized salt was introduced the incidence of goiter was reduced from its previous level of 38.6% to 1.4% in 1951. In Switzerland iodized salt was introduced as early as 1840. The subsequent incidence of goiter fell from 40% to 8.2%.[7]

The link between goiter and follicular carcinoma was demonstrated by Beahrs in 1951.[8] He compared the incidence of papillary versus follicular carcinoma in 517 patients operated on during two periods: a period of high incidence of goiter from 1907 to 1937, and a period of low incidence of goiter from 1938 to 1947. The proportion of papillary carcinoma doubled from 30 to 60% and follicular carcinoma fell from 30.4% to 17.6%. When there was a low goiter incidence the proportion of total tumors that was papillary changed from 30% to 60%; the proportion of follicular fell from 30.4% to 17.6%. Other types of thyroid carcinoma make up the difference to equal 100%.

In 1969 Cuello et al. studied 229 patients from a nonendemic goiter area (Connecticut) and 217 patients from an endemic goiter area (Cali, Colombia).[9] Approximately 75% of follicular carcinoma was associated with goiter versus approximately 55% of papillary carcinoma. Although no difference in the incidence of papillary carcinoma was found in the two areas, the incidence of follicular carcinoma was greater in Cali. In men in Cali, follicular carcinoma was seven times as common as it is in women, while in Connecticut it was only three times more common in men than in women.

Williams and Doniach compared the incidence of papillary versus follicular carcinoma in an area of high iodine intake (Iceland) with an area of low iodine intake (Northern Scotland).[10] In the area of low iodine intake the ratio of papillary to follicular carcinoma was 3.6:1, as opposed to 6.5:1 in the resion of high iodine intake.

A single contradictory study was reported from Denmark in 1976.[11] When endemic goiter area was compared with a nonendemic goiter area, the incidence of follicular carcinoma was found to be similar in both areas.

Several other factors are considered to be important in the etiology of follicular carcinoma. Although a clearly increased incidence of chronic thyroiditis has been demonstrated in patients with thyroid carcinoma,[12] it is generally agreed that chronic thyroiditis does not play a causative role, and may even be protective. Occult, grossly evident, multicentric, and metastatic thyroid carcinoma have all been found in patients with Graves' disease.[13] Although debate continues as to whether there is an increased incidence of thyroid carcinoma in patients with Graves' disease, the weight of evidence seems to point to the fact that there is,[14] furthermore, thyroid carcinoma tends to be more virulent due to the presence of TSAb (Thyroid stimulating antibody).[15]

Stanbury reported three patients with inborn errors of iodine metabolism who developed thyroid carcinoma—two follicular and one anaplastic.[16] One patient with follicular carcinoma had a peroxidase defect, goiter, and congenital cretinism. The other patient with follicular carcinoma had a goiter, with increased ^{131}I uptake in the thyroid and lung metastases. The patient's mother and 6 of his 12 siblings were goitrous. The patient was later studied by Cooper.[17] He found a leak of inorganic iodine from the gland with increased ^{131}I uptake in two of the affected patients but not three others. He mentions 15 prior cases of thyroid malignancy associated with familial goiter but only 4 had strict pathological criteria for malignancy.

A link between elevated TSH and the development of follicular carcinoma is postulated. In animals with elevated thyroid-stimulating hormone (TSH), hyperplastic thyroid tissue degenerates into follicular tumors. However, the evidence is not as clear in humans. In humans both benign and malignant thyroid tumors that develop in congenital goiter are follicular. The two patients in Cooper's study who developed follicular carcinoma both had partial thyroidectomies and were therefore exposed to increased TSH.

Although genetic abnormalities associated with thyroid cancer have been reported (Multiple Endocrine Neoplasia-Type II [MEN II] with medullary carcinoma and Gardner's syndrome with papillary carcinoma), pure follicular carcinoma has not been reported in the absence of familial goiter. However, in 1983 Riccabonna et al. reported a family in which four of eight children born of nongoitrous parents developed Hurtle cell carcinoma.[18] Another disorder associated with follicular carcinoma is Cowden's Syndrome, which consists of follicular tumors, with arrhenoblastoma and multiple hamartomas.[19,20] Finally, unknown environmental factors may play a role. Riccabonna reported three couples with thyroid cancer one of which had follicular carcinoma.[18]

Clinical Features

Although it was initially felt that follicular carcinoma was rare under the age of 40, this is no longer the case.[21] Cady reviewed the experience at the Lahey Clinic from 1935 to 1975 and found that although follicular carcinoma tended to occur in older patients prior to 1960, a shift occurred after that date.[22] More younger patients began to present with follicular carcinoma and more older patients presented with papillary and papillary–follicular carcinoma, so that the incidence became essentially the same among different age groups. Almost half the patients with follicular carcinoma were under the age of 40. Similar results were found by Young and Mazzaferri in their review of follicular carcinoma in the Armed Forces,[5] in which the mean age was found to be 35 years.

It is generally felt that follicular carcinoma occurs more commonly in women than in men. Young and Mazzaferri found that 72% of follicular carcinoma in their series occurred in women.[5] In Cady's series, follicular carcinoma was more common in men than papillary or papillary-follicular carcinoma (35% versus 22%). Men and women did not differ significantly in age or manner of presentation.

Follicular carcinoma of the thyroid generally presents as a solitary nodule in a gland that is otherwise normal to palpation, or may less commonly be found as a dominant nodule in a multinodular gland. However, it is three times more likely to be occult than other forms of well-differentiated thyroid carcinoma.[22] In Young and Mazzaferri's series, 85% presented with a thyroid nodule and 75% of those were less than three cm.[5] A follicular nodule on presention may be increasing in size or be so slowly growing that an increase in size may not be appreciated. Less commonly, hoarseness secondary to involvement of the recurrent laryngeal nerve or dysphagia secondary to esophageal compression may be a presenting symptom.

In the same series, 182 of 214 patients presented with disease apparently limited to the thyroid, 19 had palpable lymph nodes, and 7 presented with distant metastases (these are less common and appear in lung, brain, or bone). In two patients who presented with single metastases (one pulmonary and one bone), the primary lesion could not be identified. In one patient described by Boehm who had a slowly growing solitary metastasis to the skull a 3 mm lesion was found in the thyroid at surgery.[23] Less commonly, presentation may occur with signs and symptoms of spinal cord compression.[24] Finally, functioning follicular carcinoma may produce thyrotoxicosis. It is rare for the disease to present in this manner;[39] it is usual for widespread functioning metastases to be present.[25] Triiodothyronine (T_3) toxicosis has also been reported.[26]

Laboratory evaluation has not been helpful in diagnosing follicular carcinoma; thyroid function tests are generally normal. Measurement of thyroglobulin has not been found to be useful in differentiating follicular carcinoma from benign follicular adenoma or from other malignant thyroid lesions. Schaeder and his colleagues measured thyroglobulin levels in 904 adult patients who had a history of childhood radiation therapy.[27] Although levels tended to be higher in patients with nodules than without nodules, too much overlap limited its usefulness as a screening test. Mean levels in patients with benign and malignant nodules were indistinguishable. The latter were confirmed by Bascheri and his colleagues, who noted that several benign thyroid diseases, for example, Hashimoto's thyroiditis, Graves disease, and nontoxic goiter may be accompanied by high thyroglobulin levels.[28]

Of the radiological procedures ^{131}I or ^{123}I scanning is the most useful because follicular carcinoma can be virtually ruled out in a solitary nodule that is "hot," that is, autonomous. There are, however, scattered reports of follicular carcinoma in a hot nodule.[29] Of the nodules that are "cold," or take up less radioactive iodine than the rest of the gland, 10% to 20% may be carcinoma.

Ultrasound is useful in the patient with a "cold" nonfunctioning nodule on scan. It can differentiate a cyst, which has a very low probability of malignancy, from a solid lesion. Although it was initially felt that a "halo" around a solid lesion was an indication that it was probably benign, this is no longer believed to be the case; it is generally felt that sonography is not useful in determining whether a solid lesion is benign or malignant.

Computed tomographic (CT) scanning and

magnetic resonance imaging (MRI) are useful in locating metastatic lesions but have not helped in differentiating benign from malignant lesions. MRI has been used to evaluate resected tissue.[30] The T-1 was found to be higher for malignant tissue than for normal thyroid or benign adenoma; however, it could not distinguish between papillary and follicular carcinoma.

The remaining diagnostic technique in wide use is needle biopsy—either aspiration with a fine needle, or the obtaining of a core or piece of tissue using either a wider bore or cutting needle. The major areas of controversy regarding needle biopsy involves the effectiveness of the techniques and the interpretation of the results one obtains. The pitfalls one encounters with any of these techniques are best understood in terms of the specificity and sensitivity of the procedure. The latter depends on the skill used to obtain the material (i.e., sampling from the nodule and not the normal thyroid tissue adjacent to it, sampling from multiple areas of a large nodule), the manner in which the material is handled once it is obtained, the skill and experience of the pathologist, and finally the criteria used to call a smear "suspicious." In the study by Galvan et al., 13,561 patients had aspiration performed and 2744 underwent surgery.[31] Of 181 malignant neoplasms found at surgery, 93.4% were recognized by aspiration (indicating the sensitivity of the procedure), that is, 12 were missed and 20 of the 23 were follicular carcinoma. Of 2563 cases without malignancy at surgery, 1884 were read as "negative," that is, the specificity was 73.9%. One must note that the true sensitivity was not determined because the majority of the patients (80%) were not operated upon. In fact, this is a difficulty encountered in many studies: only patients with suspicious or positive biopsies are operated upon. This was also true in the study by Nishyama et al. that compared fine needle aspiration (FNA) with core biopsy (CB).[32] They studied 415 patients who were felt to be at risk for carcinoma (they had "cold" nodules on isotope scans). FNA and CB were performed on 282, FNA only on 112, CB only on 5; twenty-one had insufficient material for evaluation by either method. Pathology was reported as "negative," "suspicious," or "positive." Patients with suspicious or positive results were sent for surgery—patients with negative biopsies were not. fifty-eight of the 394 patients with adequate pathological material were read as positive; 40 (69%) had malignant nodules at surgery. Of those 58 patients, 31 had positive FNA and CB and 24 of those had malignant nodules at surgery. Eight had positive FNA and a negative CB; 3 had malignant nodules at surgery. Nine patients had negative FNAs and positive CB; 5 had a malignant nodule at surgery. The total rate of false positives was 31%. The sensitivity of aspiration alone was 85% and biopsy alone, 75%. If the number of patients with positive CB but negative FNA are added, the number of thyroid cancers found increased from 34 to 40 (an increase of 17.6%). If one adds positive FNA to negative CB, 10 additional cancers were found—an increase of 33%. Thus the advantage of doing both procedures was substantial. A similar conclusion was reached by LoGerfo and his colleagues who concluded that a combination of FNA and CB produced the greatest yield of carcinoma at surgery.[33] King and Yuen used a 21-gauge needle and prepared cell blocks and found this superior to the use of smears alone.[34]

The issue of interpretation of suspicious biopsies was studied by Gharib and his colleagues.[35] They note that 15% to 30% of aspirates obtained by FNA are reported as suspicious. The incidence in their study was 17% of 1970 patients. Ten percent to 50% of patients with suspicious FNA will have malignant nodules at surgery.

Thus, although the use of needle biopsy is still controversial, these authors concluded, and it is generally accepted, that needle biopsy (both FNA and CB) is not a useful method for differentiating a benign from a malignant follicular lesion.

Pathology

Follicular carcinoma appears as an encapsulated expansile lesion that is often difficult to differentiate from its benign counterpart—the follicular adenoma.[3] In general, carcinoma is

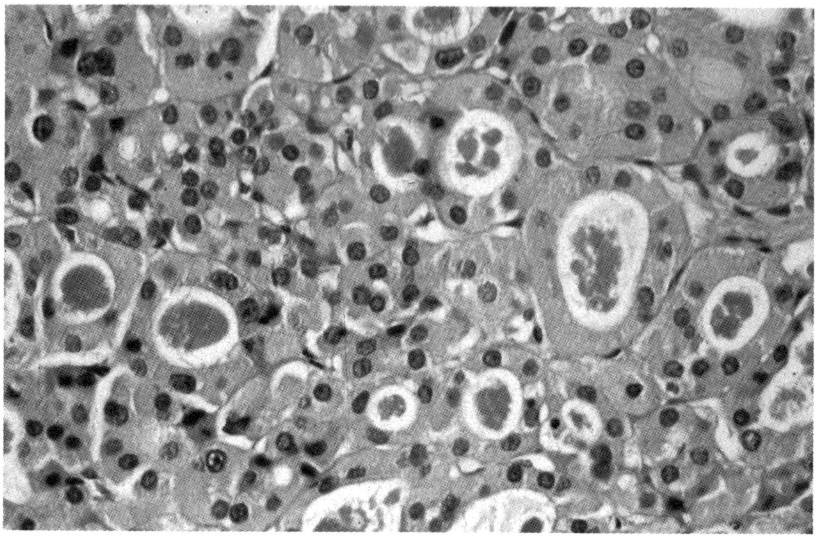

Figure 2.1. Follicular carcinoma. Well differentiated. (original magnification × 340)

characterized microscopically by large nuclei, frequent and/or atypical mitotic figures, vascular invasion, and distant metastases.[36,37] The metastases are generally osseous or pulmonary. Lymph node involvement is unusual and occurs late in the course of the disease. Two exceptions are the Hurtle cell variant in which lymph node metastases may occur early, and which generally is somewhat more aggressive than the ordinary follicular carcinoma,[38] and insular carcinoma, which is much more aggressive and follows a more rapid and often fatal course.[39]

Due to the confusion regarding the pathology of thyroid tumors in general and follicular tumors in particular, it was felt necessary in 1974 to hold an international conference to classify thyroid tumors.[40] Follicular carcinoma was believed to have two growth patterns: well-differentiated (FWD) which consisted of follicles that could not be distinguished from normal thyroid, adenomatous goiter, or adenoma (Fig. 2.1); and moderately differentiated (FMD), which consisted of solid masses of cells in a trabecular pattern, with varying degrees of differentiation into follicles (Fig. 2.2).

This classification was revised in 1988.[41] Follicular carcinoma was divided into "minimally invasive" and "widely invasive." Minimally invasive lesions were defined as grossly encapsulated and, with respect to architecture and cytology, virtually indistinguishable from follicular adenoma. The diagnosis of malignancy depends on finding vascular invasion or invasion of the full thickness of the capsule (Fig. 2.3). The diagnosis can only be made pathologically on a fixed specimen; it cannot be made on frozen section or needle biopsy. Vascular invasion is defined as invasion into veins in or beyond the capsule. Tumor in capillaries within the tumor is not considered significant.[42] However, there is debate as to what extent of capsular invasion is necessary to diagnose a tumor as being malignant. Some authors accept invasion into the capsule for this diagnosis,[43] whereas others require penetration through the capsule.[44]

The widely invasive type of follicular carcinoma is characterized by widespread infiltration of blood vessels (Fig. 2.4) or adjacent thyroid tissue (Fig. 2.5). It is often not completely encapsulated, and distant metastases are common. The distant metastasis may be better differentiated than the primary tumor and may look like normal thyroid tissue.[42] These tumors are clinically and surgically recognizable as cancer. They extend into cervical veins or through the thyroid capsule. Microscopically they are usually cellular or microfollicular.[45]

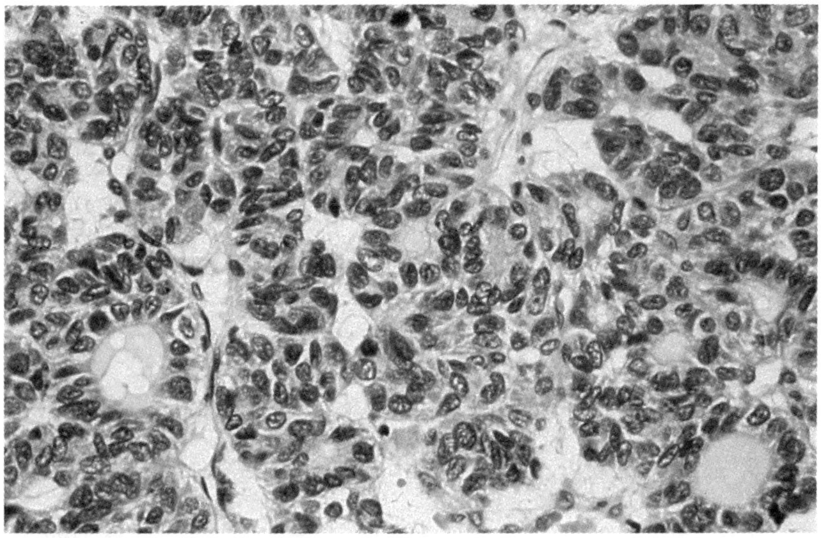

Figure 2.2. Follicular carcinoma. Moderately differentiated. Follicular and trabecular patterns. (original magnification × 220)

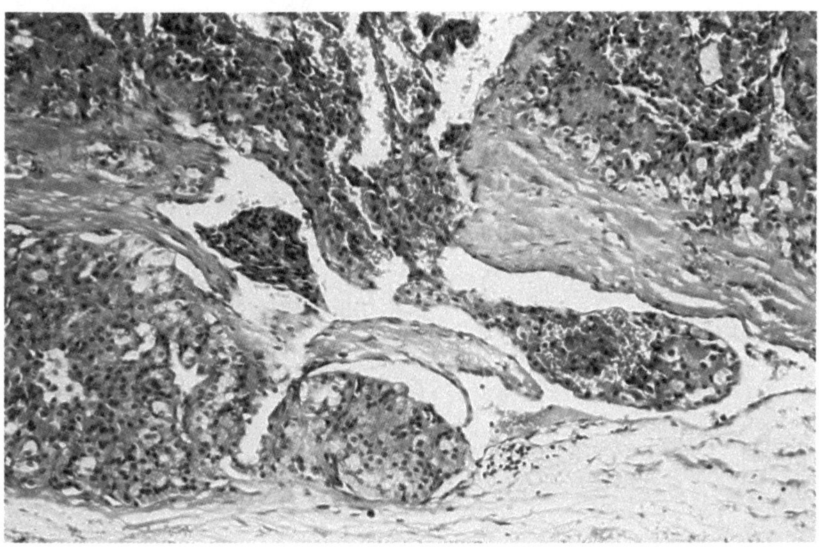

Figure 2.3. Follicular carcinoma. Capsular and vascular invasion. (original magnification × 135)

Additional changes in the classification system included the replacement of Hürtle cell carcinoma by follicular carcinoma, oxyphilic cell type (Fig. 2.6), and the description of a rare clear cell variant (Fig. 2.7).[42]

It is important to distinguish between FWD and FMD because each has a markedly different prognosis; the latter must be treated more aggressively than the former. Lang found that 80% of patients with invasive lesions developed metastases and 20 died of metastatic disease.[45] Woolner found that patients with the widely invasive type had a 50% mortality as opposed to the 3% mortality found in the minimally invasive type.[46,4]

Most recurrences occur within 5 years after

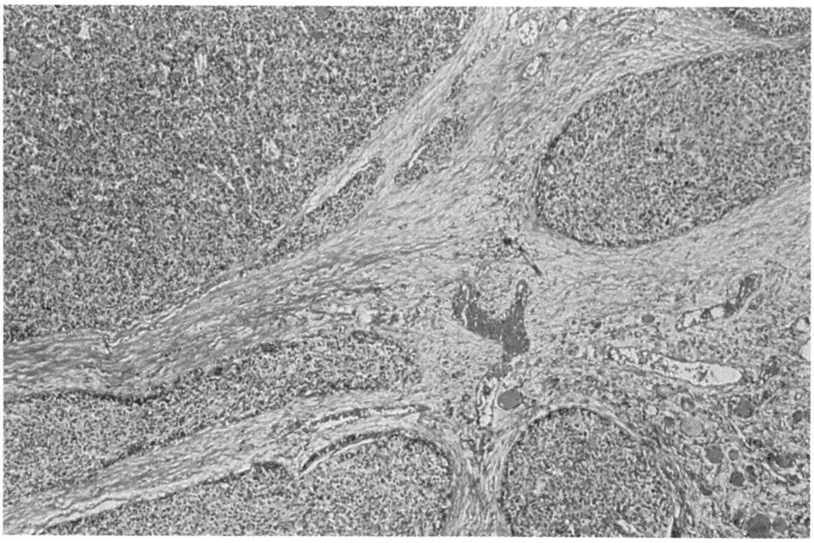

Figure 2.4. Follicular carcinoma, widely invasive. Vascular invasion. (original magnification × 55)

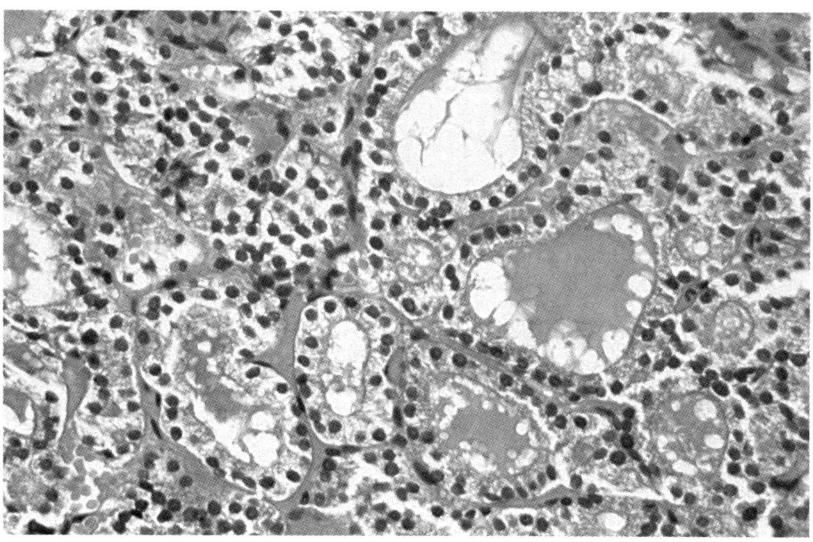

Figure 2.5. Follicular carcinoma, bone metastasis. Well-formed follicles.

surgery, although there are numerous instances of metastases becoming evident many years after surgery.

Because of the difficulty in distinguishing benign from malignant lesions by means of ordinary pathology, other techniques have been attempted. Immunostaining for thyroglobulin has been found to correlate with the degree of invasiveness of the tumor.[47,48,49] Several authors have found that ultrastructural, morphomatic, and flow cytometric analysis are not useful in differentiating benign from malignant lesions.[50,51,52] However, Grant et al. studied patients with known cases of follicular adenoma and follicular carcinoma, and found that although flow cytometry was not useful in differentiating between the two, aneuploidy was associated with a poorer prognosis.[53]

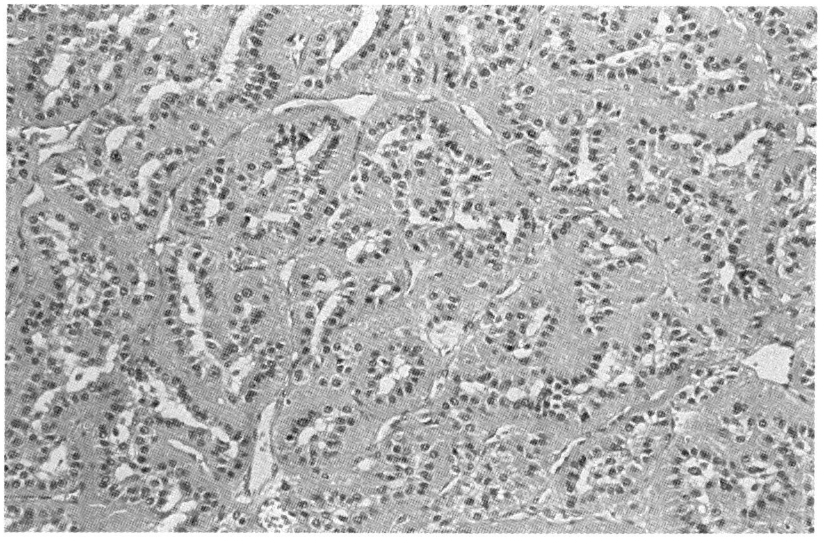

Figure 2.6. Follicular carcinoma, oxyphilic cell type. (original magnification × 135)

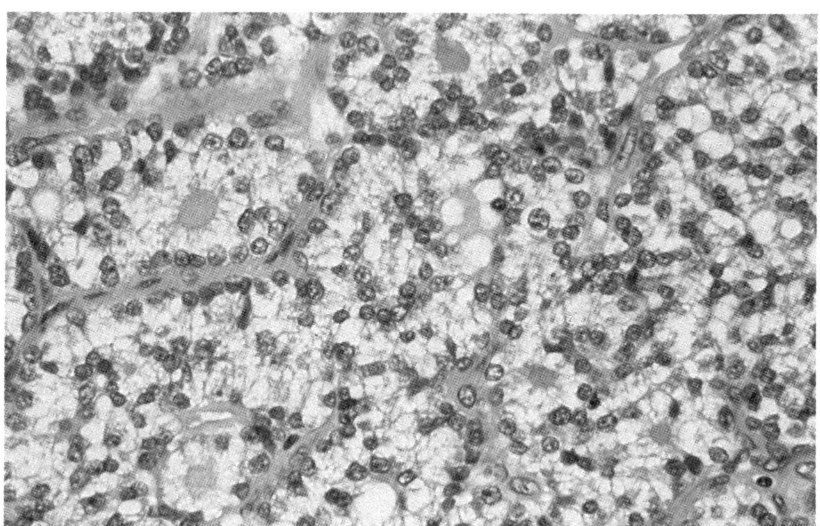

Figure 2.7. Follicular carcinoma, clear cell variant (original magnification × 340)

Treatment and Prognosis

No aspect of the understanding of follicular carcinoma is more complex than the interlocking topics of treatment and prognosis. Obviously, the results of treatment will depend on the modes and aggressiveness of treatment chosen. Yet it is also clear that the prognosis will depend on the various risk factors associated with the tumor and its interaction with its host. These difficulties are compounded by the literature, in which many studies combine follicular carcinoma (which has a more negative prognosis) with papillary or papillary follicular carcinoma (which has a better prognosis) under the single classification of "well differentiated thyroid carcinoma." In addition many of the series provide only a relatively short follow-up period for a group of tumors that tend to metastasize late and potentially kill even later. In general, prognosis is determined by various characteristics of the tumor, that is, size, histology, degree of invasiveness, and capacity to take up radioactive iodine (the prognosis is also modified by the age and sex of the host.) Negative risk factors tend to co-occur. Hence, the more invasive lesions that do not take up radioactive iodine tend to occur in men over the age of 45. Simpson and his colleagues applied multivariate analysis to 504 patients with follicular carcinoma.[54] Risk factors in order of importance were extrathyroidal invasion, distant metastases, primary tumor size, nodal involvement, and age at diagnosis. In Cady's series from the Lahey Clinic Foundation low risk patients (men under the age of 40 and women under the age of 50) did better than the high risk group (all older patients). This superseded the effects of pathologic type or degree of invasiveness.[55]

In Woolner's series noninvasive tumors were compared to invasive tumors.[4] Of 69 patients with noninvasive tumors, 92.8% were alive after 5 years and 85.5% were alive after 10 years. This compares with those patients with invasive tumors, of whom 70.3% were alive after 5 years and only 44.4% of whom were alive after 10 years. In Young and Mazzaferri's series (in which the follow-up period was too short to evaluate survival) only 7% of patients with little invasion had recurrences, as opposed to 27% in those with moderate or extensive invasion.[5] Extensive invasion was associated with early metastases; these were the only tumors that resulted in death in that series.

As compared with papillary carcinoma, in which small tumors are clearly associated with a better prognosis, there is debate as to whether size is a factor in patients with follicular carcinoma. In Cady's series, although there was a significantly greater mortality in patients with larger tumors, many patients with small tumors died.[55] In Young and Mazzaferri's series of 241 patients, there were 2 cases of patients dying in which the primary tumor was too small to find.[5] There was a 10% recurrence rate in cases in which the primary tumor was less than 1.5 cm and an 8% recurrence rate in cases in which the tumor was greater than 1.5 cm. On the other hand, size was a factor in Simpson's series,[54] in addition, Schmidt and Wang found that their patients with lesions larger than 3.5 cm did poorly compared with patients whose lesions were smaller than 3 cm.[56]

Presence of metastatic disease was, as one might expect, indicative of a poor prognosis. In Young and Mazzaferri's series patients survived an average of only 3.1 years if metastases were found at the time of presentation.[5] In a larger series of 283 patients with metastases to lung and bone from well-differentiated thyroid carcinoma, cases were followed for up to 40 years (median = almost 4 years).[57] Metastatic disease was found by conventional x-ray, measurement of thyroglobulin, and total body scans with 1 to 2 mCi of ^{131}I; after 1980, CT scans of the chest were also utilized. In patients with metastases and FWD (well-differentiated follicular carcinoma) 33% survived for 10 years while only 15% survived for 10 years if the tumor was only FMD (moderately well differentiated).

Age is also a significant prognostic factor. In Schlumberger's series, 72 patients in whom differentiated thyroid carcinama presented in childhood (age under 16 years) were followed for as long as 20 years (median = 13 years).[58] Of this group, 4 were FWD and 17 were FMD. None of the children with FWD died and only 2 with FMD died. In Young and Mazzaferri's series (all with follicular carcinoma) all 7 patients who died were 43 years old or over with an average age of 61 years.[5]

Multivariate analysis was applied to a series of 682 patients with well-differentiated thyroid carcinoma studied by Tubiani and Schlumberger.[59] Of 546 of those patients whose disease was confined to the neck the pathologic findings indicated FWD in 67 and FMD in 125. In general the patients with FWD were similar to patients with papillary carcinoma, inasmuch as the FWD patients had a 15% excess mortality at 20 years. Patients with FMD did significantly more poorly. (Fig. 2.8)

In this series age was the most important

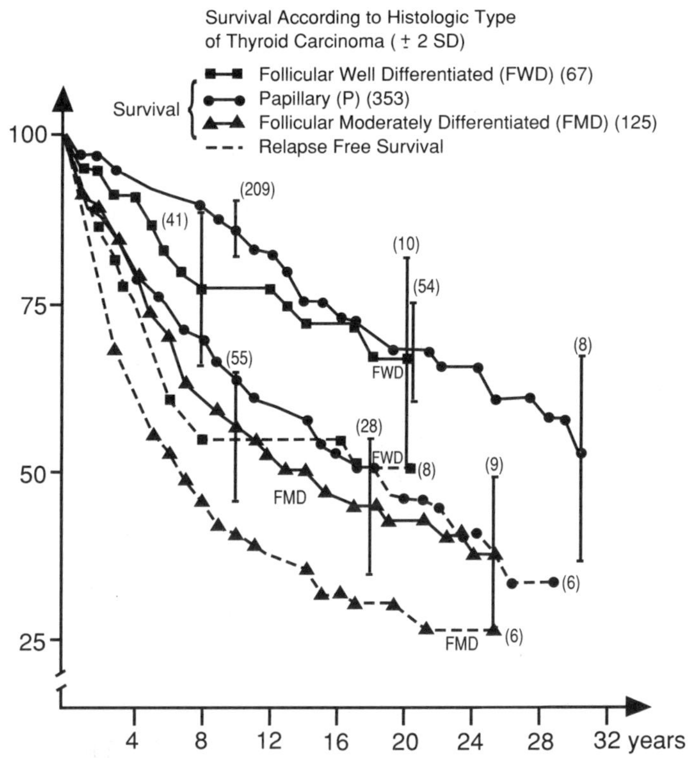

Figure 2.8. Relapse-free survival and total survival in patients with differentiated thyroid cancer of the various histologic types: papillary FWD, FMD. Reprinted, by permission, from Tubiana, M., Schlumber, M., Rougier, P., et al., 1985. (59)

prognostic factor. The mortality risk increased significantly at 45 years; however, there was no increase in mortality between 45 and 80 years of age. Age influenced the probability of relapse, as well as the interval between presentation and relapse and the length of survival after relapse. In addition older patients' metastases were less likely to take up radioiodine (RaI). Histological type was again found to be important; there was a significant difference in survival rates and probability of relapse between patients with FWD and those with FMD. Women had a better prognosis than men in terms of probability of relapse and years of survival.

Brennan and his colleagues at the Mayo Clinic recently reported their experience with 100 patients with follicular carcinoma.[60] The patients had been treated between 1946 and 1970. The mean duration of follow-up was 17.4 years and the maximum was 32 years. Of the 100 patients, whose mean age was 53 years, 57 were female and 43 were male.

They analyzed their data by both univariate and multivariate analysis. By univariate analysis, age greater than 50 years, tumor size larger than 3.9 cm, higher tumor grade, marked vascular invasion, adjacent tissue invasion, and distant metastatic disease at presentation were all associated with increased mortality. However, multivariate analysis of data revealed that only age greater than 50 years, marked vascular invasion, and distant metastasis at the time of presentation were independent predictors of cancer associated mortality.

They classified their patients as low risk if they had no more than one of these predictors of mortality, and as high risk if they had two or more. The power of these variables was demonstrated by the fact that the low-risk group

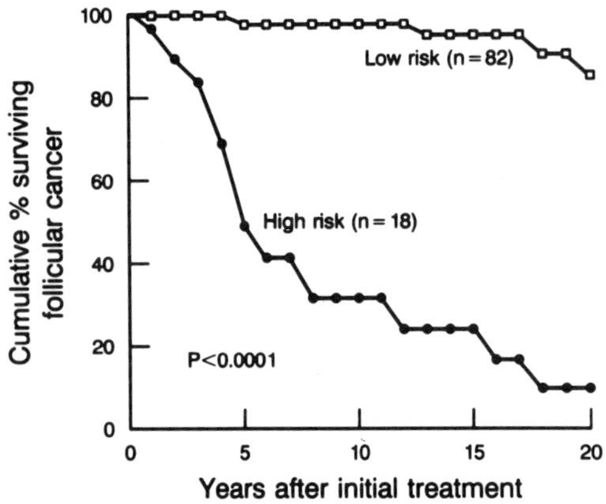

Figure 2.9. Cumulative survival among 100 patients with follicular thyroid cancer, plotted by high-risk and low-risk categories. (High risk = two or more of the following factors present: age greater than 50 years, marked vascular invasion, and metastatic disease at time of initial diagnosis.) Reprinted, by permission, from Brennan, MD., et al., 1991. (60)

had a 5-year survival rate of 99% at 5 years and 86% at 20 years, as compared with the high-risk group, which had a 5-year survival rate of only 47% and a 20-year survival rate of 8%. (Fig. 2.9)

As pointed out by Mazzaferri in an editorial accompanying his paper,[61] the survival figures must be examined in light of the fact that the patients underwent near-total, rather than total, thryoidectomy and that only a few patients received ablative radioactive iodine postoperatively.

Treatment

Follicular carcinoma of the thyroid is most often treated with surgery, radioactive iodine, and suppressive doses of thyroid hormone. External irradiation and chemotherapy are also used in certain situations.

Although subtotal thryoidectomy will almost always be curative in patients with noninvasive follicular carcinoma,[62,63] a strong argument can be made for total or near-total thryoidectomy, particularly in the case of invasive tumors. In the series of 101 patients with well-differentiated thyroid carcinoma studied by Saamen et al., (these patients were not subdivided into papillary and follicular groups) the rate of pulmonary metastasis was 9% with a less-than-total thyroidectomy and 5% with total thyroidectomy.[64] In Young and Mazzaferri's series the extent of surgery did not affect the recurrence rate, which was 11.9% in patients with limited thyroidectomy and 10.5% in patients with total thyroidectomy.[5] Young and Mazzaferri do, however, advocate total thyroidectomy for all patients with invasive disease because almost all the patients they studied who experienced a recurrence developed invasive carcinoma.

There is even more controversy regarding the surgical approach to the Hürthle cell variant of follicular carcinoma. For many years there was debate as to whether or not all Hürthle cell tumors were malignant and whether, if there was a benign type, it could be differentiated pathologically. For this reason some authors who believed that because behavior could not be predicted from gross appearance or from pathologic studies, all patients should be treated aggressively with total thyroidectomy.[38] Gundry et al. reviewed 33 years of experience with Hürthle cell tumors and concluded that size was also a factor—he advocated total thyroidectomy for histologically malignant tumors or for any tumor greater than 2 cm.[65] This was contradicted in another study, which indicated that large Hürthle cell tumors could be benign.[66] Other authors, however, believe that benign tumors can be differentiated from malignant ones and that these tumors should be handled in a fashion similar to follicular lesions.[67–70] Because Hürthle cell malignancies, unlike other follicular lesions, can metastasize to regional lymph nodes early in the course of the disease, most authors agree that a lymph node dissection is indicated in malignant lesions.[71]

Total thyroidectomy facilitates follow-up in patients with malignant follicular lesions. Thyroglobulin can be measured in order to look for recurrences. In addition, because metastatic lesions that will ultimately take up radioactive iodine may not do so in the presence of normal thyroid tissue, total thyroidectomy allows for the use of ^{131}I scans to look for recurrences and ^{131}I therapy to treat recurrences.[72,73]

It is generally accepted that suppressive

doses of thyroid hormone are efficacious in treating these patients. Well-differentiated tumors are TSH dependent—that is, TSH stimulates growth. In Young and Mazzaferri's series the overall recurrence rate over 17 years was 34% in patients who did not receive thyroid hormone versus 12% in those who received suppressive doses of thyroid hormone. Full suppression can be determined by measurement of TSH or by demonstrating failure of TSH to rise after thyrotropin-releasing hormone (TRH).[74]

The third major modality of treatment is administration of radioactive iodine. In addition to the advantage of being able to follow the cases of patients whose normal thyroid tissue has been ablated with serial thyroglobulin and ^{131}I scans, it has been well demonstrated in studies that patients treated with RaI generally have a better prognosis. In some of these studies a complete separation of patients with follicular versus papillary carcinoma is not made. In addition, the various series use different criteria for determining recurrence; that is some use the less sensitive criterion of physical exam, whereas others use more sensitive methods such as measurement of thyroglobulin and ^{131}I scanning with doses as large as 100 mCi of RaI.[64,75] Therefore, although the various series are not totally comparable it is fair to say that they demonstrate a definite trend. In 1970 Varna and Beierwaltes demonstrated that patients with follicular carcinoma who were treated with surgery and RaI did better than those treated with surgery alone.[74]

A series of 54 patients with thyroid carcinoma studied by Krishnamurthy and Blahd over 25 years demonstrated that the ability of the tumor to take up radioactive iodine was a critical factor in determining prognosis.[76] Of 44 patients in whom ablation of the metastases could be accomplished, none died of carcinoma. In the remaining 10, 7 died and 5 of those had well-differentiated carcinoma. In Young and Mazzaferri's series the patients were divided into several subgroups: those with distant metastases versus those with disease confined to the neck; those with positive nodes versus those with negative nodes; those who had total thyroidectomy versus those with less-than-total thyroidectomy; and, finally, those who did versus those who did not receive suppressive doses of thyroid hormone postoperatively.[5] All of the above benefited from RaI, with the best results (although not statistically significant) in those treated with total thyroidectomy, suppressive doses of thyroid hormone, and RaI (Fig. 2.10). The most striking benefit was demonstrated in those with invasive disease.

In Saamon's series of 101 patients with pulmonary metastases from well-differentiated thyroid carcinoma, 22 patients had follicular carcinoma.[64] Seventeen died with a 5-year survival rate of 68% and a 10-year survival rate of 36%. Sixty-four percent of the patients with follicular carcinoma had significant ^{131}I uptake by metastases. The importance of tumor burden was demonstrated as well. Those patients with a positive ^{131}I scan but a negative chest x-ray did better than those with a positive scan and a positive chest x-ray. (Fig. 2.11) This series also demonstrated that negative risk factors tend to oc-occur; patients over 60 years old had tumors that did not take up RaI and that were more poorly differentiated.

In 1986 Schlumberger et al. reported on a series of 283 patients with lung and bone metastases with well-differentiated thyroid carcinoma.[57] In this series, the patients with follicular carcinoma were divided into those with FWD and those with FMD. There were 8 remissions among the 39 patients with FWD, who had a 10-year survival rate of 33%. There were only 11 remissions among the 121 patients with FMD, who had a 15% 10-year survival rate. Once-again the effect of sensitivity of testing on recurrence rate is demonstrated. Thirty percent of the patients in this study were free of disease at 15 years using x-ray and ^{131}I scan as criteria; however, 66% of those had detectable thyroglobulin levels and 66% of those had micronodules on CT scans of the chest. Some of those did not have radioactive iodine uptake upon the administration of 1 to 2 mCi of ^{131}I but did with 100 mCi. Multivariate analysis demonstrates once again the importance of tumor burden (micronodular lung metastases with single bone metastases vs. macronodular lung metastases with multiple bone metastases)

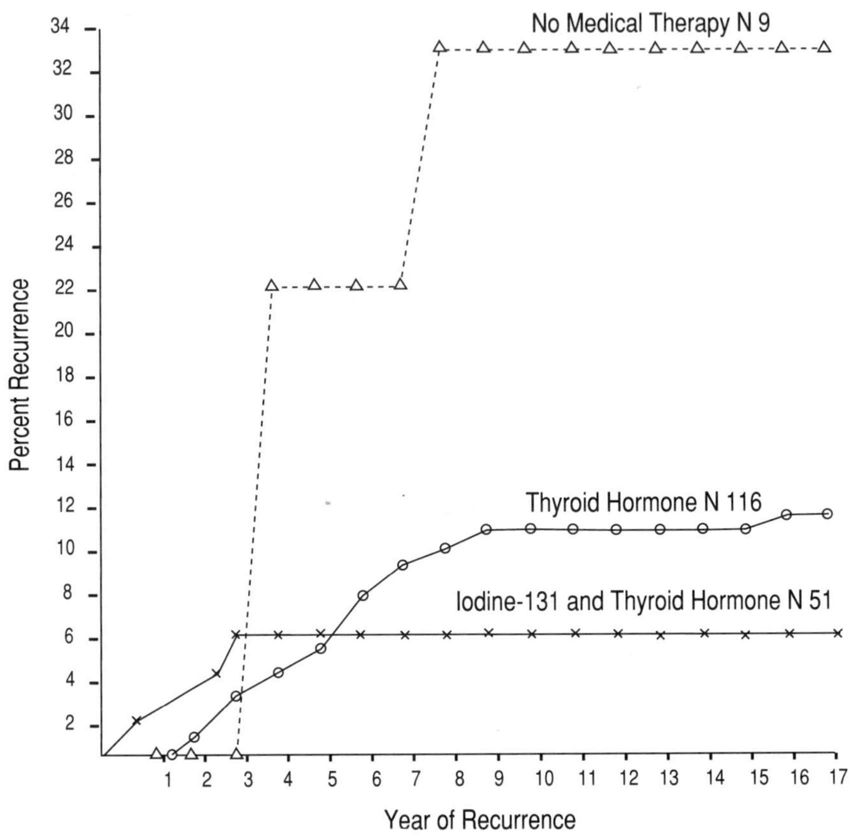

Figure 2.10. Cumulative recurrence rate, divided according to type of medical therapy used after total thyroidectomy Reprinted, by permission, from Young, R.L., Mazzaferri, E.L., Rahe, A.J., Dorfman, S.G., 1980. (5) Copyright by the Society of Nuclear Medicine, 1990.

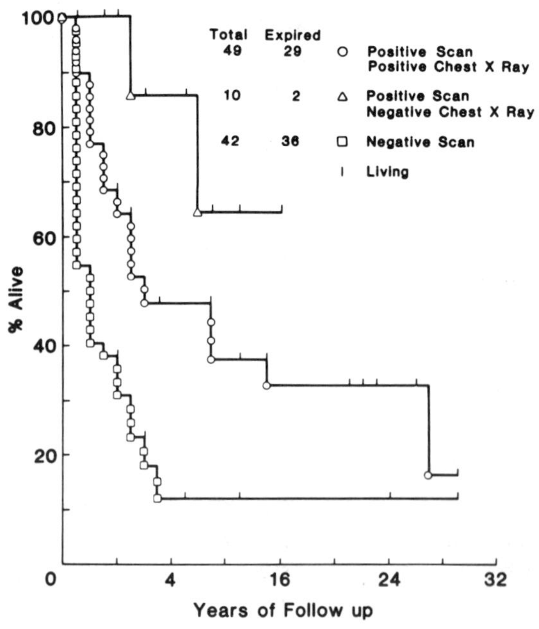

Figure 2.11. Comparison of survival from time of metastasis in patients with positive scan, positive of negative chest x-ray, and negative scan. Position scan, positive x-ray *vs.* positive scan, negative x-ray, $p < 0.04$; positive scan, positive x-ray *vs.* negative scan, $p < 0.002$; positive scan, negative x-ray *vs.* negative scan, $p < 0.002$. Reprinted, by permission, from Samaan, N.A., Schultz, P.N., Haynie, T.P., Ordonez, N.G., 1985. (64) Copyright by The Endocrine Society, 1985.

and the importance of ^{131}I uptake in survival. Of 182 patients with significant ^{131}I uptake, 77 (54%) survived for 10 years versus 94 who did not have significant uptake. The group without significant uptake had only 2 remissions and a 10-year survival rate of 9%. Again, clumping of negative risk factors was noted—older patients tended to have FMD primary lesions, and macronodular lung metastases that did not take up radioactive iodine.

References

1. Cuello C, Correa P, Eisenberg H. Georgraphic Pathology of thyroid carcinoma. Cancer 1969; 23:230–239.
2. Williams ED. Pathology and natural history. In: Duncan W, ed. Thyroid Cancer. Vol. 73. Berlin: Springer-Verlag, 1980:47–55.
3. Ingbar SH, Braverman LE. Werner's The Thyroid: a Fundamental and Clinical Text. 5th ed. Philadelphia: J.B. Lippincott Company, 1986;1329–1348.
4. Woolner LB, Beahrs OH, Black BM, McConahey WM, Keating FR. Classification and prognosis of thyroid carcinoma: A study of 885 cases observed in a thirty year period. Am J Surg 1961;102:354–387.
5. Young RL, Mazzaferri EL, Rahe AJ, Dorfman SG. Pure follicular thyroid carcinoma: Impact of therapy in 214 patients. J Nucl Med 1980;21:733–737.
6. Olin RM. Iodine deficiency and prevalence of simple goiter in Michigan. JAMA 1924;82:1328–1332.
7. Brush BE, Atland JK. Goiter prevention with iodized salt: results of a thirty-year study. J Clin Endocrinol Metab 1952;12:1380–1388.
8. Beahrs OH, Pemberton J, Black BM. Nodular goiter and malignant lesions of the thyroid gland. J Clin Endocrinol Metab 1951;1157–1165.
9. Cuello C, Correa P, Eisenberg H. Geographic pathology of thyroid carcinoma. Cancer 1969;23: 230–239.
10. Williams ED, Doriach I, Bjarnason O, Michie W. Thyroid cancer in an iodide rich area: A histopathological study. Cancer 1977;39:215–222.
11. Lindahl F. Follicular thyroid carinoma in Denmark 1943–1968. Danish Medical Bulletin 1976;23:107–119.
12. Hirabayaghi RN, Lindsay S. The relation of thyroid carcinoma and chronic thyroiditis. Surg Gynecol Obst 1965;121:243–252.
13. Shapiro SJ, Friedman WB, Perzik SL, Catz B. Incidence of thyroid carcinoma in Graves' disease. Cancer 1970;26:1261–1270.
14. Mazzaferri EL. Thyroid cancer and Graves' disease. J Clin Endocrinol Metab 1990;70:826–829.
15. Belfiore A, Garofalo MR, Giuffrida D, et al. Increased aggressiveness of thyroid cancer in patients with Graves' disease. J Clin Endocrinal Metab 1990;70:830–837.
16. Stanbury, JB. Thyroid specific metabolic incompetence and tumor development. In: Hedinger CE, ed. Thyroid Cancer. Vol. 12. New York: Springer Verley, 1969:183.
17. Cooper DS, Axelrod L, DeGroot LJ, Vickery AL, Maloof F. Congenital goiter and the development of metastic follicular carcinoma with evidence for a leak of non-hormonal iodide: Clinical, pathological, kinetic, and biochemical studies and a review of the literature. J Clin Endocrinol Metab 1981;52:294–306.
18. Riccabona G, Oberladstatter M, Fill H, Zechmann W, Fuchs D, Jenewein I. Incidence of thyroid cancer in families: Some case reports. Acta Endocrinol 1983. Suppl 252:19.
19. Lloyd KM, Dennis M. Cowden's Disease: a possible new complex with multiple system involvement. Ann Intern Med 1963;58:136–142.
20. Weary PE, Gorlln RJ, Gentry WC Jr, Comer JE, Green KE. Multiple hamartoma syndrome (Cowden's disease). Arch Dermatol 1972;106:682–690.
21. Thompson NW, Nishiyama RH, Harness JK. Thyroid carinoma: Current controversies. In: Ravitch MM, Steicher FM, eds. Current problems in Surgery 15, No. 11. Chicago: Yearbook Medical Publishers, 1978:1–15.
22. Cady B, Sedgwick CD, Meissner WA, Bookwalter JR, Romagosa V, Werber J. Changing clinical, pathologic, therapeutic, and survival patterns in differentiated thyroid carcinoma. Ann Surg 1976; 184:541–553.
23. Boehm T, Rothouse L, Wartofsky L. Metastatic occult follicular thyroid carcinoma. JAMA 1976;235:2420–2421.
24. Goldberg LD, Ditchek NT. Thyroid carcinoma with spinal cord compression. JAMA. 1981;245: 953–954.
25. McKonnon JK, Von Westap C, Mitchell R. Follicular carcinoma of the thyroid with functioning metastases and clinical hyperthyroidism. Can Med Assoc J 1975;112:724–727.
26. Sung LC, Cavalieri RR. T_3 thyrotoxicosis due to metastatic thyroid carcinoma. J Endocrinol Metab 1973;36:215–217.
27. Schneider AB, Favus MJ, Stachura ME, et al. Plasma thyroglobulin in detecting thyroid carcinoma after childhood head and neck irradiation. Ann Int Med 1977;86:29–34.
28. Bascheri L, Giani C, Taddei P, Lari R, Pinchera A. Serum thyroglobulin as a marker of thyroid carcinoma. In: Andreoli M, Monaco F, Robbins J (ed). Advances in Thyroid Neoplasia. 1981:1182–1201.
29. Smith M, McHenry C, Jarosz H, Lawrence AM, Paloyan E. Carcinoma of the thyroid in patients with autonomous nodules. Am J Surg 1988;54:448–449.
30. Miyata Y, Sasaki T, Takaya K, Taguchi Y, Kasai M. New approach for diagnosis of malignant goiter using nuclear magnetic resonance. In: Medeiros-Neto G, Gaitan E, eds. Frontiers in Thyroidology. Vol. 2. New York: Plenum 1986:1303–1307.
31. Galvan G. The value of the aspiration biopsy cytology for the diagnosis of thyroid malignancies. (Compari

son of cytology and histology in 2744 patients with hypofunctional thyroid nodules) Acta Endocrinol 1983;252:55–56.
32. Nishiyama RH, Bigos ST, Goldfarb WB, Flynn SD, Taxiarchis LN. The efficacy of simultaneous fine-needle aspiration and large-needle biopsy of the thyroid gland. Surgery 1986;100:1133–1137.
33. Lo Gerfo P, Starker P, Weber C, Moore D, Feind C. Incidence of cancer in surgically treated thyroid nodules based on method of selection. Surgery 1985;98:1197–1201.
34. Kung IT, Yuen RW. Fine needle aspiration of the thyroid. Distinction between colloid nodules and follicular neoplasms using cell blocks and 21-gauge needles. Acta Cytol 1989;33:53–60.
35. Gharib H, Goellner J, Zinsmeister AR, Grant CS, Van Heerden JA. Fine needle aspiration biopsy of the thyroid. Ann Int Med 1984;101:25–28.
36. Lang W, Georgii A, Stauch G, Kienzle E. The differentiation of atypical adenomas and encapsulated follicular carcinomas in the thyroid gland. Virchows Archiv 1980;385:125–141.
37. Hazard JB, Kenyon R. Atypical Adenoma of the Thyroid. Arch Pathol 1954;58:554–563.
38. Thompson NW, Dunn EL, Batsakis JG, Nishiyama RH. Hurtle cell lesions of the thyroid gland. Surg Gynecol Obstet 1974;139:555–560.
39. Flynn SD, Forman BH, Stewart AF, Kinder BK. Poorly differentiated ("insular") carcinoma of the thyroid gland: an aggressive subset of differentiated thyroid neoplasms. Surgery 1988;104:963–970.
40. Hedinger C, Soben LH. Histological typing of thyroid tumours. In: International Histological Classification of Thyroid Tumors. No. 11. WHO, 1974:17.
41. Hedinger C. Histological typing of thyroid tumors. 2nd ed. Berlin, Springer-Verlag 1988:1–34.
42. Franssila KO, Ackerman LV. Follicular carcinoma. Sem Diagn Pathol 1985;2:101–122.
43. Kahn NF, Perzin KH. Follicular carcinoma of the thyroid: An evaluation of the histologic criteria used for diagnosis. Pathol Annu 1983;18(Part 1):221–253.
44. Lang W, Georgii G. The differentiation of atypical adenomas and encapsulated follicular carcinomas in the thyroid gland. Virch Arch Pathol 1980;385:125–141.
45. Lang W, Choritz H, Hundeshagen H. Risk factors in follicular thyroid carcinomas. A retrospective follow-up study covering a 14 year period with emphasis on morphological findings. Am J Surg Pathol 1986; 10:246–255.
46. Woolner LB. Thyroid carcinoma: Pathologic consideration with data on prognois. Sem Uncl Med 1971; 1:481–502.
47. Harach HR, Franssila KO. Thyroglobulin immunostaining in follicular thyroid carcinoma. Histopathology 1988;13:43–54.
48. Ryff de Leche A, Staub JJ, Kohler-Faden R, Muller-Brand J, Heitz PU. Thyroglobulin production by malignant thyroid tumors. An immunocytochemical and radioimmunoassay study. Cancer 1986;57:1145–1153.
49. Mizukami Y, Michigishi T, Nonomura A, et al. Distant metastases in differentiated thyroid carcinomas: A clinical and pathologic study. Hum Pathol 1990; 21:283–290.
50. Joensu H, Klemi P, Eerola E. DNA aneuploidy in follicular adenomas of the thyroid gland. Am J Pathol 1986;124:373–376.
51. Johannessen JV, Sobrinho-Simoes M. Follicular carcinoma of the human thyroid gland. An ultrastructural study with emphasis on scanning electron microscopy. Diagn Histopathol 1982;5:113–127.
52. Lukacs GL, Balazs G, Zs-Nagy I. Cytoflourimetric measurements on the DNA contents of tumor cells in human thyroid gland. J Cancer Res Clin Oncol 1979;95:265–271.
53. Grant CS, Hay ID, Ryan JJ, Bergstrah EJ, Reunwater LM, Guillnar JR. Diagnostlc and prognostic utility of flow cytometric DNA measurements in follicular thyroid tumors. World Jnl of Surgery, 1990;14:283–289.
54. Simpson WJ, McKinney SE, Carruthers JS, Gospodarowicz MK, Sutcliffe SB, Panzarella T. Papillary and follicular thyroid cancer. Prognostic factors in 1,578 patients. Am J Med 1987;83:479–488.
55. Cady B, Rossl R, Silverman M, Wool M. Further evidence of the validity of risk group definition in differentiated thyrold carcinoma. Surgery 1985;98: 1171–1178.
56. Schmidt RJ, Wang CA. Encapsulated follicular carcinoma of the thyroid: diagnosis, treatment, and results. Surgery 1986;100:1068–1077.
57. Schlumberger M, Tubiana M, DeVathaire F, et al. Long term results of treatment of 283 patients with lung and bone metastases from differentiated thyroid carcinoma. JCEM 1986;63:960–967.
58. Schlumberger M, DeVathaire F, Travagli JP, Vassal G, et al. Differentiated thyroid carcinoma in childhood: Long term follow-up of 72 patients. J Clin Endocrinol Metab 1987;65:1088–1094.
59. Tubiana M, Schlumberger M, Rougier P, et al. Long term results and prognostic factors in patient with differentiated thyroid carcinoma. Cancer 1985;55:794–804.
60. Brennan MD, Bergstrahl EJ, Van Heerden JA, McConahay WM. Follicular thyroid cancer treated at the Mayo Clinic, 1946–1970: Initial manifestations, pathological findings, therapy and outcome. Mayo Clinic Proc. 1991;66:11–22.
61. Mazzaferri EL. Treating thyroid carcinoma: Where do we draw the line? Mayo Clinic Proc. 1991;66:105–111.
62. Woolner LB, Beahrs OH, Black BM. Classification and prognosis of thyroid carcinoma: A study of 885 cases observed in a thirty year period. Am J Surg 1961;102:354–387.
63. Brooks JR, Starnes HF, Brooks DC, Pekley JN. Surgical therapy for thyroid carcinoma: a review of 1249 solitary thyroid nodules. surgery 1988;104:940–946.
64. Samaan NA, Schultz PN, Haynie TP, Ordonez NG.

Pulmonary metastasis of differentiated thyroid carcinoma: Treatment results in 101 patients. J Clin Endocrinol Metab 1985;60:376–380.
65. Gundry SR, Burney RE, Thompson NW, Lloyd R. Total thyroidectomy for Hürthle cell neoplasm of the thyroid. Arch Surg 1983;118:529–532.
66. Gonzalez-Campora R, Herrero-Zapatero A, Lerma E, Sanchez F, Galera H. Hürthle cell and mitochondrion-rich cell tumors. A clinicopathologic study. Cancer 1986;57:1154–1163.
67. Tollefren HR, Shah JP, Huvos AG. Hürtle cell carcinoma of the thyroid. Am J Surg 1975;130:390–394.
68. Watson RG, Brennan MD, Goellner JR, McConahey WM, Taylor Wf. Invasive Hürtle Cell Carcinoma of the Thyroid: Natural History and Management. Mayo Clin Proc 1984;59:851–855.
69. Bondeson L, Bondeson AG, Ljunberg O, Tibblin S. Oxyphil Tumors of the Thyroid: Follow-up of 42 Surgical Cases. Ann Surg 1981;194:677–680.
70. LiVolsi VA. Surgical pathology of the thyroid gland. Philadelphia: WB Saunders 1990;193–212.
71. Har El G, Hadar T, Segl K, Levy R, Sidi J. Hürthle cell carcinoma of the thyroid gland. A tumor of moderate malignancy. Cancer 1986;57:1613–1617.
72. Dobyns BM, Bertozzi G. Identification of cold nodules and surgical management of carcinoma of the thyroid. Ann Surg 1970;172:703–710.
73. Pochin EE. Prospects from the treatment of thyroid carcinoma with radioiodine. Clin Radiol 1967;18:113.
74. Varma VM, Beierwaltes WH, Nofal MM, Nishiyama RH, Copp JE. Treatment of thyroid cancers: Death rates after surgery and after surgery followed by sodium iodide I-131. JAMA 1970;214:1437–1442.
75. Spies WG, Wojtowicz CH, Spies SM, Shah AY, Zimmer AM. Value of post-therapy whole-body I-131 imaging in the evaluation of patients with thyroid carcinoma having undergone high-dose I-131 therapy. Clin Nucl Med 1989;14:793–800.
76. Krishnamurthy GT, Blahd WH. Radioiodine I-131 therapy in the management of thyroid cancer. Cancer 1977;40:195–202.

3

Radiation-Induced Thyroid Carcinoma

ROBERT LLOYD SEGAL

Introduction

In the middle third of this century, from approximately 1920 to 1955, Roentgen ray therapy was used for the treatment of a variety of diseases. Many of these conditions involving the head and neck were benign lesions and/or infections (Table 3.1).[1–11] Following the observation by Duffy and Fitzgerald[12] in 1950 "of the association of prior radiation in 10 of 28 children and young adults with thyroid carcinoma," many studies have proven that radiation to the thyroid gland induces thyroid carcinoma. Though this association is noted especially in children and adolescents, it is also present in adults.[13,14] The thyroid carcinoma is associated with the Roentgen ray therapy itself. There is no association of carcinoma with the particular underlying disease or pathology for which the radiation therapy has been given.[9,15,16]

Large-scale studies were undertaken to determine the incidence of radiation-induced thyroid carcinoma in a selected population at risk, the risk factors associated with this neoplasia, treatment of radiation-induced thyroid carcinoma, and methods for follow-up of previously treated patients at risk.[14,15]

This chapter will review the incidence, risk factors, radiation factors, and treatment of radiation-induced thyroid carcinoma as well as associated nonthyroidal disorders which may develop after the head, neck, and upper thorax are exposed to radiation.

Table 3.1. Benign head, neck, and chest lesions treated with radiation

Acne valgaris
Tonsillitis—persistent or recurrent
Adenoids—enlarged or recurrent infections
Keloids
Hemangioma
Enlarged thymus
Normal thymus
Lymphadenitis
Chronic skin lesions
Congenital cardiac lesions (cardiac catheterization and angiography)
Chronic pulmonary lesions (repeated diagnostic chest x-rays)
Dermatological conditions of the scalp
Mastoiditis
Pneumonitis
Sinusitis
Impetigo
Pertussis

Definition

Radiation-induced thyroid carcinoma is a carcinoma of the thyroid gland that develops in a patient with prior radiation exposure, either direct or indirect, to the thyroid gland, as a consequence of radiation to the head, neck, face, or upper thorax.[17] There is no underlying chemical or pathologic marker for radiation-induced carcinomas that will differentiate them from naturally occurring thyroid cancer. Radiation-induced thyroid carcinoma differs from naturally occurring thyroid carcinoma in three ways: 1) radiation-induced thyroid carcinoma is often multicentric; 2) radiation-induced thyroid carcinoma may have distant metastases to the lungs more frequently than naturally-occurring carcinoma; and 3) the recurrence rate of nodularity postoperatively with an incomplete thyroidectomy may be higher in the radiation-induced thyroid carcinoma than in the naturally occurring thyroid carcinoma.[18–22]

Incidence

Determination of the incidence of thyroid carcinoma following radiation therapy may be difficult and is often inaccurate. Radiation-induced thyroid carcinoma is calculated by determining the incidence of radiation-induced thyroid carcinoma in a specific population and subtracting the incidence of naturally occurring thyroid carcinoma expected in that population.[14,22,26] The reported baseline incidence of naturally occurring thyroid carcinoma is variable; therefore, the increment due to radiation will be dependent upon the value chosen for the incidence of naturally occurring thyroid carcinoma. Naturally occurring thyroid carcinoma has an incidence of approximately 36 to 60 cases per million persons per year. It is associated with a death rate of approximately 9 per one million persons per year.[24,25] The ratio of females to males is 2:1. These tumors are extremely rare in children; however, their incidence increase with each decade in life (Fig. 3.1).

The statistics presented in autopsy surveys will in some cases include microscopic carcinomas of the thyroid gland. These carcinomas are usually less than 0.5 cm in diameter, are predominantly papillary in cell type and, with rare exceptions, are of no clinical significance. They do not require the same therapeutic approach as do the larger, clinically significant lesions. In rare cases, these minimal tumors can metastasize and become fatal.

The fact that there is such a variation in the reported incidence of thyroid carcinoma as determined by autopsy statistics affects the calculation of radiation-induced thyroid carcinoma.[26,27,28,29]

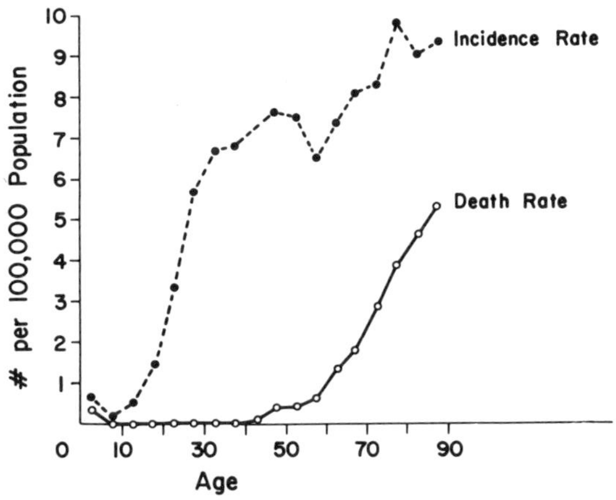

Figure 3.1. The incidence rate of thyroid carcinoma and death rate from thyroid cancer are diagrammed in relation to the experience per 100,000 population in each decade. The sharply increasing mortality occurring after age 50 is evident. (Data obtained and redrawn from Young JL Jr, Percy CL, Astaire AJ, eds. Surveillance, Epidemiology, and End Results: Incidence and Mortality Data, 1973–77. National Cancer Institute Monograph 57, NIH Publication No. 81-2330, 1981). Reprinted, by permission, from DeGroot, D., 1989. (24)

Several long-term follow-up studies using hospital records of radiation treated patients, usually children, with known doses of radiation and portals of entry have accurately been reported.[30,31] In these surveys patients were contacted and followed-up in accordance with a strict protocol. The correlation of radiation risk factors and other possible risk factors with the long-term effects of radiation, including the development of thyroid neoplasia, was evaluated. This type of study most accurately determines the factors that may be involved, not only with respect to radiation-induced thyroid carcinoma, but also with respect to other radiation-induced lesions. The chief disadvantage of this study technique is a lack of ability to contact all patients at risk.[6,9]

Because of the usual leisurely growth of most thyroid carcinomas, there is a long latent period between the radiation exposure and the development of the tumor. This long latent period, which may be as long as 41 years and may thus be a major variable in the reported

Table 3.2. Factors influencing the incidence of radiation—induced thyroid cancer

Dose of radiation.
Age of patient at the time of exposure to radiation.
Sex (females greater than males).
Duration of follow-up.
Genetic factors—rh group and blood type, HLA.
Iodine deficiency and subsequent thyroid-stimulating hormone (TSH) stimulation.
Racial and ethnic factors.
Familay history.
Thyroiditis.

incidence of radiation-induced thyroid carcinoma, must be evaluated in studies in which incidence statistics are presented.[6] Table 3.2 lists the factors which influence the incidence of radiation-induced thyroid carcinoma.

Radiation Dose Factors

It was felt that the dose of radiation received would be a priori the single most important determinant in the incidence of radiation-induced thyroid carcinoma. This assumption has been proven to be correct. A straight-line relationship between the dose of radiation and the incidence of thyroid carcinoma exists in the range between 200 and approximately 1500 rads, as shown in Fig. 3.2.[26] The frequency of thyroid cancer may be increased one hundredfold after a significant x-ray exposure. The incidence of benign nodules of the thyroid gland occurring after radiation exposure is on the order of ten times the incidence of carcinoma. Thus nodularity (both benign and malignant) is a frequent sequela of exposure of the thyroid gland to radiation.[21–23]

There is still some controversy as to whether or not there exists a radiation threshold for the induction of thyroid carcinoma.[25,26,31] A study by Modan showed an increase in the incidence of thyroid carcinoma when the radiation reaching the thyroid gland was on the order of 6 rads.[10] These investigators studied children who underwent scalp radiation for *Microsporum audouinin* infections and compared the treated children with older and younger sibling controls. A statistical increase in the incidence of thyroid carcinoma was noted in the exposed

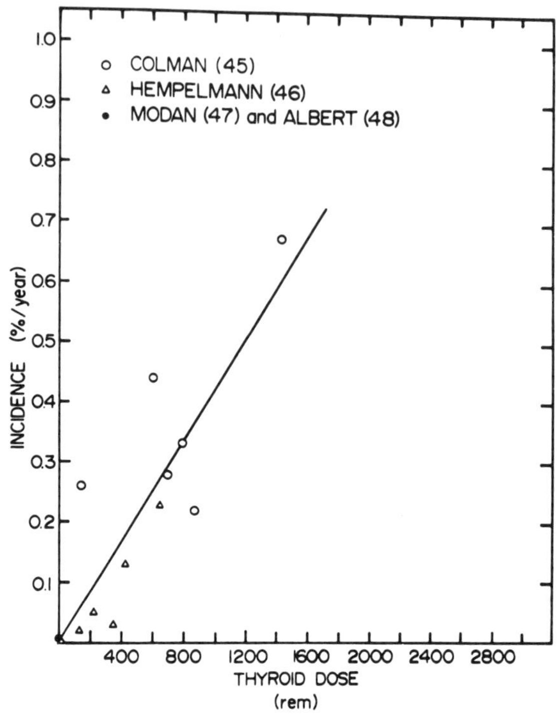

Figure 3.2. Estimated dose response for thyroid cancer and external radiation. Reprinted, by permission, from Maxon, H., Thomas, S., Saenger, E., Buncher, C., Kereiakes, J. 1977. (26)

group. The calculated dose of radiation to the thyroid gland was derived from phantom studies that reconstructed the position of the patient and the applied radiation. Though this study failed to be confirmed by dermatologists at New York University using a similar protocol, it is cited nonetheless by those who claim that there is no threshold dose necessary for the induction of thyroid neoplasms.[31] It is also cited by radiation safety and protection agencies in formulating guidelines for maximum permissible radiation exposure to the thyroid gland. Some have criticized the Modan study by noting that movement of the head would markedly increase the applied dose of radiation to the thyroid gland. If there is no threshold dose for radiation-induced thyroid carcinoma, then as little as 1 rad might induce neoplasia in some individuals; in addition, populations living at high altitudes with increased exposure to natural radiation could be expected to have a higher incidence of thyroid

Table 3.3. Estimated risk of thyroid cancer following radiation exposure in infancy and childhood—selected studies

Investigators	Radiation exposure: Time of exposure	Type of radiation	Mean thyroid dose (rad)	Number exposed	Type of controls	No. of follow-up years and (Mean)	Risk of thyroid Cancer/ 10^8 children/ rad yr
Hempelmann *et al.* (10, 9)	1926–1957	X-ray therapy	229	2,878	Siblings	6–37 (16)	2.5
Subgroup C (20, 9)	1930–1946	X-ray therapy	239	233	Siblings	17–32 (24)	5.5
Ann Arbor Study (8, 9)	1932–1954	X-ray therapy	20	958	Population rates	12–36 (29)	2.2
Modan *et al.* (16)	1949–1960	X-ray therapy	6.5	10,902	Siblings and matched population controls	12–23 (17)	6.1
Albert *et al.* (2, 1, 23)	1940–1958	X-ray therapy	6.0	2,213	Clincal controls	11–32 (21)	0
Jablon *et al.* (12)	1945	Atomic bomb blast N and γ	143	811	Unexposed and low-exposure residents	25	2.9
Conard *et al.* (4)	1954	Fallout β and γ	1,225	19	Unexposed residents	20	2.1

Reprinted, by permission, from Silverman C, Hoffman D.A., 1979. (30)

carcinoma. There are no data to support this thesis. At this time the question of whether or not a threshold dose exists is not settled.

At high doses of radiation exposure, the cytotoxic effects of radiation would theoretically include sterilization of the thyroid field. If this biological effect were to take place, one would effectively ensure the development of hypothyroidism in the exposed population. This chain of events does occur, and has been reported. This sterilizing effect of the radiation may account for the fact that thyroid carcinoma rarely develops after extremely high doses of radiation.[26,31]

The biological effects of radiation include a random track or path through tissue, chemical changes secondary to the energy released, and derangement of macromolecules, particularly in the nucleus. The energy imparted by the radiation disrupts chemical bonds of the nuclear proteins; it subsequently causes decreased reproductive capacity of the affected cells, possibly decreasing their secretory function. This implies an eventual decrease in thyroid hormone production.[32] The decrease in thyroid hormone production secondary to the biological effects of radiation on the thyroid gland will evoke the hormone-stabilizing efforts of the body; there will be increased production of thyroid stimulating hormone. This hormone acts as a growth factor and may promote tumor formation.

Because of the random nature of the distribution of radiation passing through thyroid tissue, pathologic changes may be noted in more than one region. The estimated risks of thyroid carcinoma in irradiated individuals is presented in Table 3.3.

In this table the combined effects of radiation are presented in infants and children and correlated with length of follow-up, time of exposure, type of radiation, and dosage. As can be seen, the incidence of thyroid carcinoma is highly significant. DeGroot et al. noted a peak incidence of 5% at 20 to 25 years postradiation in patients treated for acne or disease of the tonsils and adenoids with chargeteristic doses of 500 rads. Other factors influencing the inci-

Table 3.4. Estimated risk of thyroid cancer in four groups of irradiated persons

Irradiated group	Number	Observed/expected	Average dose (rad)	Risk coefficient (per 10^4/rad)
Marshall Islanders (11)*	243	7	213*	134*
Japanese survivors (74)	10,000	23	115	20
Neck irradiation	2,872	24	119	70
Tinea capitis (65)	10,402	10	10	92

*The thyroid dose has been recently reviewed, and the importance of the presence of short half-life isotpes of iodide in the fallout has been emphasized. Thus, these figures cannot now be regarded as accurate. Reprinted from Dolphin GW: Radiation Carcinogenesis. In Duncan W (ed.): Recent Results in Cancer Research, p. 27. New York: Springer-Verlag, 1980.

dence of thyroid carcinoma include the portals of entry of the radiation and the type and energy of radiation, as well as the effect of secondary filters (discussion of which is beyond the scope of this chapter).

The phenomenon of radiation-induced thyroid carcinoma is age-dependent. Infants and children are at greater risk than adults. This may be due to growth factors other than thyroid-stimulating hormone (TSH), that are operative in infants and children, but absent in adults. The growth of the thyroid from 20 mg grams at birth to 25 g in adulthood may not be mediated exclusively by thyroid stimulating hormone. The existence of other growth factors has been postulated, but not proven. The reduced sensitivity of the adult thyroid to radiation-induced thyroid carcinoma is responsible for the lower incidence of thyroid carcinoma in those exposed to atomic radiation in the Marshall Islands, Hiroshima and Nagasaki, and in those exposed to radiation in hospitals and nuclear energy facilities (Table 3.4).[32,33,34]

For unknown reasons, the incidence of carcinoma of the thyroid gland is greater in females than in males, in both irradiated and nonirradiated populations.

There is a long latent period between the time of radiation exposure of the thyroid gland and the development of carcinoma secondary to this radiation. The absolute incidence of thyroid carcinoma in radiated individuals continues to increase with time for up to 40 years.[9,32] It should be reiterated that DeGroot et al.[34] found that a maximal incidence of radiation-induced thyroid carcinoma occurs between 20 and 25 years (Fig. 3.3). These long-term studies have demonstrated that the carcinogenic effects of radiation to the thyroid are ongoing, although the relative risks decline beyond 25 years, due perhaps to the aging of the population and the increased incidence of naturally occurring thyroid carcinoma. This decrease in relative risk after 25 years is illustrated in Fig. 3.4.[33]

DeGroot and others have found that the shorter the induction period, the more clinically aggressive the carcinoma. This observation has been reported by several groups. A short latent period for the development of thyroid carcinoma may result in a large lesion. All groups have found that the prognosis of thyroid carcinoma, both radiation-induced and naturally occurring, correlates with the size of the original lesion. The shorter induction period may mean more rapid growth and a larger initial lesion.[8,9,16]

Genetic factors influencing the development of naturally occurring thyroid carcinoma include chromosomal instability in patients with medullary carcinoma, an increased incidence of HLA-DR1 in undifferentiated thyroid carcinoma and an increased incidence of HLA-DR7 in undifferentiated follicular thyroid carcinoma.[18] None of these factors has been shown to be operative in patients with radiation-induced thyroid carcinoma. One group recorded a protective effect of the blood type O phenotype and an increased incidence of radiation-induced thyroid carcinoma in patients with type A.[18,33]

There is a high incidence of endemic nodular goiter in areas where there is iodine deficiency.

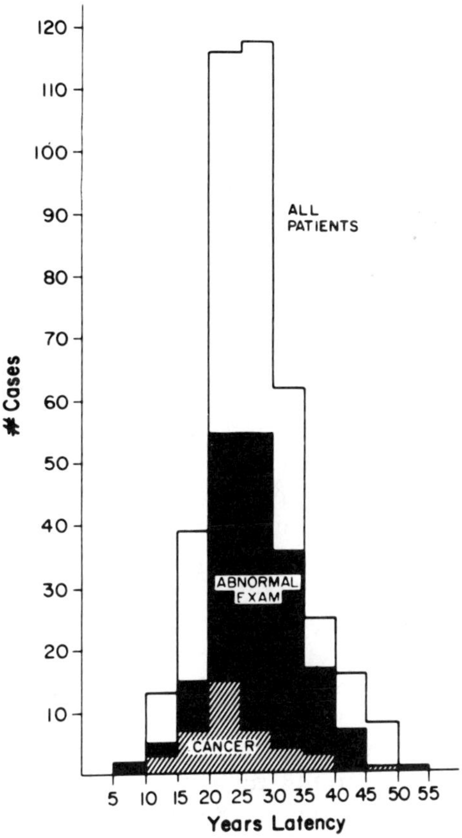

Figure 3.3. Distribution of patients with a history of irradiation to the head and neck, according to the time after irradiation at which they were examined. The majority of patients were seen 20–35 years after irradiation, but the incidence of tumors peaked 5–10 years earlier. Tumors continued to occur through 40 years after irradiation; it is not clear that there is a finite latency period. Reprinted, by permission, from "Thyroid Neoplasia" in *The Thyroid and Its Diseases* 5th ed. John Wiley & Sons.

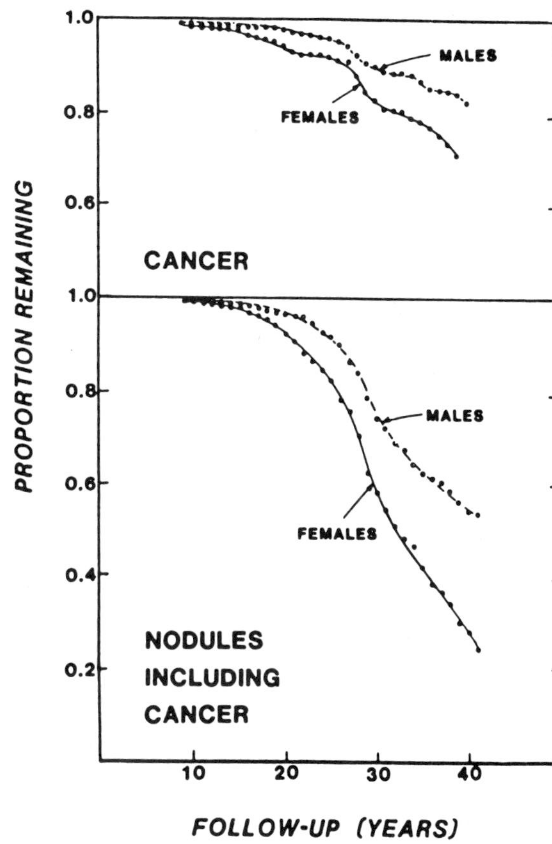

Figure 3.4. Disease-free survival curves derived from the proportional hazards model and evaluated at the average age and dose. The *points* are the actual observations. The *upper panel* shows the cancer-free survival, while the *lower panel* shows the survival without developing neoplasms (benign and malignant). Reprinted, by permission, from Perkel, U.S., Gail, M.H., Lubin, J., et al., 1988. (37) Copyright by The Endocrine Society, 1988.

These glands show an increased incidence of anaplastic carcinoma. There is no study showing an increased incidence of radiation-induced thyroid carcinoma in iodine-deficient glands in humans. Radiation-induced thyroid carcinoma occurs in mice and rats following the use of propylthiouracil and thiourea derivatives to induce hyperplasia and hypertrophy of the thyroid gland. Even minimal doses of radiation in these animals will cause a high incidence of thyroid cancer.[35]

There are no reports of ethnic or racial predisposition to the development of thyroid carcinoma following radiation. The Japanese have a high incidence of microscopic sclerosing carcinomas that are not clinically significant. The incidence of these carcinomas was the same in the control population as in those exposed to radiation in Hiroshima and Nagasaki and, indeed, in the Japanese raised in Hawaii.[36]

There is evidence that with naturally occurring thyroid carcinoma a positive family history is an additional risk factor for the development of well-differentiated thyroid carcinoma.[33,37]

Conversely, there is no evidence that in patients with radiation-induced thyroid carcinoma there is an increased risk for the development of thyroid carcinoma in their offspring. There is, however, evidence that radiation may induce medullary carcinoma in patients who have a family history of the disease and are genetically predisposed (see Chapter 8). These tumors may appear at an earlier age in those exposed to radiation than in those family members not exposed to radiation.

The incidence of thyroiditis in the general population is variable. This disease may impair thyroid function and invoke TSH stimulation of the thyroid gland in an attempt to maintain hormonal stasis. This TSH stimulation may sensitize the thyroid gland to the biologic effects of radiation and predispose one to develop radiation-induced thyroid carcinoma.[38] As previously noted, TSH stimulation is a factor in the induction of thyroid carcinoma in experimental animals.[33]

Pathology

Given the multiple biologic effects of radiation upon cells and the tumorigenic quality of this radiation, one would expect that there might be a difference between the behavior of radiation-induced carcinoma and naturally occurring carcinoma.[20] This possibility has been investigated by several groups. One approach to this question is to compare those patients with thyroid carcinoma who have not had a history of radiation either in childhood or in infancy and who develop thyroid carcinoma, with those who have naturally occurring thyroid carcinoma and have no previous history of radiation.[20,21] It should be noted that historically up to 80% of children and teenagers who develop thyroid carcinoma have a history of previous radiation.

Naguib and Samaan[21] et al. compared thyroid carcinoma in radiated and nonradiated patients. The prevalence of different histologic types of thyroid carcinoma was almost identical in the irradiated and nonirradiated groups. Bilateral abnormalities of the thyroid gland were found in a significantly greater number of patients who had been irradiated than in the control group: 51% versus 35%, with a probability of more than 0.005. Spitalnik[19] et al. found that 88% of their irradiated patients showed focal epithelial hyperplasia, with a large proportion showing moderate to severe involvement throughout the thyroid. A control group of nonirradiated patients showed only a 12% incidence of minimal focal hyperplasia. One half of the irradiated cases who had focal hyperplasia also had associated adenomas within the gland. Eighty-five percent of the patients showing carcinoma exhibited this extensive hyperplasia.[20] Adenomas, both single and multiple, and adenomatous hyperplasia were found in over half (51%) of the radiated thyroids. These adenomas were mainly of the microfollicular type. Small microfollicular adenomas were found in only 2% of the nonirradiated cases. A large proportion (68%) of the irradiated thyroids contained mild-to-moderate infiltration with lymphocytes or thyroiditis, often with the formation of germinal centers. No changes of this kind were found in the control population. Colloid nodule formation was found in 51% of the irradiated thyroids; the control thyroids showed minimal colloid nodule formation (32%). Oxyphilic cell change was seen in 42% of the irradiated thyroids. None of the controls showed oxyphilic changes. One quarter of the irradiated thyroids showed mild diffuse fibrosis, which presented as thickening of the supportive lobular stroma, not as broad areas of dense collagen. No similar fibrosis was observed in the control glands. Sixty-two percent of the irradiated glands were found to have well-differentiated carcinoma. The size ranged from 0.1 cm to 5.5 cm in the greatest dimension; the average diameter was 1.6 cm. Nearly 60% of the adenocarcinomas were of the mixed papillary–follicular type; pure papillary carcinoma was the next most frequent malignancy. No undifferentiated carcinomas were present in this series. The high incidence of focal hyperplasia in this group of irradiated patients was interpreted as being due to the effect of TSH stimulation on the gland. Thyroiditis with the oxyphilic cell changes suggested the development of a cellular autoimmune reaction in the irradiated glands, possibly caused by physical damage to the epithelial cells with the release of thyroglobulin and microsomal antigen. Colloid nodular change that was present in these glands may represent prolonged intermittent stimulation of the gland by TSH. Low-dose radiation of the thyroid did not lead to widespread destruction of the parenchyma with subsequent fibrous replacement. Instead, the fibrosis was of the mild, diffuse, interstitial type.[19,23]

All groups have found that childhood radiation to the thyroid gland causes marked changes in the morphology of the gland, including multiple nodules of varying histologic type, extensive fibrosis and, less commonly, the changes characteristic of thyroiditis in addition to those characteristic of thyroid cancer. Komorowski[22,22A,22B] and others found that almost all the glands removed at surgery following radiation had multiple nodules ranging from 0.1 cm to several centimeters in diameter. The adenomatous nodules were of varying histologic types including follicular, fetal and Hürthle cells; most glands contained all three types. These features presented difficulties in both the clinical evaluation of the patients and the evaluation of glands during surgery because the irradiated thyroid gland may contain multiple small nodules that are not detectable by gross observation prior to surgery. DNA content of radiation-associated carcinoma was not different from naturally occurring thyroid cancer.[22A] In a number of cases it was only after microscopic examination of sections of the thyroid gland that numerous small nodules became apparent.[18] In 8 of the 12 cases cancer was found in an area other than the large gross nodule that presented clinically. Furthermore, the gross appearance of the malignant nodules in these irradiated glands was not sufficiently characteristic to aid in identifying suspicious areas for frozen sections.[18] The standard histologic criteria for diagnosis of thyroid cancer apply to irradiated patients. The significance of the one case of medullary carcinoma following childhood radiation reported by this group remains speculative. There was no evidence of multiple endocrinopathy in that patient.[23] Others have reported on the development of medullary carcinoma in irradiated individuals. In addition, one case of anaplastic thyroid cancer has been reported.[18]

Several groups have studied the pathology of the irradiated versus nonirradiated thyroid gland in both the presence and absence of carcinoma. Radiation biology would predict that the irradiated gland would have multiple areas of involvement. Aside from cancer, the effects of radiation on the thyroid gland include hyperplasia, benign adenomas, colloid nodules (usually microfollicular in type), and oxyphilic cell changes (perhaps secondary to autoimmunity) involving the release of thyroglobulin and microsomal fractions. Invasion of the thyroid gland by lymphocytes occurs, producing a clinical picture consistent with thyroiditis. Fibrosis occurs; although in most glands it is found to be minimal, with thickening of the septa. These changes occur in multiple areas of the thyroid gland and give rise to multiple nodules within the gland.[22] These irradiated glands, when compared to controls, contain multiple nodules that may range from 0.1 cm to 1.6 cm. Identification of thyroid carcinoma in the irradiated glands is enhanced if multiple sections are taken, owing to the multicentricity of radiation effects.[21]

The pathology of lymph gland involvement depends on the size of the original lesion. The incidence of local lymph gland involvement is not greater than that of corresponding carcinomas in the nonirradiated group that are in size equal. The presence of psammoma bodies in all the cases of papillary carcinoma was noted by one group.[21]

There is disagreement between groups as to whether or not the multifocal carcinomas secondary to radiation are more aggressive than naturally occurring thyroid carcinomas.[9] The types of local and distant metastases in radiation-induced thyroid carcinoma are reported by one group as being quite different from those of a control group. In this report, the incidence of lung involvement was found in all patients who had distant metastases. Lung metastases were present in just over half the patients who had a naturally occurring thyroid carcinoma. This difference in the distribution of metastasis may influence therapy.[21]

Diagnosis and Treatment

The diagnosis of radiation-induced thyroid carcinoma is dependent on knowing the history of exposure of the thyroid gland to radiation. In the patient who presents with a thyroid mass, it is routine to obtain this vital piece of medical history. However, the historical information may be inadequate or erroneous. In a series of patients who had had irradiation of the neck for tuberculous adenitis, 36% did not mention or recall this aspect of their medical history. In a group of 128 patients with thyroid lesions, Schneider found that many did not initially mention their prior exposures to radiation.[9] Because the exposure to radiation may have taken place in infancy or childhood, patients may not be aware that it had occurred. Repeated questioning during follow-up visits may increase the accuracy of this aspect of the patient's medical history. Parental consultation and ancillary historical facts may aid in determining whether or not radiation therapy was given. Questioning whether shielding was used, whether other people were in the room at the same time, and so on, may also aid in identifying a history of radiation exposure. Occasionally a false positive radiation history may be obtained, usually from those who have received Grenz ray or ultraviolet therapy for acne.

Patients whose thyroid glands have been radiated may present with a normal gland, a diffuse goiter, a solitary nodule, a multinodular thyroid gland, or a metastatic thyroid carcinoma.[9,16] In addition to a history of radiation exposure, the basic exam of a radiation-exposed patient should consist of evaluation of the thyroid gland and the neck based on a careful exam by a clinician experienced in examination of the thyroid. Thyroid function is evaluated by administering chemical tests that measure thyroid hormone levels (and sensitive TSH assay). In addition, antithyroid antibody tests should be performed.[39]

In addition, a baseline ^{123}I scan should be done.[9] We believe that this test is of value in delineating a "cold" or nonfunctioning area, which may be either a nonpalpable abnormality or a lesion missed on physical examination. The use of ^{123}I is necessary to minimize the additional radiation exposure of the thyroid gland and to accurately delineate the functioning and nonfunctioning areas within the gland. Radioactive iodide preparations are more accurate than technetium for thyroid scanning.

Sonography may not be helpful in the evaluation of irradiated thyroid glands because of its extreme sensitivity, which may delineate clinically insignificant lesions. Annual or biannual examinations are indicated for all patients with a history of thyroid radiation exposure.

If a solitary nodule is present, fine needle aspiration biopsy of the thyroid may be undertaken. Some believe that the presence of a solitary nodule in an irradiated thyroid may be predictive of neoplastic transformation in other portions of the gland. Observation of the nodule for a short period under thyroxine (T_4) suppression may result in complete supression of those few nodules that are not significant.[41] A solitary nodule may be a marker for carcinomatous transformation in other areas of the gland. In many instances, a nodule that appears to be solitary on clinical investigation is found not to be solitary at surgery. In our opinion, if the nodule either does not regress, or enlarges under thyroxin suppression, or if it is initially greater than 2.5 cm, then surgery is necessary. Additional indications for surgical intervention include a fine needle aspiration or other biopsy positive for carcinoma, esophageal or tracheal compression, or evidence of local or distant metastasis.[42]

We believe that the treatment of differentiated thyroid carcinoma in the irradiated patient should be somewhat different from that of naturally occurring thyroid carcinoma. If the gland has been radiated and carcinoma is present, we favor a total thyroidectomy.[43] This surgical procedure will obviate the risk of a recurrence of thyroid cancer or an occurrence of a new neoplastic lesion in residual thyroid tissue due to radiation. If there is definite carcinoma present, and total thyroidectomy is not undertaken for technical surgical reasons, we suggest a near-total thyroidectomy with subsequent radioiodine ablation of residual thyroid tissue. This accomplishes the goal of ablation of all residual radiation-exposed thyroid tissue, which is a potential source of neoplastic transformation in the future. Postoperatively, patients who have had a total thyroidectomy require the use of replacement levothyroxine therapy to maintain a euthyroid state. In particular, when a total thyroidectomy has not been performed, suppressive use of levothyroxine should be encouraged to reduce the incidence of recurrence. There is no proof as yet that the extent of the surgical procedure affects prognosis.

The prognosis for naturally occurring thyroid carcinoma and radiation-induced thyroid carcinoma appears to be similar.[9,16,39] The main prognostic factor is the size of the initial lesion. Since radiation-induced thyroid carcinoma occurs in younger people and may have been present for longer periods of time before the diagnosis is made, in age-matched controls the prognosis is less favorable for the larger lesion than for the smaller ones.

Most patients who were treated with radiation to the head and neck are now between 35 to 45 years posttherapy. Because thyroid carcinoma may be more aggressive in older patients, it is necessary that ongoing follow-up studies be conducted with strict adherence to a protocol in the postradiated patients, no matter how old, so that the carcinomas that may develop will be diagnosed early, before the prognosis becomes unfavorable.

In the years since 1955, when radiation-induced neoplastic change in the thyroid was first recognized, the use of radiation therapy to the head, neck, and face for benign conditions has been virtually discontinued. With time, the entity of radiation-induced thyroid carcinoma should disappear. This trend is already evident, as can be seen in Ceccareli's 1988 report on 78 patients with childhood thyroid carcinoma.[43] Only four of these patients gave a history of prior radiation. In previous series of childhood thyroid malignancies similar to this, over 80% of the patients gave a history of prior radiation.

There is widespread use of radioactive iodine in the diagnosis and treatment of thyroid disease. The radiation from ^{131}I, ^{123}I and technetium, which are commonly used diagnostically or therapeutically, is listed in Table 3.5.[44] As can be seen, a significant amount of radiation is delivered to the thyroid gland from diagnostic studies that use these isotopes. This radiation could theoretically lead to the occurrence of radiation-induced thyroid carcinoma. In extensive studies in the United States, Denmark and Iceland, no increase in the incidence of thyroid carcinoma has been noted. Maxon[26,31] has calculated the risk for the development of thyroid cancer from diagnostic and therapeutic use of isotopes and has shown that there is minimal risk, if any.

Table 3.5. Thyroid and whole body radiation secondary to isotopic studies of thyroid gland*

Isotope	Dose	Thyroid radiation (rem)	Whole-body radiation (rem)
^{123}I	100 μCi	0.5–2	0.0003
^{99}Te	2.5 mCi	0.2–1.8	0.003
^{131}I	50 μCi	25–100	0.04

* Assumes normal thyroid function and uptake

Reprinted, by permission, from Atkins, Harold L., "The Thyroid" in *Clinical Radionuclide Imaging*, 3rd Ed. Freeman, Leonard M., ed. Philadelphia W.B. Saunders, 1986.

It has been previously noted that in patients receiving more than 2000 rads to the thyroid gland from external radiation, the incidence of carcinoma is minimal. As previously noted, this is due to the sterilizing effect of the radiation on the thyroid gland; cytotoxic effects essentially cause an absence of viable thyroid tissue. Nevertheless, there have been occasional reports of patients who have had more than 2000 rads administered to the thyroid gland who did develop carcinoma.[45]

In the treatment of hyperthyroidism or other thyroid conditions treated with radioactive iodine, the amount of radiation delivered to the thyroid gland is usually above 2000 rads. Therefore, therapeutic doses of radioactive iodine are not accompanied by neoplastic transformation of the gland, except in rare instances.[46–56]

Radiation to the head, neck, face, or upper thorax is obviously not limited to the thyroid gland. Therefore, it is not surprising that tumors of other organs in close proximity to the thyroid gland may be associated with thyroid neoplasia. For example, both benign and malignant salivary gland tumors have been reported following radiation in this area. Carotid body tumors, neuromas and other rare tumors such as esophagal carcinoma have been reported to occur with thyroid cancer following external radiation.

Hyperparathyroidism may occur after radiation to the head or neck, usually developing approximately a decade later than radiation-induced thyroid carcinoma does. Radiation-induced hyperparathyroidism may be due to hyperplasia, adenoma formation, or in a small number of cases, carcinoma of the parathyroid glands. The incidence of hyperparathyroidism in postirradiated patients may be higher than thyroid carcinoma. The treatment of this condition is usually surgical.[56–67]

Thyroid and breast carcinoma has been reported in patients in whom the radiation field has included the upper thorax.[68]

Conclusion

The number of people at risk for the development of radiation-induced thyroid carcinoma who are now entering a period 40 to 50 years after exposure to radiation is estimated to be over one million. At this particular time, such cancers may be more aggressive in this age group. The molecular basis of this transformation has been postulated as being partially due to the activation of oncogenes,[69] or to the inactivation of antitumor genes or suppressor agents. Neither of these theories, however, has been proven, despite extensive investigation. The clinician must constantly be aware of the potential danger of carcinogenesis in post-irradiated patients and must provide systematic ongoing follow-up for all patients known to be at risk.

References

1. Thomson D, Grammes C, Starkey R, Sunderlin F. Thyroid abnormalities in patients previously treated with irradiation for acne vulgaris. Southern Medical Journal 1984;77:21–23.
2. Talmi Y, Kalmanovitch M, Zohar Y. Thyroid carcinoma, cataract and hearing loss in a patient after irradiation for facial hemangioma, J Laryngol Otol 1988;102(1):91–92.
3. Martin EC, Olson AP, Steeg CN, Casarella WJ. Radiation exposure to the pediatric patient during cardiac catheterization and angiocardiography—Emphasis on the thyroid gland. Circulation 1981; 64:153–158.
4. Waldman HD, Rummerfield PS, Gilpin EA, Kirkpatrick SE. Radiation exposure to the child during cardiac catheterization. Circulation 1981;64:158–163.
5. Gustafsson M, Mortensson W. Radiation exposure and estimate of late effects of chest roentgen examination in children. Acta Radiol. Diagnosis 1983;24:309–314.
6. Schneider AB. Thyroid nodules following childhood irradiation: A 1989 Update. Thyroid Today; 1989;12(2):1–8.
7. DeGroot L, Paloyan E. Thyroid carcinoma and radiation: A Chicago Epidemic. JAMA 1973;224:487–491.
8. Favus MJ, Schneider AB, Stachura ME, et al. Thyroid cancer occurring as a late consequence of head-and-neck irradiation. N Eng J Med 1976;294:1019–1025.
9. Schneider AB, Shore-Freedman E, Ryo UY, et al. Radiation-induced tumors of the head and neck following childhood irradiation: Prospective studies. Medicine 1985;64:1–15.
10. Ron E, Modan B. Benign and malignant thyroid neoplasms after childhood irradiation for tinea capitis. JNCI 1980;65:7–11.
11. Shore RD, Woddard E, Hildreth N, et al. Thyroid tumors following thymus irradiation. J Natl Cancer Inst 1985;74:1177–1184.
12. Duffy BJ, Fitzgerald PJ. Thyroid cancer in childhood and adolescence: Report on 28 cases. Cancer 1950;3:1018–1032.
13. Wang JX, Boice JD, Li BX, et al. Cancer among medical diagnostic x-ray workers in China. JNCI 1988;80:344–350.
14. McTiernan AM, Weiss NS, Daling JR. Incidence of thyroid cancer in women in relation to previous exposure to radiation therapy and history of thyroid disease. JNCI 1984;73:575–581.
15. Pifer J, Hempelmann L. Radiation-induced thyroid carcinoma. Annals NY Academy of Sciences 1948;838–847.
16. DeGroot L, Frohman L, Kaplan E, Refetoff S. Radiation-Associated Thyroid Carcinoma. New York: Grune & Stratton; 1977.
17. Ingbar SH & Braverman LE, Werner's. The Thyroid: A Fundamental and Clinical Texts, 5th ed. Philadelphia: J.D. Lippincott Co.; chap. 17, p. 436.
18. Wilson S, Komorowski R, Cerletty J, Majewski J, Hooper M. Radiation-associated thyroid tumors: Extent of operation and pathology technique influence the apparent incidence of carcinoma. Surgery 1983;94:663–669.
19. Spitalnik PF, Straus II FH. Patterns of human thyroid parenchymal reaction following low-dose childhood irradiation. Cancer 1978;41:1098–1105.
20. Hanson G, Komorowski R, Cerletty J, Wilson S. Thyroid gland morphology in young adults: normal subjects versus those with prior low-dose neck irradiation in childhood. Surgery 1983;94:984–988.
21. Naguib A, Samaan P, Schultz N, Ordonez R, Hickey R, Johnston D. A comparison of thyroid carcinoma in those who have not had head and neck irradiation in childhood. J Clin Endocrinol Metab 1987;64:219–223.
22. Komorowski R, Hanson G. Morphologic changes in the thyroid following lose-dose childhood radiation. Arch Pathol Lab Med 1977;101:36–39.

22A. Komorowski R, Deaconson T, Vetsch R, Cerletty J, Wilson S. DNA content in radiation-associated thyroid cancer. Surgery 1988;104:992–996.

22B. Komorowski R, Hanson G, Garancis J. Anaplastic thyroid carcinoma following low-dose irradiation. Am Soc of Clin Pathologists 1978;70:303–307.

23. Wilson S, Platz C, Block G. Thyroid carcinoma after irradiation. Arch Surg 1970;100:330–337.

24. Endocrinology. DeGroot LJ (ed.); Endocrinology, 2nd ed., 1989, chap. 49. Thyroid Neoplasia, Philadelphia: WB Saunders & Co., Vol. I, pp. 764–766.

25. Young J, Percy C, Astaire A. Surveillance, epidemiology, and end results: Incidence and mortality data. 1973–1977 National Cancer Institute Monograph 57, NIH Publication No. 81-2330, 1981.

26. Maxon H, Thomas S, Saenger E, Buncher C, Kereiakes J. Ionizing irradiation and the induction of clinically significant disease in the human thyroid gland. Am J Med 1977;63:967–978.

27. Farunaga F. Occult thyroid cancer. In DeGroot LJ, et al., eds. Radiation-Associate Thyroid Carcinoma. New York: Grune & Stratton, 1977:161–174.

28. Sampson RJ. Prevalence and significance of occult thyroid cancer. In DeGroot L, Frohman LA, Kaplan EL, Refetoff S, eds. Radiation Associated Thyroid Carcinoma. New York: Grune & Stratton, 1977:137–153, 175–181.

29. Nishiyama R, Ludwig F, Thompson N. The prevalence of small papillary thyroid carcinomas in 100 consecutive necropsies in an American population. In DeGroot L, et al., eds. Radiation-Associated Thyroid Carcinoma. New York: Grune & Stratton; 1977:123–135, 501–503.

30. Silverman C, Hoffman DA. Thyroid Tumor Risk from Radiation During Childhood. Preventive Med 1979;4:100–105.

31. Goldschmidt H, Sherwin W. Reactions to ionizing radiation. J Am Acad Dermatol 1980;3:551–569.

32. Smallridge R, Wartofsky L, Burman R. Thyroid carcinoma and Hodgkin's disease (letter). Ann Intern Med 1981;94:412–413.

33. Doniach J. Pathology of irradiation thyroid damage. In: DeGroot L, et al., eds. Radiation-Associated Thyroid Carcinoma. New York: Grune & Stratton; 1977:199–212.

34. Wood J, Tamagaki H, Neriishi S, Sato T, Sheldon W, Archer P, Hamilton H, Johnson K. Thyroid carcinoma in atomic bomb survivors of Hiroshima and Nagasaki. Am J Epidemiology 1969;89:4–14.

35. Rallison M, Dobyns B, Keating F, Rall J, Tyler F. Thyroid disease in children: A survey of subjects potentially exposed to fallout radiation. Am J Med 1974;56:457–568.

36. Johnson C. Before Chernobyl: Hanford, Savannah River and Rocky Flats. JAMA 1987;257–191.

37. Perkel VS, Gail MH, Lubin J, et al. Radiation-induced thyroid neoplasms: Evidence for familial susceptibility factors. J Clin Endocrinol Metab 1988;66:1316–1322.

38. Al-Hindawi A, Black E, Brewer D, Griffiths S, Hoffenberg R. Thyroid hormone measurements in experimental thyroid cancer in rats. In DeGroot L, et al., eds. Radiation-Associated Thyroid Carcinoma. New York: Grune & Stratton; 1977:215–216.

39. Sampson R, Key C, Buncher C, Iijima S. Thyroid carcinoma in Hiroshima and Nagasaki: Prevalence of thyroid carcinoma at autopsy. JAMA 1969;209:65–70.

40. Rimoin D, Schimke RN. Genetic Disorders of the Endocrine Glands. New York: Mosby., 1971:127–149.

41. DeGroot, LJ. Diagnostic approach and management of patients exposed to irradiation to the thyroid. J Clin Endocrinol Metab 1989;69:925–928.

42. Razack M, Katsutaro S, Sako K, Rao U. Suppressive therapy of thyroid nodules in patients with previous radiotherapy to the head and neck. Am J Surg 1988;156:290–292.

43. Segal R, Cobin R, Futterweit W, Fiedler R, Sirota D. Thyroid nodules in the irradiated patient: an indication for total thyroidectomy. J Surg Oncol 1985;28:126–130.

44. Ceccarelli C, Pacini F, Lippi F, Elisei R, Arganin M, Miccoli P, Pinchera A. Thyroid cancer in children and adolescents. Surgery, December 1988;104:1143–1148.

45. Weshler Z, Krasnokuki D, Peshin Y, Biran S. Thyroid carcinoma induced by irradiation for Hodgkin's disease. Radiologica Oncol 1978;17:383–386.

46. Maxon H, Thomas S, Chen I. The role of nuclear medicine in the treatment of hyperthyroidism and well-differentiated thyroid adenocarcinoma. Clinical Nuclear Medicine 1971;7:87–98.

47. Sheline G, Lindsay S, McCormack R, Galante M. Thyroid nodules occurring late after treatment of thyrotoxicosis with radioiodine. JCEM, 1962;22:8–18.

48. Holm L. Thyroid treatment and its possible influence on occurrence of malignant tumors after diagnostic 131I. Acta Radiol. 1980;19:445–459.

49. Hennemann G, Krenning E, Sankaranarayanan K. Place of radioactive iodine in treatment of thyrotoxicosis. Lancet, June 14, 1986;1:1369–1372.

50. Graham G, Burman K. Radioiodine treatment of Graves' Disease: diagnosis and treatment. Annals Intern Med 1986;105:900–905.

51. Freitas J, Swanson D, Gross M, Sisson J. Iodine-131: Optimal therapy for hyperthyroidism in children and adolescents? J Nuclear Med, 1979;20:847–850.

52. Spencer R, Chapan C, Rao H. Thyroid carcinoma after radioiodine therapy for hyperthyroidism: analysis based on age, latency and administered dose of I-131. Philadelphia: J.B. Lippincott.

53. Socolow E, Hashizume A, Neriishi S, Niitani R. Thyroid carcinoma in man after exposure to ionizing radiation. N Eng J Med 1963;268–8, 406–410.

54. McDougall I, Kennedy J, Thomson J. Thyroid carcinoma following Iodine-131 therapy. Report of a case and review of the literature. J Clin Endocrinol Metab 1971;33:287–292.

55. Safa A, Schumacher O, Rodriguez-Antunez A. A long term follow-up results in children and adolescents treated with radioactive iodine (131-I) for hyperthyroidism. N Eng J Med 1975;292:167.

56. Wiener J, Thijs L, Meijer S. Thyroid carcinoma after 131-I treatment for hyperthyroidism. Acta Med Scand 1975;198:329–330.
57. Christmas TJ, Chapple CR, Noble JG, Milroy EJG, Cowie AGA. Hyperparathyroidism and neck irradiation. Am J Surg 1988;156:873–874.
58. Christmas TJ, Chapple CR, Noble JG, Milroy EJG, Cowie AGA. Hyperparathyroidism and Neck Irradiation. Br J Surg 1988;75:873–874.
59. Hedman I, Tisell L. Associated hyperparathyroidism and nonmedullary thyroid carcinoma: The etiologic role of radiation. Surgery 1984;95:392–397.
60. Sivula A, Ronni-Sivula, H. Natural history of treated primary hyperparathyroidism. Surg Clin North Am 1987;67:329–341.
61. Linos D, VanHeerden J, Edia A. Primary hyperparathyroidism and nonmedullary thyroid cancer. Am J Surg 1982;143:301–303.
62. Prinz R, Barbato A, Braithwaite S, Brooks M, Lawrence A, Paloyan E. Prior irradiation and the development of coexistent differentiated thyroid cancer and hyperparathyroidism. Cancer 1982;49:874–877.
63. Prinz R, Barbato A, Braithwaite S, Brooks M, Emanuele M, Gordon D, Lawrence A, Paloyan E. Simultaneous primary hyperparathyroidism and nodular thyroid disease. Surgery 1982;92:454–458.
64. Hedman I, Tisell L. Associated hyperparathyroidism and nonmedullary thyroid carcinoma. Surgery 1984;95:392–397.
65. Rao S, Frame M, Miller M, Kleerekoper M, Block M, Para M. Hyperparathyroidism following head and neck irradiation. Arch Intern Med 1980;130:205–207.
66. Shore-Freedman E, Abrahams C, Recan W, Schneider A. Neurilemomas and salivary gland tumors of the head and neck following childhood irradiation. Cancer 1983;51:2159–2163.
67. Van Den Berg C, Edis A. Multicentric thyroid carcinoma, parathyroid adenomas, and vagal neurilemmoma in a young man with antecedent tonsillar radiation. Mayo Clin Proc 1980;55:648–650.
68. Shinizu T, Matsui T, Kimura O, Maeta M, Koga S. Radiation induced esophageal carcinoma—case report and review of literature. Japan J Surg 1990;20–1, 97–100.
69. Fusco A, Brieco M, Santoro M, et al. A new oncogene in human thyroid papillary carcinomas and their lymphnodal metastases. Nature 1987;328:170–172.

4

Thyroid Cancer in the Pediatric Patient

JEFFREY I. MECHANICK

Introduction

Thyroid carcinoma in children and adolescents is rare. When a juvenile presents with a neck mass or swelling, the clinical evaluation is particularly challenging to the endocrinologist. In general, thyroid neoplasms in the pediatric population are distinguished from those in the adult condition by (1) a strong association with previous neck irradiation (Chapter 3); (2) a predominance of the papillary form (Chapter 1); (3) a presentation with cervical lymph node metastases; and (4) a need to specially consider the therapeutic effects of initial surgical approaches and the subsequent effects of thyroid function on growth and development (Table 4.1). These distinguishing features justify consideration of pediatric thyroid cancer as being a separate entity from the adult form.

Table 4.1. Distinguishing features of pediatric thyroid cancer compared to the adult condition

Greater association with prior irradiation
Less % female
More common presentation with cervical lymph node metastases
Greater chance of malignancy in a nodular thyroid
Less association with thyroiditis
Greater prevalence of papillary cancer
Less prevalence of undifferentiated cancer
Less bone metastases
More bilaterality
Greater efficacy of radioiodine therapy
Better survival

Anatomic Variants in the Pediatric Thyroid Gland

Unlike adults, in children the presence of thyroid nodularity, single or multiple, is unusual (0.22% to 1.8% prevalence rate)[1–4] and is frequently associated with malignant neoplasms.[5] This principle applies not only to the hypofunctioning ("cold") nodule but to the functioning and hyperfunctioning/autonomous ("hot") nodule as well.[6] Nevertheless, suspicious neck masses in the pediatric patient may represent not only thyroid nodularity, but also anatomical variants resulting from a developmental abnormality. During embryogenesis, the median anlage of the thyroid gland migrates caudally along the thyroglossal duct in association with the heart. Mechanical aberrations can lead to a final midline location of the gland that ranges from a sublingual to an intracardiac site. Virtually all cases of "lateral aberrant thyroid" represent metastases of thyroid cancer to a lymph node. In rare cases, normal thyroid tissue may be found in such nodes. In cases of metastatic thyroid cancer in the pediatric patient, early involvement of the upper pretracheal lymph node superior to the isthmus, the Delphian node, is frequently demonstrated. However, involvement of this node can be easily confused with an enlarged pyramidal lobe.

In a series of 6 girls aged 5 to 15 years with thyroid masses, 4 had demonstrable autonomy (1 with papillary adenocarcinoma), 1 had hemiagenesis with the viable lobe enlarged due to lymphocytic thyroiditis, and 1 had an ectopic thyroid with chronic inflammation.[7] It should be noted that thyroid carcinoma has been described in patients with thyroidal hemiagenesis[8] and ectopic (thyroglossal duct) thyroid tissue.[9,10] An incidental finding of ectopic thyroid tissue is found in 1% to 5% of children undergoing surgery for thyroglossal duct cyst or subhyoid median neck cyst.[11]

In addition, the differential diagnosis of a neck mass in a child or adolescent must also include nontoxic goiter. This condition has been referred to by other names such as "dyshormonogenetic goiter" and "recurrent carcinoma of childhood." This anatomic variant results from abnormally rapid trapping of perchlorate dischargeable ^{131}I and is treated with thyroxine or iodine. Childhood nontoxic goiter is often found in association with a family history of goiter and deafness. However, children with this anomaly must still be monitored closely for cancer since 15% of children with thyroid cancer and no previous history of radiation have a prior history of nontoxic goiter.[12]

General Survey

Since the first reported case of thyroid cancer in a child in 1902,[13] there have been numerous clinical studies designed to identify recognizable risk factors for early detection, accurate diagnostic strategies in the evaluation of a neck mass, and the natural history of pediatric thyroid cancer. Although these studies primarily involve different methodologies—retrospective studies with varying sample populations and geographic areas—important conclusions can be drawn from the data.

Demographics

Thyroid cancer has been estimated to account for 0.5% of all cancers for all ages in both sexes; approximately 10% of all cases of thyroid cancer occur in patients under the age of 21 years.[14] Cancer of the thyroid accounts for 1% to 1.5% of all childhood cancers and about 6% of all childhood neck cancers.[15] In table 4.2, 22 clinical series comprising data from 1267 children and adolescents are presented.[16–36] Data are broken down into five geographic regions with the respective prior exposure of patients in those regions to head or neck radiation because many of the features of pediatric thyroid cancer are influenced by environmental and genetic factors. All patients were studied after the advent of the atomic age and were 21 years of age or younger.

Identification of Risk Factors

Perhaps the best studied and most widely recognized risk factor for thyroid cancer is radiation to the head, neck, or upper chest. Since the original suggestion[37] and description of this association[38,39] in 1949 to 1950, many large studies have confirmed this observation. In a series of 19 children irradiated as infants during the 1940s and 1950s, 18 (95%) developed thyroid neoplasia 5.5 to 17 years later: 78% were carcinomatous and the remainder adenomatous.[16] In the past, a variety of malignant and nonmalignant conditions have been treated with x-ray therapy. These include obstructive respiratory symptoms ascribed to an enlarged thymus, tonsillitis, adenitis, eczematous rashes, enlarged mediastinal or neck lymph nodes, mastoiditis, pneumonitis, sinusitis, allergic rhinitis, facial acne, hemangiomata, lymphoma, medulloblastoma, and nasopharyngeal carcinoma.

The mid-1950s represent the peak years during which such irradiation was performed. In 18 consecutive cases of children with thyroid cancer aged 3 to 15 years reported by the Cleveland clinic, none presented with the disease during 1924 to 1939, 3 during 1939 to 1950, and 15 during 1950 to 1958.[21] Similarly, there were no cases of thyroid cancer in 57 children with a nodular thyroid presenting to the Mayo Clinic during 1900 to 1930; however 41 of 72 children (57%) with a nodular thyroid presenting during 1930 to 1955 had thyroid cancer.[5,40] Furthermore, from 1960 to 1975 there was a decline in the incidence of carcinomatous thyroid nodules to 17%.[41]

Despite the observation that neck irradiation increases the risk of thyroid cancer, there does not appear to be a clear difference in the rate of

Table 4.2. Clinical presentation of pediatric thyroid cancer in selected series

	Sample populations					
Parameter	USA[5,16–21,38–40]	Europe[12,24–26,28,29,36]	Canada[23]	Israel[33,34]	Japan[32]	Combined[35]
N	289	242	63	48	149	476
Number of series reviewed	8	8	2	2	1	1
Prior irradiation (%)	56	7	5	17	3	76
% female	57–71	60–75	70	78	75	62
Time from first symptoms to diagnosis (years)	2	2	—	—	—	2
Interval from radiation to diagnosis (years)	8–10	6	—	8	—	8
Neck exam: thyroid mass alone (%)	7–38	4–33	87	38–53	—	—
Enlarged cervical lymph node(s) alone (%)	36–56	35–96	13	43–63	10	—
Both (%)	57	0–35	0	5	—	—
Histology: differentiated (%)	97	88–94	65–92	100	97	90
Papillary elements (%)	53–94	51–90	48–67	62–73	73	72
Pure follicular (%)	9–29	6–33	17–25	28–31	25	18
Undifferentiated (%)	0–3	0–11	0	0–7	3	3
Medullary (%)	3	1–15	8–15	0–4	0	3
Stage:						
No spread (%)	16–46	33	—	—	—	—
Cervical nodes and/or local spread (%)	62–88	65–75	33	48–88	—	74
Pulmonary (%)	12–46	6–25	40	0	17	14
Bone (%)	0–7	0	0	0	0	2

Sources for data; USA: refs. 5, 16–21, 38–40; Europe: refs. 12, 24–26, 28, 29, 30, 36; Canada: ref. 23; Israel: refs. 33, 34; Japan: ref. 32; combined: ref 35.

presentation of thyroid cancer in irradiated and nonirradiated children (Table 4.2). Although childhood head and neck irradiation is at present relatively infrequent, a careful history must be taken, and if positive or suspicious with respect to exposure to radiation, examinations must continue to be performed on a yearly to bi-yearly basis.

Because thyroid nodularity is less common in children as compared with adults, its presence in a child suggests a greater likelihood of malignancy than in the adult, whether or not there is a history of neck irradiation. Desjardins et al.[23] performed a retrospective study of 58 patients aged 3 to 20 years, who during the 1970s and 1980s, had thyroid nodules, 91% of which were solitary. They found scintigraphic evidence of nonfunctioning, cold nodules in 73% of the solitary cold nodules, and malignancy in 30%. This latter figure is slightly higher than a previous figure of 14% reported by Hung et al. in 1982[42] and 10% reported by Belfiore et al.[31] in 1989, in which there was no history of irradiation, but substantially less than the figures of 39% to 83% (mean = 49%) reported of children with nodular goiters who were studied before the early 1970s, when neck irradiation was more common.[15,16,34,43–46] In comparison, approximately 5% of solitary thyroid nodules in adults studied by Belfiore[31] were carcinomatous. Thus, regardless of the prior history of neck irradiation, if a thyroid nodule is found in a young patient there is an increase risk that it harbors a cancer. This may be related to an increased susceptibility of the juvenile nodular gland to carcinogenic stimuli; therefore, definitive diagnostic evaluation is necessary.

The association of autoimmune thyroiditis with thyroid cancer in children and adolescents has been well described[47,48] although a causal relationship has not been established. The cooccurence of thyroid carcinoma and autoimmune thyroiditis ranges from 3% to 50% in reported series.[15,22,49,50] Thus, whether or not a child is on thyroxine replacement therapy for Hashimoto's thyroiditis, careful and long-term follow-up for the development of thyroid nodules must be undertaken. Indeed, up to 10% to 15% of children with Hashimoto's thyroiditis present with thyroid nodules composed of lymphoid or hyperplastic tissue.[51] In a recent study of nine patients with papillary carcinoma under the age of 20 years, lymphocytic infiltration of the thyroid gland was most pronounced near the primary lesion and correlated with the degree of intrathyroidal spread of the cancer.[52] The apparent immunomechanism in juvenile thyroid cancer is antibody-dependent cellular cytotoxicity (ADCC), which is similar to that in autoimmune thyroiditis.[51]

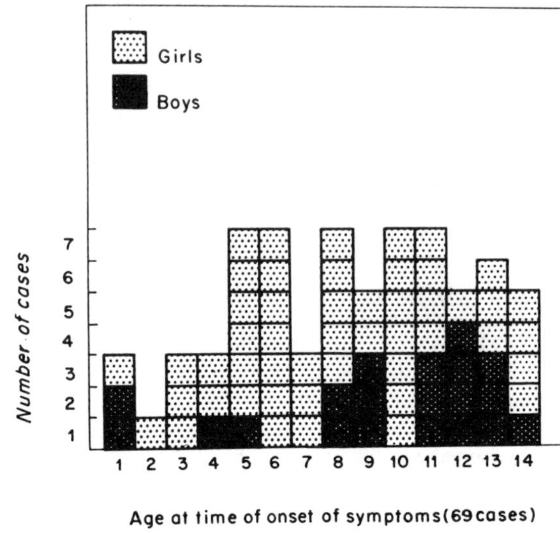

Figure 4.1. Age at onset of symptoms or signs of thyroid cancer in 69 children. Reprinted, by permission, from Hayles, 1963. (40)

Other risk factors for pediatric thyroid cancer include female sex and familial history of childhood thyroid cancer (familial papillary carcinoma[53], multiple endocrine neoplasia type IIa[54] and IIb[55], Von Hippel-Lindau syndrome[56], Gardner's syndrome[57], Cowden's syndrome[58], or Pendred's syndrome[59,60]).

Clinical Presentation

A child may present with the disease anytime from a few days to over a decade (average latency = 2 years) following the appearance of symptoms ultimately referable to thyroid cancer (Fig. 4.1). This latency period reflects the lack of concern often generated by a painless neck mass. In over 98% of cases, the predominant complaint is the presence of a neck mass or masses not associated with a preceding infection or systemic illness. In rare cases, a child may present with vocal cord paralysis due to tumoral involvement of the recurrent laryngeal nerve. A particularly rare entity is congenital thyroid cancer, five cases of which were described by Winship.[61]

A distinguishing feature of pediatric thyroid cancer compared to the adult form is the very high frequency with which cervical lymph nodes are found to be enlarged at presentation. One should bear in mind, however, that cervical lymphadenopathy may be found in a variety of benign pediatric thyroid conditions including mature teratoma, follicular adenoma, and Hashimoto's thyroiditis, as well as other nonthyroidal illnesses.[23] Approximately one third to one half of children with thyroid cancer will present with cervical lymphadenopathy alone. As mentioned above, this does not represent a "lateral aberrant" thyroid gland but rather, nodal metastases. Lymph nodes that are involved are firm, irregular, movable, and nontender, with fixation/matting being a late finding. There are usually 3 to 4 metastatic lymph nodes on presentation with a diameter of 1 to 2 cm each. Bilateral palpable nodal metastases occur in 14% to 46% of patients and are most common with the papillary type of thyroid cancer.[17,20,26] Occasionally, nodal metastases are mistaken in children for branchial-cleft cysts or adenitis. The most commonly involved lymphatic chains are the deep jugular and the tracheoesophageal. Anterior superior mediastinal involvement is associated with recurrent laryngeal nodal metastases.

Local spread of thyroid cancer beyond the cervical lymph node chains occurs in 2% to 30% of cases and is suggested by nonproductive cough (tracheal involvement), hoarseness (invasion of the larynx or recurrent laryngeal nerve), and dysphagia (esophageal involvement).[20,35] In addition, 30% to 80% of children with thyroid cancer of both papillary and follicular types will have intrathyroidal metastases, invasion of the thyroid capsule, and micro-invasion of blood vessels.[19,25,33,62,63] Therefore, the physical finding of unilateral thyroid involvement is unreliable: in 11 children studied by Kodama et al.[32] unilateral primary lesions were palpated preoperatively in 82% of cases; however at surgery, 78% of glands had bilateral involvement.

Symptoms referable to distant metastases are infrequent. Of 28 patients with thyroid cancer aged 4 to 18 years studied at Memorial Sloan-Kettering Hospital, 13 (46%) presented with pulmonary metastases.[39] Of the 13, eleven (85%) were asymptomatic; the other two complained of cough or hemoptysis. The chest roentgenograms were deceptive since they depicted a diffuse, miliary/micronodular process and not large solitary masses, and were therefore confused with tuberculosis and fungal infections. Schlumberger et al. have suggested that involvement of the laryngeal nerve lymph node chain heralds pulmonary involvement. Distant metastases may also involve the mediastinum and myocardium. Bone metastases, even in children exposed to neck irradiation, are exceedingly rare (0% to 7%) in comparison with adults (20%).[64]

Papillary cancers tend to be smaller and often nonpalpable, although more frequently multicentric in thyroid tissue than are follicular cancers. The overall prevalence of "microsopic" contralateral thyroidal metastases in all differentiated thyroid cancers is as low as 10% to 15%[65] and as high as 62% to 87%.[33,62,63] Pure papillary or "papillary-follicular" cancers are associated with autoimmune thyroiditis in 8% to 45% of cases.[22,35] In a retrospective study of 23 cases of childhood thyroid cancer in which 15 were well-differentiated with postoperative follow-up ranging from 8 months to 20 years (average = 7.5 years), Desjardins et al.[22] concluded that (1) the presence of psammoma bodies suggests intrathyroidal metastasis but less aggressiveness and a better prognosis, regardless of nodal metastases and (2) the presence of Hürthle cells suggests a more aggressive evolution. Psammoma bodies are also found in Hashimoto's thyroiditis.[32] In general, distant metastases are rare in childhood papillary thyroid cancer although unilateral lymph node metastases and bilateral lymph node metastases are found in 54% of cases and 46% of cases, respectively.[26]

In children, pure follicular thyroid cancers account for 6% to 33% of all types of thyroid cancer. They tend to metastasize via a hematogenous route to the lungs. These cancers nearly always present with an abnormal thyroid on examination, in contrast to papillary cancers, which present with cervical adenopathy in 50% of cases.[26] As mentioned above, bone metastases in follicular cancer are rare in children. Histologically, microinvasive follicular cancer is indistinguishable from the benign follicular adenoma.[29]

Diagnostic Approach

The diagnostic evaluation of a child or adolescent with a neck mass is primarily based on (1) assessment of established and suspected historical risk factors and (2) physical findings on neck examination (Table 4.3). Certainly, any child with a suspicious lymph node (failure of regression following adequate appropriate antiinflammatory or antibiotic therapy) should undergo lymph node biopsy. Compliance with this principle would minimize the latency between onset of symptom and diagnosis (above) without introducing significant morbidity.

Biochemical markers (calcitonin, chromogranin A, carcinoembryonic antigen, etc.) for medullary carcinoma of the thyroid (MCT; see chapter 8) must be obtained in any child with a family history of MCT or multiple endocrine neoplasia syndrome, or in cases in which cytologic investigation is suspicious for MCT. Calcium-pentagastrin stimulation testing is indicated in children at risk for MCT when baseline studies are nondiagnostic.

Thyroid anatomy is best delineated by the use of ^{123}I, ^{131}I or ^{99m}Tc scintigraphy (to exclude aberrancies) and ultrasonography (to confirm physical findings). ^{123}I has the advantage of emitting less radiation and may be more

Table 4.3. General guidelines for management of differentiated thyroid cancer in children and adolescents

Initial evaluation
- History of neck irradiation, familial involvement of thyroid cancer, viral infections, and neck trauma
- Immunization status
- Detailed neck examination
- Thyroid function tests
- Biopsy of suspicious cervical lymph node
- Fine needle aspiration of suspicious thyroid nodule

Additional diagnostic methods
- Serum tumor markers
- Scintigraphy
- Ultrasonography
- Chest roentgenogram
- Quantitative cytology

Initial therapy
- Subtotal or near-total thyroidectomy
  - Less surgery: unilateral, small, encapsulated follicular cancer
  - More surgery: extensive local involvement where symptomatic relief is expected as result of the procedure or when high-does (>150 mCi) radioactive iodine may be avoided by increasing amount of tissue resected
- No prophylactic neck dissection
  - Modified neck dissection for gross nodal involvement

Postoperative management
- Whole body radioiodine scintigraphy 6 weeks postoperatively to identify residual neck tumor and distant metastases
- Adjuvant ablative radioiodine treatment 7 weeks postoperatively for thyroid remnant, nodal involvement, and/or distant metastases
- Annual chest roentgenograms
- Periodic whole-body radioiodine scintigraphy to identify distant metastases:
  - First follow-up 6–12 months, then
    - Every 1–2 years (if disease present)
    - Every 2–5 years (if disease-free; ?lifelong)
- High-dose radioiodine treatment for distant metastases
- Lifelong L-thyroxine suppression
- Lifelong regular thyroglobulin levels to monitor for recurrence
- Lifelong regular thyroid function testing and neck examination in addition to routine evaluation of growth and development

suitable for children. The presence of unilateral functioning thyroid tissue most often represents a developmental abnormality rather than an autonomous nodule in a normal gland. Negative scintigraphic results should not be interpreted as arguing against further evaluation, inasmuch as 30% of children with thyroid cancer have been reported to have entirely normal scans.[19]

A routine chest roentgenogram must be obtained for any child with a suspicious neck mass to detect pulmonary metastatic involvement. Bone scanning does not need to be performed routinely in light of the rarity of osseous metastases.

Features suggesting the need for surgical exploration for thyroid neoplasm include positive history of neck irradiation, suspicious cervical lymphadenopathy, and rapidly growing, solitary nonfunctioning thyroid nodules. Any palpable thyroid nodule is a candidate for fine needle aspiration (FNA) though situations that are particularly deserving include: multinodular or uninodular (functioning and/or nonfunctioning) thyroid in an otherwise low-risk patient, simple cystic lesions detected by ultrasonography in any child, and follow-up of nonsuppressible nodularity in a low-risk patient. FNA is more difficult technically in prepubertal children owing to noncompliance with positioning efforts, pain control, and smaller neck and nodule size. Therefore, when possible, FNA should be performed by a physician experienced with pediatric cases. Many endocrinologists suggest surgical exploration of high-risk children with suspicious nodules or lymph nodes without utilizing FNA. However, because benign lesions may currently account for up to 90% of suspicious nodules,[31] at a time when pediatric neck irradiation is not generally performed, FNA is generally recommended and assists decision making regarding surgery.[66–68]

Two drawbacks of FNA, however, are the relatively high false negative rate (10% to 37%) and reproducibility rate (2% to 37%).[69,70] Recently, quantitative cytological methods, for example, flow cytometry for DNA-ploidy determination, have been applied to FNA samples; however, attempts to discriminate between malignant and benign tissue, and not simply individual cells, remain unsuccessful.[71–75] Nevertheless, in certain instances, like follicular carcinoma, DNA aneuploidy provides major prognostic value. Moreover, it appears that children have a lower rate of aneuploidy in thyroid tumors (10%) than adults (25%), which may explain the more indolent course observed in pediatric thyroid cancer.[76] Compared to nonirradiated adults, there is also significantly less aneuploidy in DNA content from thyroid cancers in adults exposed to neck irradiation.[77]

Surgical exploration is indicated for a positive or suspicious FNA. If the FNA is negative for malignancy, suppressive therapy with thyroxine and observation may be undertaken. If significant regression of the nodule does not occur after 3 to 6 months of adequate suppression, then the child should be surgically explored. Overall, management decisions in pediatric thyroidology are not algorithmic, but require simultaneous consideration of the patient's history, physical examination, imaging and cytologic studies, and most importantly, full discussion with the child's parents or guardians about the risks and benefits of a surgical procedure.

Surgical Findings

Thyroid exploration enables histopathologic diagnosis to be performed as well as providing a means of gauging the degree of local spread either by extension or by lymphogenous/hematogenous metastasis. Nearly all pediatric thyroid cancers are of the differentiated thyroid epithelial type (65% to 100%); of these, the majority have papillary elements (51% to 94% of all types). To a degree, the more favorable prognosis observed with pediatric thyroid cancer compared to the adult form is due to the higher incidence of papillary carcinoma in the younger age group;[35] however, other factors also play a role since adult papillary cancer is more lethal than the pediatric form.

In roughly one-third of cases, neck exploration in children with thyroid cancer reveals no evidence of metastases. In the remaining cases, spread may be limited to the lymph nodes, or involve direct extension and invasion of perithyroidal tissue. Overall, unilateral nodal involvement is seen in approximately 50% to 70% and bilateral involvement in 30% to 50% of cases.[26,40] The deep jugular and recurrent laryngeal nerve lymph node chains are most commonly affected.[36] Local invasion occurs in 5% to 33% of cases.[25,33] In decreasing order of frequency the structures affected are: thyroid capsule, trachea/esophagus, recurrent laryngeal nerve, and straight neck muscles.[12,17,26,30,33,35,36]

Natural History and Cause of Death

Based on the findings of Winship and Rosvoll[35] who reviewed 878 cases of pediatric thyroid cancer that occurred before 1970, the cause of death in 75% of this group was respiratory obstruction/asphyxiation or respiratory infection. Four patients died of tumor hemorrhage but only 18 from wide-spread metastases to (in decreasing order of frequency) cervical lymph nodes, lungs, mediastinum, bone, liver, adrenal, or brain.[35] The most lethal cancer type was undifferentiated, followed by medullary, "unknown", "unclassified," and finally well-differentiated (papillary and follicular were essentially equal).[35]

Varieties of Pediatric Thyroid Cancer

Well-Differentiated Thyroid Cancer

The overwhelming majority of pediatric cases of thyroid cancer are of this type. Controversial management decisions involve the extent

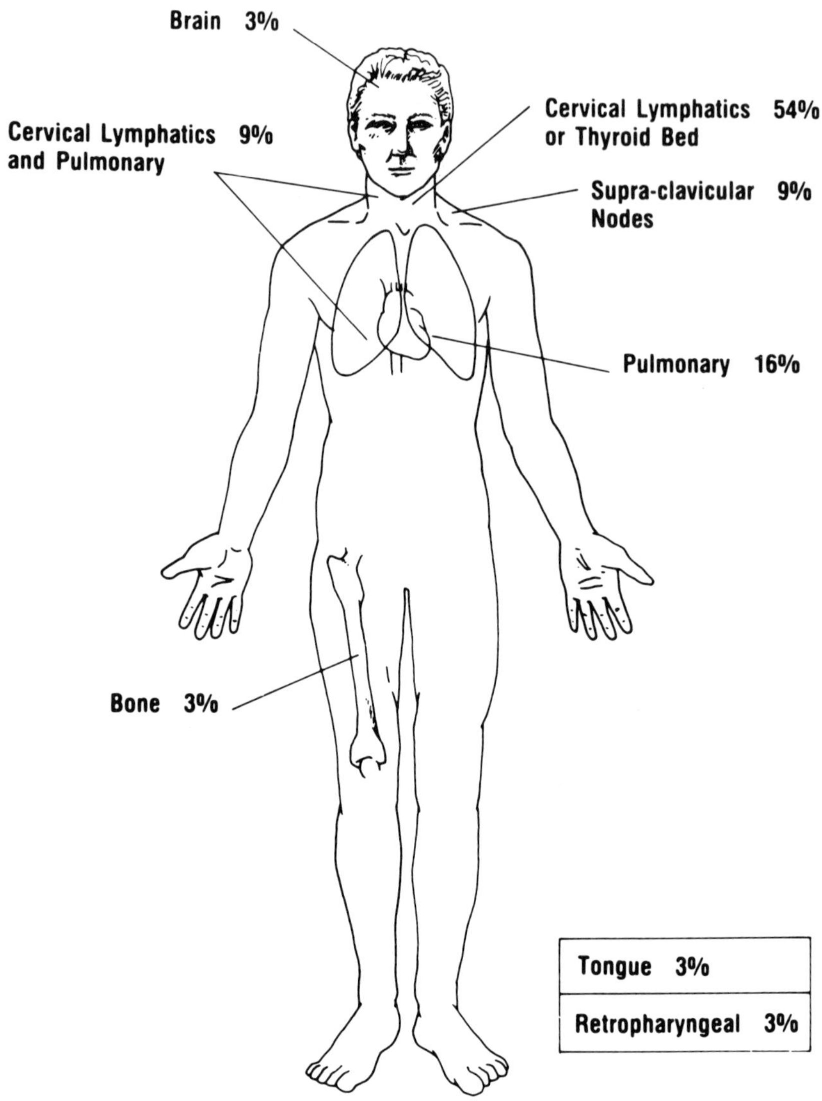

Figure 4.2. Sites of recurrence of differentiated thyroid cancer in children. Reprinted, by permission, from MP La Quaglia et al, 1988. (79)

of surgery, the utilization of adjuvant radioiodine therapy, and the use of thyroxine suppressive therapy.

Surgical Approach

Perhaps the most significant issue in the management of children with thyroid cancer concerns the choice of surgical procedure. This decision is based primarily on the patient's risk factors, the extent of local and distant involvement, and knowledge of the natural history of the tumor.

Children with thyroid cancer have extensive disease on presentation. This was assumed to have a negative impact on survival and led to the assumption that aggressive initial surgery was indicated. However, in 1967, Klopp et al.[78] raised considerable doubt about the notion that extensive surgical intervention in pediatric thyroid cancer was necessary. They reported a "relatively favorable outcome

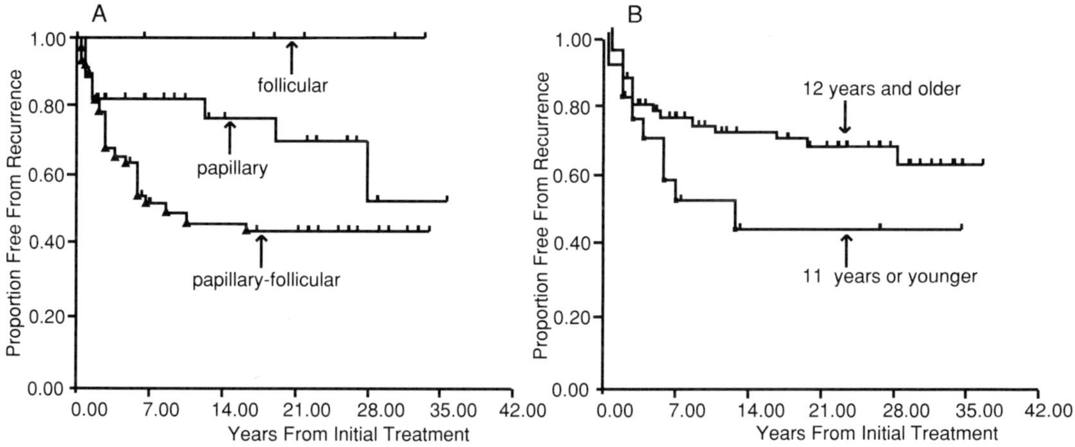

Figure 4.3. Effect of histology and age on recurrence rate following thyroid surgery in children. Panel A: Effect of histological type; Panel B: Effect of age at presentation. Reprinted, by permission, from MP La Quaglia et al, 1988. (79)

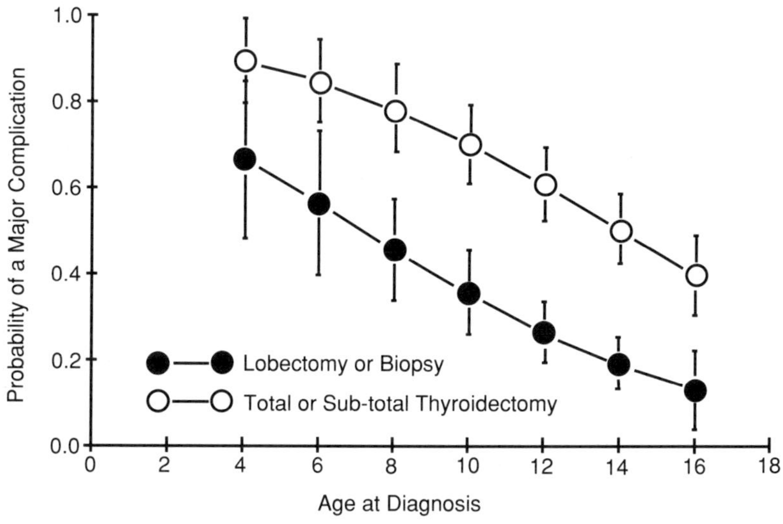

Figure 4.4. Effect of age and procedure on major morbidity following thyroid surgery in children. Reprinted, by permission, from MP La Quaglia et al, 1988. (79)

irrespective of treatment, or at least despite lack of what is considered adequate therapy."[78] La Quaglia et al.[79] performed a retrospective analysis of 100 patients under the age of 18 from 1949 through 1986 at the Memorial Sloan-Kettering Cancer Center, New York City and found an overall recurrence rate of 34% up to 25 years after initial surgical treatment. The type of thyroid surgery and lymphatic dissection had no significant effect on the length of the period before recurrence.[79] Age and histologic subtype were predictive of length of the period before recurrence (Fig. 4.2 and 4.3), but age and extent of thyroid surgery determined major morbidity (Fig. 4.4).[79] The authors concluded that in children, total thyroidectomy or radical neck dissection does not have a significantly lower recurrence rate compared to less extreme surgery. They recommended that the more aggressive procedures be avoided because of the higher complication rates.

The conservative approach,* however, continues to be challenged. Some investigators specifically advocate total thyroidectomy for bilateral disease and near-total thyroidectomy for unilateral disease in light of the high frequency of intrathyroidal metastases.† It should be noted, however, that in children, the risk of hypoparathyroidism is as high as 26% and injury to the recurrent laryngeal nerve as high as 37% when radical surgery is performed.[14,30]

At present, conservative surgical therapy is recommended. A general principle is to perform bilateral resection consisting of ipsilateral total lobectomy, isthmectomy, and contralateral subtotal or near-total lobectomy, with special care to preserve the laryngeal nerves, and at least one parathyroid gland and its vascular supply in situ (Table 4.3).[83] This approach is applicable to papillary cancer in which occult thyroidal metastases are frequent, as well as to invasive follicular cancer. Ipsilateral lobectomy and isthmectomy may be reserved for a small (<1.5–2.0 cm) unilateral, noninvasive, encapsulated follicular cancer because multicentricity is less frequent.[84]

Performing a modified neck dissection, with preservation of the sternocleidomastoid muscle, when cervical lymph node involvement is suspected or established, is also debatable. It has been suggested that in children the presence of lymph node metastases has little or no effect on the overall prognosis[36,85–87]; therefore, elective or prophylactic neck dissection would be unwarranted.[26] Since the majority of differentiated thyroid cancers in children take up radioactive iodine, and are particularly sensitive to it, adjuvant therapy with ^{131}I can provide the benefit of ablating residual thyroidal and nodal tumor without the risks of total thyroidectomy and neck dissection.

Aggressive treatment, such as total thyroidectomy with or without radical neck dissection, must be reserved for exceptional cases with extensive local involvement in which additional resection is expected to provide commensurate improvement. When distant metastases are known to exist, total or near-total thyroidectomy for unilateral or bilateral disease is a reasonable alternative to minimize any residual tumor that may be competing for radioiodine. If parathyroid tissue is found in a resected thyroidectomy specimen, it may be autotransplanted within the neck or to the forearm to avoid lifelong vitamin D and calcium therapy for hypopituitarism.

Adjunctive Radioactive Iodine Therapy

Radioiodine is not recommended as single-modality therapy for pediatric thyroid cancer. In children who have had less than a total thyroidectomy, in which there is a remnant and, therefore, a possibility of residual tumor, nodal involvement, or distant metastases; ablative ^{131}I treatment is indicated. Conversely, if the entire primary tumor has been resected and there is no evidence of local spread or distant metastasis, radioiodine treatment may be deferred. The complications of ablative radioactive iodine preclude its routine use after adequate initial surgery in children.[86,88] These complications include leukemia, chromosomal injury, restrictive lung disease due to fibrosis, sterility, and pancytopenia.[89]

A major concern of physicians considering radioactive iodine as part of their treatment plans for thyroid cancer in a child is the effect on the gene mutation rate and the immediate effect on chromosomes in the gonads. In general, an administered dose of 150 mCi ^{131}I would double the natural mutation rate.[90] This translates to 240 children per 100,000 live births having a deleterious mutation.[90] Furthermore, this same dose would be responsible for about 50 live births with a congenital abnormality due to a ^{131}I-induced reciprocal translocation.[90] Overall, 150 mCi would be expected to produce a genetic abnormality in 0.3% of live births and 500 mCi in 1.0% of live births.[90]

The frequency of acute myelogenous leukemia after ^{131}I treatment is 0.5% but usually occurs only with very high doses (>900 mCi)[90,91]; however, it must be noted that thyroid carcinoma is only one of several forms of solid second malignancies that occur after acute lymphoblastic leukemia in children.[92] The risk of developing one of these complica-

* References 7, 19, 22, 29, 32, 35, 65, 80, 81
† References 12, 19, 20, 25, 28, 33, 36, 82

tions is significant because of the long-term survival of these patients.[93]

The efficacy with which radioiodine destroys metastases depends on the amount of thyroid tissue that remains to trap and sequesters the administered dose. The thyroid-stimulating hormone (TSH) level should be allowed to increase over 30 mIU/l for optimal scanning. An adequate ablative dose can be computed from the ^{131}I uptake in the neck, which should be measured by means of whole-body radioiodine scintigraphy approximately 6 weeks postoperatively; the patient should not be receiving thyroid hormone replacement or suppressive therapy. Follow-up whole-body scans should be performed at regular intervals, depending on whether distant metastases are present (Table 4.3). Thyroid replacement or suppression must be restarted immediately after scanning or radioiodine treatment to minimize the duration of hypothyroidism in children. Currently, there is insufficient data to warrant the discontinuation of scintigraphic follow-up in children. Therapeutic radioiodine dosing should continue every 6 to 12 months from the time bone marrow recovery is demonstrated until the time ^{131}I uptake is undetectable.

The benefits[19,20,27,28,35] and risks[94] of adjuvant radioiodine have been discussed by several authors. Thyroid remnants usually respond to doses of 30 to 100 mCi, although two patients reported by Ceccarelli[28] required 150 and 160 mCi. Nodal metastases require larger and multiple doses (up to 300 mCi) and pulmonary metastases require still larger doses (up to 600 mCi).[28] Approximately 90% of childhood pulmonary metastases trap radioiodine,[36] although 79% of the pediatric patients with pulmonary involvement studied by Ceccarelli[28] had pulmonary metastases that were resistant to large doses of radioiodine (185 to 500 mCi). However, ln Winship and Rosvoll's series,[35] 31% of patients experienced complete regression of pulmonary metastases following radioiodine.

When one fully evaluates the above risks and benefits, it appears that a sound general approach consists of conservative surgery followed by adjuvant radioiodine therapy. Following conservative surgery, the majority of thyroid remnants and local nodal metastases will respond to a dose of radioactive iodine at levels below those that one would expect to produce unwanted genetic effects. If extensive thyroidal or resectable nodal metastases are demonstrated, then a more aggressive surgical approach may be considered, in order to obviate the need for high-dose adjuvant radioiodine. This issue is at present far from settled. What may be ultimately determined is that, in light of the less aggressive course of pediatric thyroid cancer as compared with the adult thyroid cancer, conservative surgery and radioiodine dosing, or no radioiodine dosing at all, may be the preferred regimen.

External irradiation is not recommended for the routine treatment of differentiated thyroid cancer. In children, its usefulness is essentially limited to those cases refractory to the combination of surgery and radioiodine, in which there is significant metastatic or nonresectable, nonfunctioning tissue. This situation is one in which there is usually extreme tumor involvement of the trachea, esophagus, recurrent laryngeal nerve, or lungs.

Thyroid Suppression Therapy

There is general agreement in the literature that L-thyroxine therapy must be instituted and continued lifelong in patients with childhood thyroid cancer following initial surgery. The rationale for thyroid hormone therapy postoperatively is twofold. First, replacement therapy is required following extensive resection of the thyroid gland to prevent hypothyroidism and its attendant deleterious effects on growth and development of the child. Second, suppression of endogenous TSH is mandatory. The usual starting dose in children is 1 to 2 μg/kg/day. The dose is then titrated to as high as 150 to 200 μg daily to suppress TSH below detectable levels, using a sensitive immunoradiometric or chemiluminescent assay system (0.2–0.3 mIU/l). There is currently no evidence that suppression therapy is detrimental to growth and development. The availability of sensitive TSH assays obviates the need for thyrotropin-releasing hormone (TRH)-stimulation studies.

It has been postulated that the actively growing juvenile thyroid gland is particularly sensitive to TSH.[95] It has been suggested that, in theory, increased TSH levels are associated with the transformation of differentiated thyroid cancer into undifferentiated thyroid cancer in children. However, in a large pediatric series, papillary cancer changed to undifferentiated cancer in less than 1% of cases.[95,96] Cady et al.[97] reported significantly improved mortality rates with thyroid suppression in patients who have cancers with papillary elements but not in low-risk patients with pure follicular cancer.

In practice, suppression enables the clinician to monitor for recurrence by following serum thyroglobulin (TG) levels every 6 months.[98] If TG is detectable when the patient is on suppression, or is greater than 10 ng/ml when the patient is off suppression, then the probability of recurrence or metastases must be considered. Schlumberger et al.[98] found that 56% of patients with TG of less than 15 ng/ml had no recurrence and that 44% of patients with TG of greater than 26 ng/ml had a recurrence 3 to 6 months after initial surgery. Elevated TG levels necessitate discontinuation of suppression therapy and follow-up whole-body ^{131}I scintigraphy after the TSH reaches a level of greater than 30 mIU/l. Sometimes, an elevated TG indicates the presence of metastases that do not trap iodine. In these infrequent cases, technicium^{99m} bone scanning, thallium^{201} whole body scanning, or magnetic resonance imaging or computerized tomography of the chest and neck are useful. The presence of antithyroglobulin antibodies confounds the TG assay; however, a novel immunoradiometric TG assay has been developed, but is not yet commercially available in the United States, which reliably detects TG in the presence of such antibodies.[99]

Attention must be given to the potential noncompliance with medical therapy in this age population. The endocrinologist should schedule therapy (either dosing of medicine or time off for surgery) with minimal interruption in schooling. Adolescent patients are liable to avoid taking medicines that do not have an immediate or noticeable effect. As compliance is of utmost importance, suppressive therapy may not be easy to employ if the child is uncooperative or has ineffective parental support.

Prognosis

Although childhood thyroid cancer presents with more extensive involvement than the adult form, the prognosis is very good, with overall survival rates ranging from 80% to 100% in large series. As in the case of adult thyroid cancer, boys tend to have a poorer prognosis than girls ($p = 0.09$; Table 4.4).[100] Therefore, one might argue that boys should be treated more aggressively than girls. Klopp et al.[78] reviewed the records of 46 patients diagnosed with thyroid cancer between 1926 and 1955 who were treated with "less than accepted therapy." They found 10-year and 20-year survival rates of 82.6% and 73.9%, respectively, which compare favorably with an overall 5-year survival rate of 70% and 10-year survival rate of 80% from patients with regional disease receiving "accepted therapy" at Memorial Sloan-Kettering Hospital, New York City from 1949 to 1957.[101] Though reports of surgical mortality are rare,[30,80] major complication rates following initial surgery in children have been reported to range as high as 15% to 50%.* In addition, there may be an increased risk of osteoporosis following total thyroidectomy combined with radioiodine treatment. Cady et al.[94] noted a reduction in serum calcitonin and bone density with an increase in pathologic fractures.

In young patients with differentiated thyroid cancer treated with near-total thyroidectomy, modified radical neck dissection, postoperative radioiodine to ablate residual thyroid tissue when present, and thyroid suppressive therapy, Ceccarelli et al.[28] reported "cure" in 22 (61%) and "relapse" in 28% of those "successfully treated."

In a large retrospective study performed at the Mayo Clinic by Zimmerman et al.,[76] children with papillary cancer were found to have more postoperative cervical nodal metastases,

*References 19, 20, 35, 36, 40, 43, 61, 63, 65, 95, 102–104

Table 4.4. Association of clinical presentation and initial surgical management with remission, relapse, and metastases rates in 72 children with differentiated thyroid cancer.*

	Number	Remission (%)	Replase (%)	Early metastases (%)	Late Metastases (%)	*p*-value‡
Male	21	48	40	—	—	.09
Female	51	65	18	—	—	
Palpable thyroid tumor	67	57	26	—	—	.07
Nonpalpable thyroid tumor	5	100	0	—	—	
Palpable lymph nodes	53	51	30	—	—	.03
Nonpalpable lymph nodes	19	84	12	—	—	
Initial lung metastases	13	8	0	—	—	.002
No initial lung metastases	59	71	24	—	—	
Papillary elements	50	60	30	—	—	not
No papillary elements	21	62	8	—	—	significant
Extracapsular tumor	36	—	—	28	25	.04
No extracapsular tumor	18	—	—	6	0	
Isthmus involvement	28	—	—	39	25	.0001
No isthmus involvement	15	—	—	7	7	
Unilateral tumor	23	—	—	9	4	.0004
Bilateral tumor	23	—	—	39	30	
Unifocal tumor	10	—	—	0	0	.02
Multifocal tumor	43	—	—	26	21	
Rec. laryng nodal involvemt	39	—	—	26	21	.06
No Rec. laryng. nodal involvemt	7	—	—	0	0	
Age < 7 years	11	—	—	55	27	.001
Age between 7 and 13 years	29	—	—	10	31	
Age > 13 years	32	—	—	12	16	
No thyroid surgery	3	0	0	0	67	—
Tumorectomy alone	4	25	0	50	0	—
Lobectomy + Isthmectomy + neck dissection	31	77	21	13	13	—
Total thyroidectomy + neck dissection	27	52	36	37	19	—

Reprinted, by permission, from M Schlumberger, F De Vathaire, JP Trauagli, G Vassal, J Lemerle, Parmenter C, et al. Differentiated thyroid carcinoma in childhood: long term follow-up of 72 patients. J Clin Endocrinol Metab 1987;65:1088–1094. Copyright by The Endocrine Society, 1987.

*Surgical managment based on standard protocol designed to resect all evident tumor both macroscopic and microscopic (see text).

†Early: within 1 year after initial treatment; late: after 1 year

‡Log-rank test *p*-value comparing observed and expected total number of patient metastasis or patients without remission + those with relapse

but not local recurrences or distant metastases, as compared with adults. Interestingly, the 15-year mortality rate in patients diagnosed with distant metastases was significantly lower in children (14%), than in adults (68%).[76] This finding has been confirmed by Zohar et al.[34] The authors attribute this difference to the lower frequency of aneuploidy in pediatric thyroid cancers compared to thyroid cancers in adults. Surprisingly, even though younger patients present with more advanced disease than adults, only 9.3% have residual tumor after definitive surgery compared with 16.1% of adults.[14] Other comparisons between the prognosis in children versus the prognosis in adults are shown in Table 4.5. The overall 30-year survival rate of children with papillary cancer is not significantly different from that of normal children.[76,34]

The clinical presentation, therapeutics, and prognosis of 72 children with thyroid cancer were studied by Schlumberger et al.[36] in 72 children (Table 4.4). Only eight patients (11%) had a history of neck irradiation. Significant differences between observed and expected remission rates occurred when palpable lymph

Table 4.5. Prognosis following initial surgery in 54 children and 350 adults with differentiated thyroid cancer

	Children*					Adults				
	N	Residual Tumor (%)	Relapse (%)	Hypopara-thyroidism (%)	Vocal Cord Paresis (%)	N	Residual Tumor (%)	Relapse (%)	Hypopara-thyroidism (%)	Vocal Cord Paresis (%)
Partial thyroidectomy										
No neck dissect	10	10	10	0	0	62	27	21	0	8
Partial neck dissection	2	50	0	0	0	8	12	50	0	12
Radical neck dissection	0	—	—	—	—	4	50	0	0	0
Lobectomy										
No neck dissection	11	10	10	0	0	108	6	6	0	3
Partial neck dissection	1	0	10	0	0	10	10	0	0	0
Radical neck dissection	3	0	0	0	0	18	6	11	0	22
Near-total thyroidectomy										
No neck dissection	5	20	0	20	0	70	27	16	10	17
Partial neck dissection	4	25	0	25	0	16	31	0	25	19
Radical neck dissection	11	0	6	28	17	54	15	15	20	11
Total	54	9	7	13	6	350	16	13	6	5

Reprinted, by permission, from JA Buckwalter, Thomas CG, Freenan JB. Is childhood thyroid cancer a lethal disease? Ann Surg 1975;181:635.
*Children: under 21 years

nodes and initial lung metastases were present. Others have not been able to demonstrate an influence of cervical nodal metastases on prognosis.[85–87] The presence of papillary elements did not affect the remission rate. Metastases were associated with extracapsular tumor, isthmus involvement, bilaterality, and age less than 7 years. Based on a standard surgical protocol at Institut Gustave-Roussy (IGR),[36] it was determined that in patients without metastases on presentation, the failure rate of initial surgical management was five times greater in patients with macroscopically incomplete surgery than in those undergoing complete tumor resection ($p < 0.00001$). Limited surgery was only performed when there was no evidence of involvement of the proximal third of the contralateral lobe on frozen section.

The overall recurrence rate following complete remission was 17% at 10 years and 34% at 20 years; the overall survival was 98% at 10 years, 90.3% at 20 years, and 78% at 25 years, even though the standardized mortality ratio was 8:1 (Fig. 4.5).[36] Interestingly, brain metastases were noted in two patients previously treated for lung metastases. Lung metastases were found in association with involvement of the recurrent laryngeal nodal chain, which supports the concept of lymphatic spread between the thyroid bed and lungs, particularly behind the sterno-clavicular joint.[105]

It was concluded from the Schlumberger et al.[36] study that complete resection of macroscopically apparent tumor must be attempted with a modified neck dissection if ipsilateral jugulocarotid chain involvement is demonstrated on intraoperative frozen section. Nevertheless, as pointed out above, it is the surgical complication rate, and not necessarily the remission rate, that increases with more extensive resection in children.

It should be stressed that recommendations for the treatment of thyroid cancer in children are based on ongoing studies that, for the most part, have not followed patients long enough to detect what may be significant differences in mortality, recurrence, or even complication rates. This is due primarily to the fact that pediatric thyroid cancer has such an indolent course. Therefore, in the future, when more long follow-up intervals have elapsed, recommendations regarding surgical management, use of radioiodine, and the value of long-term

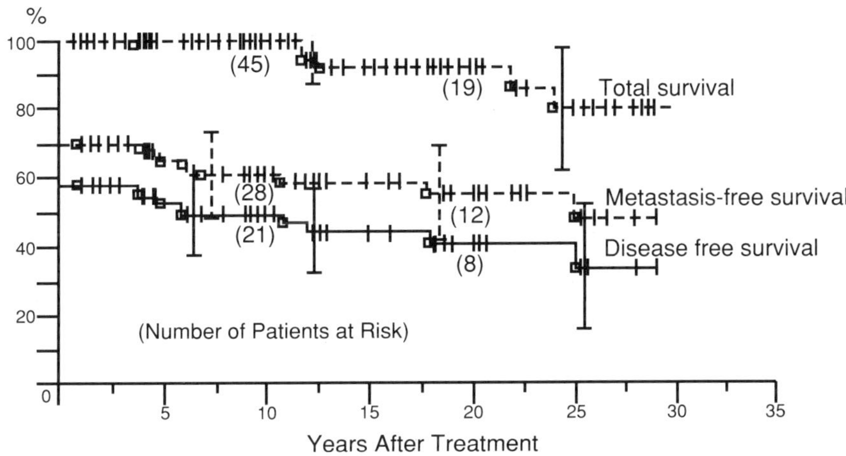

Figure 4.5. Survival of 72 children with differentiated thyroid cancer. Reprinted, by permission, from M Schlumberger et al, 1987. (36) Copyright by The Endocrine Society, 1987.

thyroxine suppression may differ somewhat from current recommendations. For now, conservative therapy as outlined above is recommended, based on what is known about the natural history of pediatric differentiated thyroid cancer and the risks and benefits of various surgical modalities (Table 4.6).

Uncommon Thyroid Neoplasms

Thyroid neoplasms may be derived from the epithelial tissue or from other constituents of the gland. Although the majority of malignant thyroid neoplasms are of the well-differentiated epithelial type, less-differentiated epithelial cancers may develop that are more aggressive and have a greater potential for malignancy and lethality. These types include insular, poorly differentiated, Hürthle cell, mucinous, columnar cell, and "tall-cell variant of papillary" carcinoma.[106,107] Fortunately, these variants are very rare in the pediatric age group.

Other thyroid neoplasms, such as medullary

Table 4.6. Summary of controversy over initial surgical management of pediatric differentiated thyroid cancer

THEORY: Pediatric differentiated thyroid cancer presents with more extension involvement but has a more indolent course compared to the adult condition.

PROCEDURE	*ADVANTAGES*	*DISADVANTAGES*
Conservative:		
Less than total thyroidectomy with resection of grossly involved cervical lymph nodes, post-operative radioiodine therapy, and lifelong suppression	lower major surgical complication rate	theoretical risk of higher metastatic rate (insufficient data to prove this currently) may need to deliver high-dose radioiodine
Aggressive:		
Total thyroidectomy with modified radical neck dissection when microscopic nodal metastases are found on intraoperative frozen section, radioiodine if there is residual tissue, and life-long suppression	superior survival rates (conficting data—unresolved at present) avoid high-dose radioiodine undless extranodal metastases are present	cosmesis major surgical complications

carcinoma (Chapter 8), teratoma, and sarcoma, have natural histories and morbidities that are very different from papillary and follicular cancers. This makes it imperative that all thyroid masses in children be studied pathologically. In fact, most of the mortality in children with thyroid cancer is due to the relatively uncommon instances of medullary and undifferentiated carcinoma. It should be noted that primary lymphoma of the thyroid gland, seen most often in adults, is extremely uncommon in children and adolescents.[108]

Undifferentiated (Anaplastic) Thyroid Cancer

Since undifferentiated thyroid cancer is a highly lethal malignancy, it must be excluded in every child or adolescent presenting with a thyroid mass. Although undifferentiated thyroid cancer is infrequent in children, there have been studies of European cases that have reported a frequency as high as 11% in children with neck masses (Table 4.1). In addition to the aforementioned risk factors for all thyroid cancers in children, there is also the risk (the degree of which is debated) of undifferentiated neoplasms arising from, or being associated with, differentiated neoplasms, possibly under the influence of elevated TSH levels.[14,96,98,109]

In Winship and Rosvoll's[35] series of 606 cases of pediatric thyroid cancer, 16 (3%) were undifferentiated. Of these, 14 (88%) were the small cell variety and 2 (12%), the spindle and giant cell varieties. The former are composed of sheets of small cells with large hyperchromatic nuclei. In terms of clinical appearance, childhood small cell cancers grow rapidly and extend aggressively into the soft tissues of the neck. Spindle and giant cell undifferentiated cancers are extremely malignant but fortunately very rare. These tumors can have a variable mix of spindle cells with giant, bizarre cells having pyknotic nuclei.

A preponderance of undifferentiated carcinomas in Europe (supporting the data in Table 4.1) in all age groups was discussed by Winship and Rosvoll.[35] Specifically, 70% of cases reported from Glasgow had "anaplastic carcinoma and 'relatively few' had papillary cancer."[110] This interesting disparity may be related to geographic differences in pathologic interpretation of specimens or to the fact that neck irradiation is less frequently used in Europe.

The reported survival rates for undifferentiated thyroid cancer in children range from 9 months to 1 year after diagnosis.[29] Among all thyroid cancer deaths in children reported by Winship and Rosvoll,[35] the highest mortality rate (81%) was found in patients with undifferentiated cancer. Unlike the case of differentiated thyroid cancer where children fare better than adults, undifferentiated thyroid cancers in children and adults exhibit the same hehavior. The rare cases of childhood undifferentiated cancer ought to be treated aggressively with total thyroidectomy, radioiodine to ablate any remaining tissue or functioning metastases, suppression, and chemotherapy and external radiation as indicated.

Teratoma

These neoplasms are virtually always benign but require surgical extirpation because of their tendency to eventually cause compressive symptoms. The true primary thyroid teratoma, presenting in stillborn or newborn infants,[111,112] is extremely rare. When it occurs, it is medially situated, with thyroidal vascularization. Occasionally, when it presents in late adolescence, the potential for malignancy is high, as it is in adults. Frequently, teratomas are in the lateral portion of the neck and involve the thyroid gland secondarily. Again, their removal is necessary to exclude a malignant thyroid lesion.

The treatment of choice is total or near-total thyroidectomy with thyroid hormone replacement therapy so that growth and development occur normally. In children, malignant teratomas have a very agressive clinical course. Despite total thyroidectomy, external radiation, and chemotherapy, survival rarely exceeds 1 year.[113]

Conclusions

Thyroid cancer in the pediatric age group differs from that in adults. When a child or adolescent is found to have a neck mass, any history of previous neck irradiation or occurrence of thyroid cancer in other family members must be obtained. Diagnostic evaluation should include a thyroid scan, sonogram, and fine-needle aspiration in order to exclude the possibility of a malignant neoplasm. If there is a high risk of thyroid cancer, then explorative surgery is warranted. When intraoperative frozen sections indicate the presence of a differentiated cancer, conservative resection with less-than-total thyroidectomy followed by radioiodine and TSH suppression is a reasonable approach. More aggressive initial surgery must be performed in cases of undifferentiated and medullary cancer. Fortunately, the outlook for youngsters with thyroid cancer is generally favorable. Nevertheless, more clinical trials with longer follow-up intervals are required to better identify optimal treatment regimens.

References

1. Gharib H, Goellner JR. Evaluation of nodular thyroid disease. Clin Endocrinol Metab 1988;17:511–526.
2. Stoffer RP, Welch JW, Hellwig CA, Chesky VE, McCusker EN. Nodular goiter. Arch Int Med 1960;106:10–14.
3. Vander JB, Gaston EA, Dawber TR. The significance of nontoxic thyroid nodules. Ann Int Med 1968;69:537–540.
4. Rallison ML, Dobyns BM, Keating R, Rall JE, Tyler FH. Thyroid nodularity in children. JAMA 1975;233:1069–1072.
5. Hayles AB, Kennedy RLJ, Woolner LB, Black BM. Nodular lesions of the thyroid gland in children. J Clin Endocrinol Metab 1956;1580–1594.
6. Sussman L, Librik L, Clayton GW. Hyperthyroidism attributable to a hyperfunctioning thyroid carcinoma. J Pediatr 1968;84:104–107.
7. Hopwood NJ, Carroll RG, Kenny FM, Foley TP. Functioning thyroid masses in childhood and adolescence. J Pediatr 1976;89:710–718.
8. Hamburger JI, Hamburger SW. Thyroidal hemiagenesis. Arch Surg 1970;100:319–320.
9. LiVolsi VA, Perzin KH, Sevetsky L. Carcinoma arising in median ectopic thyroid (including thyroglossal duct tissue). Cancer 1974;34:1303–1315.
10. McNicoll MP, Hawkins DB, England K, Penny R, Maceri DR. Papillary carcinoma arising in a thyroglossal duct cyst. Otol Head Neck Surg 1988;99:50–54.
11. Gharieb M. Angeborene form- und lageanomalie der schilddruse im kindesalter. Z Kinderchir 1972; 11:194–201.
12. Merrick Y, Hansen HS. Thyroid cancer in children and adolescents in Denmark. European J Surg Oncol 1989;15:49–53.
13. Eirhardt O. Zür anatomie und klinik der struma maligna. Beitr Klin Chir 1902;35:342–464.
14. Buckwalter JA, Nelson JG, Thomas CG. Cancer of the thyroid in youth. World J Surg 1981;5:15–25.
15. Kirkland RT, Kirkland JL. Solitary thyroid nodules in 30 children and report of a child with thyroid abscess. Ped 1973;51:85–90.
16. Hagler S, Rosenblum P, Rosenblum A. Carcinoma of the thyroid in children and adults: iatrogenic relation to previous irradiation. Pediatrics 1966;38:77–81.
17. Goepfert J, Dichtel WJ, Samaan NA. Thyroid cancer in children and teenagers. Arch Otol 1984;110:72–75.
18. Halpern S. Thyroid carcinoma in childhood. Med Ped Oncol 1981;9:143–151.
19. Liechty RD, Safaie-Shirazi S, Soper RT. Carcinoma of the thyroid in children. Surg Gynecol Obstet 1972;134:595–599.
20. Harness JK, Thompson NW, Nishiyama RH. Childhood thyroid carcinoma. Arch Surg 1971;102:278–284.
21. Crile G. Carcinoma of the thyroid in children. Ann Surg 1959;150:959–964.
22. Desjardins JG, Bass J, Leboeuf G, Di Lorenzo M, Letarte J, Khan AH, et al. A twenty-year experience with thyroid carcinoma in children. J Ped Surg 1988;23:709–713.
23. Desjardins JG, Khan AH, Montupet P, Collin PP, Leboeuf G, Polychronakos C, et al. Management of thyroid nodules in children: a 20-year experience. J Ped Surg 1987;22:736–739.
24. Pfister-Goedeke L, Stauffer UG. Thyroid carcinoma in childhood. Prog Ped Surg 1983;16:29–37.
25. Lamberg BA, Karninen-Jaaskelainen M, Franssila KO. Differentiated follicle-derived thyroid carcinoma in children. Acta Paediatr Scand 1989;78:419–425.
26. Doci R, Pilotti S, Costa A, Semeraro G, Cascinelli N. Thyroid cancer in childhood. Tumori 1978;64:649–657.
27. Jereb B, Lowhagen T. Carcinoma of the thyroid in children and young adults. Acta Radiol Ther Phys Biol 1972;2:411–421.
28. Ceccarelli C, Pacini F, Lippi F, Elisei R, Arganini M, Miccoli P, et al. Thyroid cancer in children and adolescents. Surgery 1988;104:1143–1148.
29. Richardson JE, Beaugie JM, Brown CL, Doniach I. Thyroid cancer in young patients in Great Britain. Br J Surg 1974;61:85–89.
30. Andersson A, Bergdahl L, Boquist L. Thyroid carcinoma in children. Am Surg 1977;43:159–163.
31. Belfiore A, Giuffrida D, La Rosa GL, Ippolito O, Russo G, Fiumara A, et al. Acta Endocrinol 1989;121:197–202.
32. Kodama T, Fujimoto Y, Obara T, Hidai K. Justification of conservative surgical treatment of childhood thyroid cancer: report of eleven cases and analysis of

Japanese literature. Jpn J Cancer Res 1986;77:799–807.
33. Segal K, Levy, R, Sidi J, Abraham A. Thyroid carcinoma in children and adolescents. Ann Otol Rhinol Laryngol 1985;94:346–319.
34. Zohar Y, Strauss M, Laurian N. Adolescent versus adult thyroid carcinoma. Laryngoscope 1986;96:555–559.
35. Winship T, Rosvoll RV. Thyroid carcinoma in childhood: final report on a 20 year study. Clin Proc Child Hosp 1970;26:327–348.
36. Schlumberger M, De Vathaire F, Travagli JP, Vassal G, Lemerle J, Parmenter C, et al. Differentiated thyroid carcinoma in childhood: long term follow-up of 72 patients. J Clin Endocrinol Metab 1987;65:1088–1094.
37. Quimby EH, Werner SC. Late radiation effects in roentgen therapy for hyperthyroidism. JAMA 1949;140:1046–1047.
38. Duffy BJ, Fitzgerald PJ. Cancer of the thyroid in children: a report of 28 cases. J Clin Endocrinol 1950a;10:1296–1308.
39. Duffy BJ, Fitzgerald PJ. Thyroid cancer in childhood and adolescence: a report on twenty-eight cases. Cancer 1950b;3:1018–1032.
40. Hayles AB, Johnson ML, Bears OH, Woolner LB. Carcinoma of the thyroid in children. Am J Surg 1963;106:735–743.
41. Scott MD, Crawford JD. Solitary thyroid nodules in childhood: is the incidence of thyroid carcinoma declining? Pediatrics 1976;58:521–525.
42. Hung W, August GP, Randolph JG, Schisgall RM, Chandra R. Solitary thyroid nodules in children and adolescents. J Ped Surg 1982;17:225–229.
43. Adams HD. Carcinoma in nodular goiter of childhood. Postgrad Med 1968;43:136–139.
44. Dailey ME, Lindsay S. Thyroid neoplasms in youth. J Pediatr 1950;36:460–465.
45. Sanfelippo MM, Bears OH, Hayles AB. Indications for thyroidectomy in the pediatric patients. Am J Surg 1971;122:472–476.
46. Horn RD, Ravdin IS. Carcinoma of the thyroid gland on youth. J Clin Endocrinol 1951;11:1166–1170.
47. Mauras N, Zimmerman D, Goellner JR. Hashimoto's thyroiditis associated with thyroid cancer in adolescent patients. J Pediatr 1985;106:895–898.
48. Hirabayashi RN, Lindsay S. Thyroid carcinoma and chronic thyroiditis of the Hashimoto type: a statistical study of their relationship. In: Appaix A, ed. Tumors of the Thyroid Gland. New York: American Elsevier;1966:272–291.
49. Shlicke CP, Hill JE, Schultz GF. Carcinoma in chronic thyroiditis. Surg Gynecol Obstet 1960;111:552–556.
50. Crile G, Hazard JB. Incidence of cancer in struma lymphomatosa. Surg Gynecol Obstet 1962;115:101–103.
51. Fisher DA, Oddie TH, Johnson DE, Nelson TC. The diagnosis of Hashimoto's thyroiditis. J Clin Endocrinol Metab 1975;40:795–801.
52. Kamma H, Fujii K, Ogata T. Lymphocytic infiltration in juvenile thyroid carcinoma. Cancer 1988;62:1988–1993.
53. Stoffer SS, Van Dyke DL, Bach JV, Szpunar W, Weiss L. Familial papillary carcinoma of the thyroid. Am J Med Genet 1986;25:775–782.
54. Sipple JH. The association of pheochromocytoma with carcinoma of the thyroid gland. Am J Med 1961;31:163–166.
55. Williams ED, Pollack DJ. Multiple mucosal neuromata with endocrine tumors: a syndrome allied to Von Recklinghausen's disease. J Pathol Bacteriol 1966;91:71–80.
56. Carney JA, Go VLW, Gordon H, Pearse AGE, Sheps SG. Familial pheochromocytoma and islet cell tumor of the pancreas. Am J Med 1980;68:515–521.
57. Camiel MR, Mule JE, Alexander LI, Benninghoff DL. Association of thyroid carcinoma with Gardner's syndrome in siblings. New Engl J Med 1968;278:1056–1059.
58. Friedman JM, Fialkow PJ. Genetic factors in thyroid disease. In: Ingbar SH, Braverman LE, eds. Werner's The Thyroid, Chapter 30. Philadelphia: JB Lippincott; 1986;634–650.
59. Stanbury JB. Thyroid-specific metabolic incompetence and tumor development. In: Hedinger CE, ed. Thyroid Cancer. UICC Monogr Series, Vol 12. New York: Springer-Verlag; 1969:183–192.
60. Elman DS. Familial association of nerve deafness with nodular goiter and thyroid carcinoma. New Engl J Med 1958;259:219–223.
61. Winship T. Carcinoma of the thyroid in childhood. Pediatrics 1956;18:459–466.
62. Clark RL, White EC, Russel WO. Total thyroidectomy for cancer of the thyroid; significance of intraglandular dissemination. Ann Surg 1959;149:858–866.
63. Tawes RL, DeLorimier AA. Thyroid carcinoma during youth. J Ped Surg 1968;3:210–218.
64. Frazell EL, Foote FW. The natural history of thyroid cancer; a review of 301 cases. J Clin Endocrinol 1949;9:1023–1030.
65. Pollock WF, Juler G. Thyroid carcinoma in children. Am J Dis Child 1963;105:59–64.
66. Hamburger JI, Husain M. Fine-needle biopsy: extended observations. In: Hamburger JI, ed. Diagnostic Methods in Clinical Thyroidology. New York: Springer-Verlag; 1989:221–253.
67. Harsoulis P, Leontsini M, Economou A, Gerasimidis T, Smbarounis C. Fine needle aspiration biopsy cytology in the diagnosis of thyroid cancer; comparative study of 213 operated patients. Br J Surg 1986;73:461–464.
68. Ramacciotti CE, Pretorius HT, Chu EW, Barsky SH, Prennan MF, Robbins J. Diagnostic accuracy and use of aspiration biopsy in the management of thyroid nodules. Arch Intern Med 1984;144:1169–1173.
69. Hamburger JI, Husain M. Fine-needle biopsy: extended observations. In, Hamburger JI, ed. Diagnostic Methods in Clinical Thyroidology. New York: Springer-Verlag; 1989:221–253.

70. Frable WI, Frable MA. Fine-needle biopsy of the thyroid: histopathologic and clinical correlations. In: Feneglio C and Wolff M, eds. Progress in Surgical Pathology. Masson: New York; 1980:105–115.
71. Liautaud-Roger F, Dufer J, Pluot M, Delisle MJ, Coninx P. Contribution of quantitative cytology to the cytological diagnosis of thyroid neoplasms. Anticancer Res 1989;9:231–234.
72. Luck JB, Mumaw VR, Frable WJ. Fine needle aspiration biopsy of the thyroid. Differential diagnosis by videoplan image analysis. Acta Cytol 1982;26:793–796.
73. Lukacs GL, Miko TL, Fabian E, Zs-Nagy I, Csaky G, Balazs Gy. The validity of some morphologic methods in the diagnosis of thyroid malignancy. Acta Chir Scand 1983;149:759–766.
74. Hay ID. Prognostic factors in thyroid carcinoma. Thyroid today 1989;12:1–9.
75. Bronner MP, Cleverger CV, Edmonds PR, Lowell DM, McFarland MM, LiVolsi VA. Flow cytometric analysis of DNA content in Hurthle cell adenomas and carcinomas of the thyroid. Am J Clin Pathol 1988;89:764–769.
76. Zimmerman D, Hay ID, Gough IR, Goellner JR, Ryan JJ, Grant CS, et al. Papillary thyroid carcinoma in children and adults: long-term follow-up of 1039 patients conservatively treated at one institution during three decades. Surgery 1988;104:1157–1166.
77. Komorowski RA, Deaconson TF, Vetsch R, Cerletty JM, Wilson SD. DNA content in radiation-associated thyroid cancer. Surgery 1988;104:992–996.
78. Klopp CT, Rosvoll RV, Winship T. Is destructive surgery ever necessary for treatment of thyroid cancer in children. Ann Surgery 1967;165:745–751.
79. La Quaglia MP, Corbally MT, Heller G, Exelby PR, Brennan MF. Recurrence and morbidity in differentiated thyroid carcinoma in children. Surgery 1988;104:1149–1156.
80. Exelby PE, Frazell EL. Carcinoma of the thyroid in children. Surg Clin North Am 1969;49:249–259.
81. Leeper RD. Treatment of thyroid cancer. In: Soto RJ, Sartorio de Forteza I, eds. New concepts in Thyroid Disease. New York: Alan R Liss; 1983:139–153.
82. Joppich I, Roher HD, Hecker WCh, Knorr D, Daum R. Thyroid carcinoma in childhood. Prog Ped Surg 1983;16:23–28.
83. Grant CS, Hay ID, Gough IR, Bergstrahl EJ, Goellner JR, McConahey WM. Local recurrence in papillary thyroid carcinoma: is extent of surgical resection important? Surgery 1988;104:954–962.
84. Franssila K. Value of histologic classification of thyroid cancer. Acta Path Microbiol Scand Section A (Suppl 225):1971;1–76.
85. Carcangiu ML, Zampi G, Pupi A, Castagnoli A, Rosai J. Papillary carcinoma of the thyroid. A clinicopathological study of 241 cases treated at the university of Florence, Italy. Cancer 1985;55:805–828.
86. Tubiana M, Schlumberger M, Rougier P, LaPlanche A, Benhamov E, Gardet P et al. Long-term results and prognostic factors in patients with differentiated thyroid carcinoma. Cancer 1985;55:794–804.
87. Mazzaferri EL, Young RL. Papillary thyroid carcinoma: a 10-year follow-up report of the impact of therapy in 576 patients. Am J Med 1981;70:511–517.
88. Varma VM, Beierwaltes WH, Nofal MM, Nishiyama RH, Copp JE. Treatment of thyroid cancer. Death rates after surgery and after surgery followed by sodium iodide ^{131}I. JAMA 1970;214:1437–1442.
89. Byrne J, Mulvihill JJ, Myers MH, Connelly RR, Naughton MD, Krauss MR, et al. Effects of treatment on fertility in long-term survivors of childhood or adolescent cancer. New Engl J Med 1987; 317:1315–1321.
90. Maxon HR, Smith HS. Radioiodine-131 in the diagnosis and treatment of metastatic well-differentiated thyroid cancer. Endocrinol Metab Clin North Am 1990;19:685–718.
91. Korff JM, Degroot LJ. The management of radiation-induced tumors of the thyroid. Endocrinol Metab Clin North Am 1981;10:299–315.
92. Hosoya R, Eiraku K, Saiki S, Nishimura K. Thyroid carcinoma and acute lymphoblastic leukemia in childhood. Cancer 1983;51:1931–1933.
93. Clayton GW, Kirkland RT. Thyroid carcinoma. In: Gardner LI, ed. Endocrine and Genetic Disease of Childhood and Adolescence. Philadelphia: WB Saunders;1975:325–329.
94. Cady B. The case against total thyroidectomy in differentiated thyroid cancer. In: Najarian JS, Delany JP, eds. Advances in Breast and Endocrine Surgery. Chicago: Year Book Medical; 1986:281–287.
95. Buckwalter JA, Thomas CG, Freeman JB. Is childhood thyroid cancer a lethal disease? Ann Surg 1975;181:632–639.
96. Crile G. The endocrine dependency of certain thyroid cancers and the danger that hypothyroidism may stimulate their growth. Cancer 1957;10:1119–1137.
97. Cady B, Sedgwick CE, Meissner WA, Buckwalter JA, Romagosa V, Werber J. Changing clinical, pathologic, therapeutics and survival patterns in differentiated thyroid carcinoma. Ann Surg 1977; 184:541–553.
98. Schlumberger M, Tubiana M, De Vathaire F, Hill C, Gardet P, Travagli JP, et al. Long-term results of treatment of 283 patients with lung and bone metastases from differentiated thyroid carcinoma. J Clin Endocrinol Metab 1986;63:960–967.
99. Piechaczyk M, Baldet L, Pau B, Bastide J-M. Novel immunoradiometric assay of thyroglobulin in serum with use of monoclonal antibodies selected for lack of cross-reactivity with autoantibodies. Clin Chem 1989;35:422–424.
100. Winship T, Rosvoll RV. Cancer of the thyroid in children. Proc Natl Cancer Conf 1968;6:677–681.
101. Statistical Report of End Results, 1949–1957. Memorial Hospital for Cancer and Allied Diseases and the James Ewing Hospital of the City of New York. 1965;103.
102. Tallroth E, Backdahl M, Einhorn J, Lundell G, Lo-

whagen T, Silfversward C. Thyroid carcinoma in children and adolescents. Cancer 1986;58:2329–2332.
103. Zabransky S. Das Schilddrusenkarzinom beim Kind. Arch Kinder-heilk 1969;179:236–241.
104. Withers EH, Rosenfield L, O'Niell J, Lynch JB, Holcomb G. Long-term experience with childhood thyroid carcinoma. J Ped Surg 1979;14:332–335.
105. Tubiana M, Lacour J, Monnier JP, Bergiron C, Gerard- Marchant R, Roujeau J, et al. External radiotherapy and radioiodine in the treatment of 359 thyroid cancers. Br J Radiol 1975;48:894–907.
106. Flynn SD, Forman BH, Stewart AF, Kinder BK. Poorly differentiated ("insular") carcinoma of the thyroid gland: an aggressive subset of differentiated thyroid neoplasms. Surgery 1988;104:963–970.
107. Har-el G, Hadar T, Segal K, Levy R, Sidi J. Hürthle cell carcinoma of the thyroid gland. Cancer 1986; 57:1613–1617.
108. Gorlin JB, Sallan SE. Thyroid cancer in childhood. Endocrinol Metab Clin North Am 1990;19:649–662.
109. Thomas CG. Progression in thyroid cancer. Clin Endocrinol 1968;11:26–38.
110. Jackson IMD, Thomson JA. The relationship of carcinoma to the single thyroid nodule. Br J Surg 1967;54:1007–1009.
111. Numanoglu J, Aksu Y, Mutaf O. Teratoma of thyroid gland in new-born infant. J Ped Surg 1970;5:381–382.
112. Suzuki H, Kato T, Yabe K. Teratoma of the thyroid in a 2-month old infant. Z Kinderchir 1974;15:340–344.
113. Fisher JE, Cooney DR, Voorhess ML, Jewett TC. Teratoma of the thyroid gland in infancy: report of the literature and two case reports. J Surg Oncol 1982;21:135–140.

5

Surgery for Well-Differentiated Thyroid Carcinoma

ARTHUR E. SCHWARTZ and EUGENE W. FRIEDMAN

A wide spectrum of cancers arise in the thyroid gland. These range from well-differentiated, slow-growing malignancies to relentless and almost inevitably lethal anaplastic cancers (see Table 5.1). Parafollicular thyroid cells give rise to medullary carcinoma that may be familial or sporadic. In addition, the thyroid may be the seat of lymphomas or the site of metastases from the kidney, breast, lung, or other organs. Although there is a standard accepted approach to a potentially malignant thyroid mass, specific management will depend on the histology, extent of disease, age of the patient, and other factors. Most important is the experience and judgement of the surgeon.

The protracted and generally favorable course of well-differentiated thyroid cancer complicates the evaluation of different treatment methods. There are no long-term prospective studies of the treatment of this disease. The clinical management of well-differentiated thyroid cancer rests on retrospective studies and individual clinical experience.

Classification

Thyroid cancer can be roughly divided into four major categories of which well-differentiated carcinomas (papillary and follicular malignancies) constitute approximately 90%.

Papillary thyroid cancer is by far the most common type of well-differentiated thyroid malignancy. These tumors have an indolent course and a cure rate well over 90%, even when managed conservatively. They tend to metastasize to regional neck nodes and the lungs. As in follicular cancer, they become much more aggressive with advancing age of the patient, increasing size, and penetration beyond the thyroid capsule. The outlook is worse in men.[1] Thyroid cancers arising in patients with a history of previous radiotherapy to the head and neck are almost always papillary;[2] in these patients the disease has essentially the same rate of local recurrence and survival as in those in whom the disease appears spontaneously.[3,1]

Table 5.1. Distribution of thyroid cancer by type

Well-differentiated thyroid cancer	90%
Papillary	75%
(includes Papillary–follicular carcinoma and papillary variant of follicular carcinoma)	
Follicular	15%
(includes Hürthle cell carcinoma)	
Medullary	5%
Undifferentiated	5%

Pure follicular malignancies constitute a separate group with a different pattern of behavior and a poorer prognosis; they characteristically disseminate through the bloodstream to lung, bone, and brain. They are not as common as the varieties of papillary cancer; their number appears to be decreasing, paralleling the decline in nodular goiter that occurred after the widespread introduction of iodized salt in the United States. The sex of the patient does not appear to affect survival.[4] Regional lymph node metastases are much less frequent than they are in papillary carcinoma.

If enough sections are taken, the great majority of papillary and follicular tumors will prove to be mixed papillary–follicular cancers. These behave like papillary carcinomas, offering a longer survival, with metastases to regional lymph nodes rather than the systemic dissemination found in follicular cancers. In the past, follicular thyroid carcinomas were overdiagnosed; on multiple sections and after diligent search, a great many of these prove to have papillary elements and are properly classified as mixed papillary–follicular cancers. They behave as papillary cancers and share their excellent prognosis.

In addition, in recent years the papillary variant of follicular carcinoma has been separated from true follicular cancer. These tumors mimic the acinar structure of follicular carcinoma, but the cells retain the characteristic vacuolated nuclei ("Orphan Annie cells") of papillary carcinoma. Most importantly, they behave as papillary cancers and should be managed in the same way. Perhaps 25% of previously reported follicular carcinomas are, in fact, follicular variants of papillary cancer.[5]

Clinically, the subgroups of papillary carcinoma of the thyroid have the same biological behavior. Certain papillary cancers containing "tall cells" are an exception; these are a more aggressive, and fortunately, rare variant.[6]

Hürthle cell tumors are a distinctive variant of follicular neoplasms that have a serious malignant potential. When malignant, they are more aggressive than other follicular carcinomas.[7,8] As Hürthle cell tumors become larger than 2 cm in diameter, the incidence of malignancy increases. The clinical course has been difficult to predict on a histologic basis; some authors suggest that all Hürthle cell tumors are potentially malignant.[8] Our pathologists, however, like most others, make a distinction between benign and malignant Hürthle cell tumors that we have found to be largely correct.[7] Total thyroidectomy is recommended as initial treatment for malignant Hürthle cell tumors because of their aggressive behavior.

It is usually possible to cure well-differentiated thyroid cancer. Surgery offers the only practical method. Radiotherapy is rarely useful for palliation; no drug is currently available for effective chemotherapy.

Significance of Microscopic Disease

Although surgery is often curative, it is an illusion to assume that success is directly related to the removal of all microscopic disease. Predicting the clinical behavior of well-differentiated thyroid cancer on the logical assumption that it will correspond to the extent of microscopic cancer has not proved valid. The relevance of microscopic malignancy to clinical cancer is difficult to evaluate. The concept that the high incidence of occult neck node metastases validates prophylactic neck dissection in papillary cancer, has been replaced by the realization that this procedure offers no increase in survival.[9]

In a patient with papillary carcinoma, the incidence of microscopic foci of carcinoma in the lobe that is not clinically involved is 58% when serial sections are performed,[10] and 30% on routine examination.[11] This high incidence of occult carcinoma gave rise to clinical recurrence in the opposite lobe in only 4.2% of 164 patients who had a thyroid lobectomy for papillary carcinoma that was confined to one lobe of the gland, and who were followed for 14 years.[11]

A similar contradiction is seen in the behavior of microscopic metastatic disease in the jugular lymph nodes of the neck. Two reports showed the presence of metastases in the neck nodes of patients who had thyroid operations for papillary cancer, and who, in the absence of palpable neck nodes, were subjected to elective neck dissections. Metastases were present in these nodes in 68.7% of 115 patients in one of the reports[12] and in 50% of 76 patients in the other.[9] In spite of these statistics, the development of clinical neck node metastases in patients with papillary thyroid cancer who have not had neck dissections is not common: 11 of 88 patients (12.5%) who did not have initial neck dissections later developed neck node metastases.[9] Other authors state that the incidence is from 5% to 20%,[13] and report that these patients are almost always salvaged by surgical treatment. It is no surprise that surgeons have discarded the prophylactic neck dissections that were previously routine in well-differentiated thyroid cancer.

The differences in the behavior of these foci of malignancy recognized over a long follow-up period, is the source of most of the controversy in the management of well-differentiated thyroid cancer. It is apparent that much of the microscopic disease in lymph nodes of the neck and in the thyroid gland does not progress to clinical cancer. The behavior of well-differentiated thyroid cancer cannot be extrapolated from the presence of microscopic disease. It is well established that biologic features such as the age of the patient, type, grade, size and extent of the primary tumor, and other unknown factors play prominent roles in the prognosis. Surgery is a modifying, but far from definitive influence on the course of the disease.

Needle Biopsy

Fine needle biopsy has become a valuable diagnostic tool in the evaluation of thyroid tumors. It is a safe, highly accurate test that can be performed as either an outpatient or an office procedure. It is easy to carry out, can be repeated if required, does not require local anesthesia, and is inexpensive. It differentiates between cystic and solid lesions immediately and provides material for histologic and immunochemical study. Before the use of needle biopsy, thyroid cancer was found at surgery in 14% of solitary thyroid nodules at the Mayo Clinic; after the introduction of this test, the incidence of cancer in a similar setting increased to 29%.[14]

We perform fine needle biopsies using a 22-gauge needle mounted on a 10-cc syringe. The patient lies on his or her back, supported by a pillow under the shoulders and with the neck extended. The needle is inserted into the thyroid nodule and passed back and forth through the mass while maintaining suction on the syringe. Suction in the syringe is released prior to the withdrawal of the needle from the neck to prevent loss of cellular material from the needle into the syringe. After removal, the needle is detached from the syringe, the syringe is filled with 2 to 3 cm^3 of air, the needle is replaced and the contents of the needle and syringe are expelled with air onto a glass slide. A second slide is placed over on the first and the specimen spread between both. The slides are separated and immediately treated with spray fixative, prepared with a modified Papanicolaou stain, and read. If fluid is obtained it is mixed with an equal amount of alcohol and centrifuged; the sediment is then stained and examined.

Although fine needle biopsy is an invaluable diagnostic tool, serious shortcomings must be noted. The biopsy only samples a limited area; it is possible to miss the lesion entirely. False positive and false negative results are encountered. In 92 patients who were later surgically explored, we found 3.3% of the reports to be false positives and 6.5% to be false negatives. The overall accuracy was 90.2%.[15] Fine needle biopsy cannot discriminate between the follicular cells of adenoma and follicular carcinoma.[16] In this situation, surgical excision with examination of the architecture of the lesion is required. Although fine needle biopsy is the single most valuable diagnostic test available, it is essential that clinical judgment prevail in the decision whether or not to operate upon a thyroid mass. A negative biopsy does *not* rule out malignancy.

Surgical Approach to the Thyroid Nodule

Most thyroid operations are performed as exploratory diagnostic procedures, although clinical characteristics, a history of radiation exposure, or a preoperative needle biopsy may suggest a diagnosis of malignancy. Which is the proper approach: biopsy of the lesion itself, removal of the nodule, or excision of the entire lobe or isthmus? It is almost always preferable to remove the entire thyroid lobe or isthmus than to perform an incisional biopsy because of the difficulty in establishing a definitive diagnosis on frozen section and the hazards of reoperating on a thyroid lobe. It is appalling to receive a final diagnosis of malignancy two days after a frozen section has been reported benign—a not unusual occurrence. Should the final report indicate malignancy, the surgeon who initially has performed only an incisional biopsy or a partial lobectomy is faced with a far more difficult operation that poses much greater risk to the recurrent nerve and the parathyroid glands. It is far better to remove the entire lobe or isthmus, often obviating the need for further surgery. If the opposite lobe later requires removal, the surgeon will have a virgin field to dissect and the best opportunity to preserve the recurrent nerve and the parathyroid glands.

Limitations of Frozen Section

Papillary or papillary–follicular carcinoma can usually be recognized on frozen section because of its distinct structure. Even so, it is not unusual to find small foci of papillary cancer on later, final sections. It is the diagnosis of follicular carcinoma, however, that presents the most vexing problem. Most pathologists require capsular or blood vessel invasion to be present to justify a diagnosis of follicular malignancy, although increased thickness of the capsule has been recently proposed as a criterion.[17] These features are usually difficult to establish on frozen section examination. Even on paraffin section distinguishing between benign and malignant follicular lesions can be trying. The surgeon often suspects the existence of malignancy, but cannot prove this during the operation. Removal of paratracheal nodes may establish a diagnosis in well-differentiated thyroid carcinoma, particularly papillary cancer, if they are found to contain metastases. These nodes are less frequently involved in follicular cancer, but it is worth the effort to remove them in order to make a frozen section examination. If the paratracheal nodes do not contain metastases the surgeon is often offered a diagnosis of "atypical follicular adenoma, await permanent sections." Unless there is nodularity in the opposite lobe, no further procedure can be justified. Total removal of the thyroid lobe, isthmus, and pyramidal lobe will complete the surgical management on the ipsilateral side. This area need not then be disturbed, even if the final report is changed to malignancy and a later decision is made to remove the opposite lobe.

Amount of Thyroid that should be Removed for Thyroid Carcinoma

The ideal treatment for well-differentiated thyroid cancer is total thyroidectomy. It removes the entire primary tumor as well any other foci of malignancy within the gland.

Were it not for the specter of hypoparathyroidism, total thyroidectomy would be the standard treatment for all thyroid carcinomas. The risk of injury to the recurrent laryngeal nerve in the hands of an experienced surgeon is 1% or less. The real deterrent to the routine use of total thyroidectomy is the 3% to 15% incidence of permanent hypoparathyroidism. This lifelong affliction requires continuous daily medication and lifelong surveillance. In spite of treatment, cataracts occur in 70% of patients.[18,19] Fatigue, parasthesias and muscular irritability are continuing problems.

It is difficult to evaluate whether the complete removal of the opposite thyroid lobe in patients with well-differentiated cancer confined to one thyroid lobe makes a significant contribution to survival. In an update of his original series, Tollefsen reported that 4.6% of 216 patients who had thyroid lobectomies for papillary carcinoma confined to one lobe developed a recurrence in the opposite lobe. These patients had been followed for at least 5 years (including the 164 original patients now followed for at least 14 years). Half of these patients were salvaged by further surgery. Of the nine patients who expired, seven died of metastatic disease and two with recurrent papillary carcinoma succumbed to other causes.[11]

In a series of 102 patients who had thyroid lobectomies for well-differentiated thyroid cancer confined to one lobe and followed for over 15 years, we observed four patients who developed a recurrence in the opposite lobe (Fig 5.1). One patient was salvaged by further surgery; three patients died of local recurrent disease. Two of these had tumors involving the

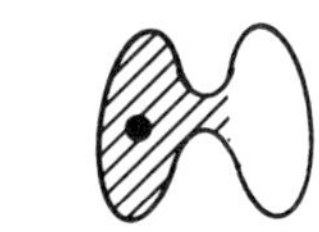

	Patients	Recurrence Opposite Lobe
Mixed P-F	70	3
Follicular	32	1
TOTAL	102	4 (3.9%)

Figure 5.1. Incidence of recurrent clinical disease in the opposite lobe of 102 patients with well-differentiated thyroid cancer confined to one lobe, treated by thyroid lobectomy and excision of the isthmus and followed-up for more than 15 years. Reprinted, by permission, from Friedman EW and Schwartz AE. Well-differentiated thyroid cancer. In: Current Therapy in Endocrinology 1983–1984. Krieger DT and Bardin WD eds. Toronto: BC Decker Publisher, 1983.

trachea that could not be completely resected during the original procedure. The other patient died of local recurrence of papillary carcinoma in the opposite lobe, 11 years after the original surgery. In this study the rate of recurrence in the opposite lobe was 3.9%. Only one death can be directly attributed to the failure to initially perform a total thyroidectomy.

Most patients who die of follicular cancer succumb to distant metastatic tumor; 50% of those with papillary carcinoma die of disseminated disease, mostly pulmonary.[20] How much of this is present at the time of original surgery and can be affected by performing a total thyroidectomy has not been adequately evaluated. Young reported that the mortality in follicular carcinoma is greatly reduced by using a combination of total thyroidectomy, radioactive iodine, and thyroid hormone. However, he notes that no mortality occurred in those patients who had no evidence of distant metastases when originally seen.[4]

Excellent long-term survival (i.e., no deaths in patients followed for 25 years) has been achieved by excising the thyroid lobe and isthmus in patients with papillary carcinoma less than 1.5 cm confined to one lobe.[21] In a review of 576 patients published in 1977, Mazzaferri reported decreased survival rates for those patients who had undergone limited resections, as compared with those who had undergone total thyroidectomy for papillary carcinoma of the thyroid gland.[22] In 1981, in a 10 year follow-up study of the same patients, these findings were confirmed. It was noted, however, that in the subgroup of patients with primary tumors of less than 1.5 cm, there was no improvement in the recurrence or survival rates of those patients who had undergone total thyroidectomy compared with those who were given thyroid hormone, and had undergone a less extensive procedure.[23] Furthermore, in this series the incidence of permanent hypoparathyroidism for those patients who had total thyroidectomies was 13.5%.[22]

As the size of the lesion increases, results of treatment become less satisfactory. Despite having an obvious theoretical advantage, the routine use of total thyroidectomy for papillary carcinoma confined to only one lobe of the thyroid gland remains controversial. Although some authors report increased survival rates in patients treated by total thyroidectomy or total thyroidectomy followed by radioactive iodine,[24,25] others find no difference in those patients managed by lobectomy and excision of the isthmus or lobectomy and partial or near total lobectomy on the opposite side.[26–28]

Multicentricity is not a prominent feature in pure follicular carcinoma. Tollefsen[29] reports a rate of 13% and Harness, 16%.[5] However, because of the increased aggressiveness of follicular cancer, and the greater risk of metastases to lungs, bones, and brain; many authors, including ourselves, advocate total thyroidectomy followed by radioactive iodine ablation of the remnant if the 24-hour uptake in the neck is more than 1–1.5%.

Total thyroidectomy for well-differentiated thyroid cancer reduces the risk of local recurrence in the gland itself. In addition, some authors report that one added benefit is a diminished incidence of pulmonary metastases, particularly in cases in which supplemental radioactive iodine is given to eliminate all residual thyroid tissue.[23–25] These advantages must be balanced against the debilitating effects of permanent hypoparathyroidism, reported to be 12.8% in one series of total thyroidectomies,[30] and 13.5% in another.[22] Acceptance of total thyroidectomy depends on the degree of risk; the incidence of permanent hypoparathyroidism in total thyroidectomy ranges from 2.8%[31] to 32%.[1] Because there is a greater understanding of the blood supply of the parathyroid glands and the importance of its preservation, the frequency of this complication has decreased significantly. Nonetheless, in spite of surgical expertise and experience, the hazard of permanent hypoparathyroidism remains inherent in the performance of the procedure. We recently reported a series of 183 patients who had total thyroidectomy: the incidence of permanent hypoparathyroidism was 3.3% and permanent nerve injury 0.55%.[32] It is our experience that although careful and consistent technique has substantially reduced the risk of hypoparathyroidism, it still remains a sporadic complication. No operative technique completely removes the danger.

We feel that when total thyroidectomy can be performed with safety, it is a valuable addition to the management of papillary thyroid cancer, particularly when the lesion is more than 1.5 cm in diameter. We agree with most authorities that total thyroidectomy followed by radioactive iodine ablation of any remaining thyroid tissue is the preferred treatment for follicular thyroid carcinoma.

Technique of Thyroidectomy

The essence of thyroid surgery for malignancy is the removal of the gland with preservation of the recurrent laryngeal nerves, superior laryngeal nerves, and the parathyroid glands. The initial approach is a total lobectomy and excision of the thyroid isthmus on the side of the malignancy. In some cases this may be sufficient.

We emphasize visualization of the recurrent nerves and the parathyroid glands. With experience it becomes possible to demonstrate the glands and conserve their blood supply. Careful hemostasis is required so that the distinctive appearance of the parathyroid glands will not be altered and the recurrent laryngeal nerve be seen clearly.

The incision is placed transversely across the anterior neck, at a level inferior to the cricoid cartilage and above the sternal notch (Fig. 5.2). A higher location in the neck produces a more pleasing appearance; a scar closer to the sternum tends to spread. Elevating the incision on the side of the thyroid mass allows the redundant skin to settle downward evenly and results in a level scar. A more superiorly placed incision also facilitates a cosmetic extension of the wound laterally and upward should a neck dissection be required (Fig. 5.3).

Good exposure is vital; it can usually be obtained by separating the strap muscles in the midline and retracting them laterally. Additional access can be provided by transecting the medial portion of the sternohyoid muscle near its insertion, or dividing the sternothyoid muscle, completely or partially, at the upper pole level (Fig. 5.4.). If required, there should be no hesitation in transecting both strap muscles transversely at their lower third; if they are adherent to tumor, they are removed with the thyroid gland. Direct extension of thyroid malignancies into the strap muscles is not unusual.

After the thyroid gland has been exposed, the middle thyroid vein is divided. This vessel drains directly into the jugular vein; failure to secure it can result in considerable hemorrhage, making it more difficult to visualize the parathyroid glands and recurrent nerve. Once the vein is severed and ligated, it is possible to mobilize the thyroid lobe safely, often by blunt dissection, to facilitate dissection of the superior pole vessels.

Division of the superior pole vessels is the next objective. The increased mobility this maneuver produces will make it possible to retract the lobe medially and upward, enhancing the exposure of the parathyroid glands and their blood supply, as well as placing the recurrent nerve on a stretch, assisting in its identification and dissection.

The superior pole is mobilized by entering the area between the superior pole vessels and the cricothyroid muscle. By clearing this space, the superior and recurrent laryngeal nerves, close companions of the muscle, are avoided.

The superior laryngeal nerves are at risk

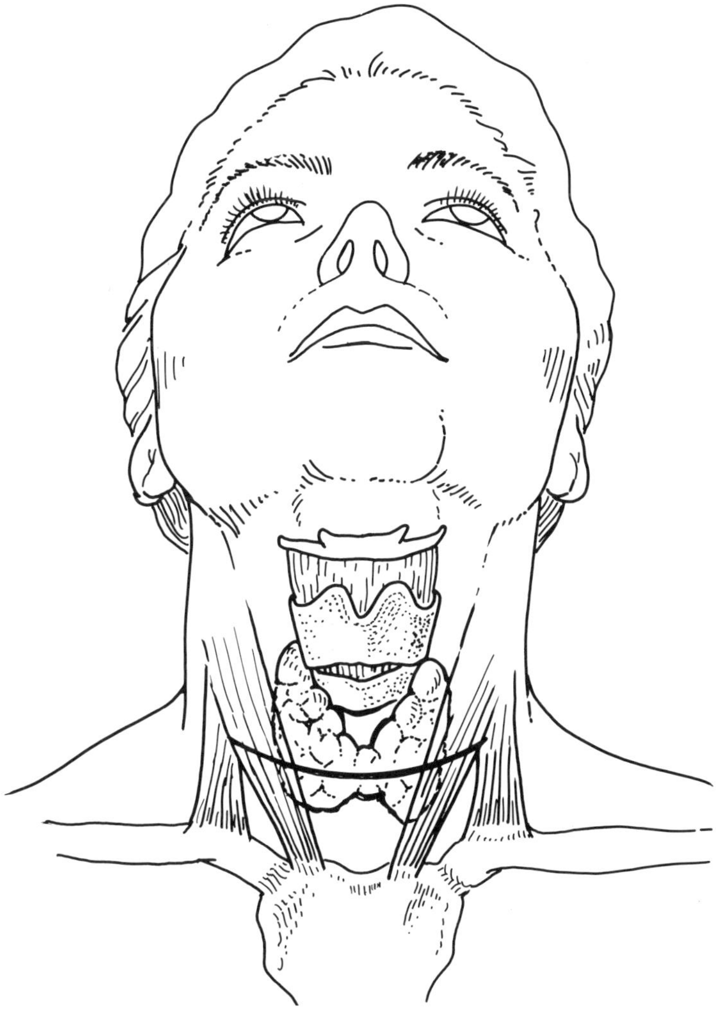

Figure 5.2. Incision for thyroidectomy.

when the superior pole vessels are divided. They are tensors of the vocal cords, enabling the patient to sustain a higher pitch and enriching the quality of speech. After injury, the diminished quality of the voice is noted quickly by those who depend upon it: singers, lawyers, and teachers. The nerve is best preserved by an awareness of its presence, dividing and ligating the superior pole vessels individually, as close to the upper pole of the thyroid gland as possible. Sometimes the nerve can be seen and avoided as it descends with the vessels, but usually it is not visualized. Once the vessels are transected, the thyroid lobe can be rotated medially to look for the inferior thyroid artery and recurrent laryngeal nerve. Dissection of the upper pole is discontinued. This avoids injury to the parathyroid gland, which, if not already located, may be present posterior to the superior pole vessels or behind Berry's ligament.

Identification of the lower parathyroid gland and the recurrent nerve is the next endeavor. The inferior thyroid artery is the guide to both; usually it can be found at a right angle to the common carotid artery entering the midportion of the thyroid lobe (discounting enlargements and distortions). The recurrent laryngeal nerve courses upward under the vessel in 80% of the patients (it lies above in 20%)

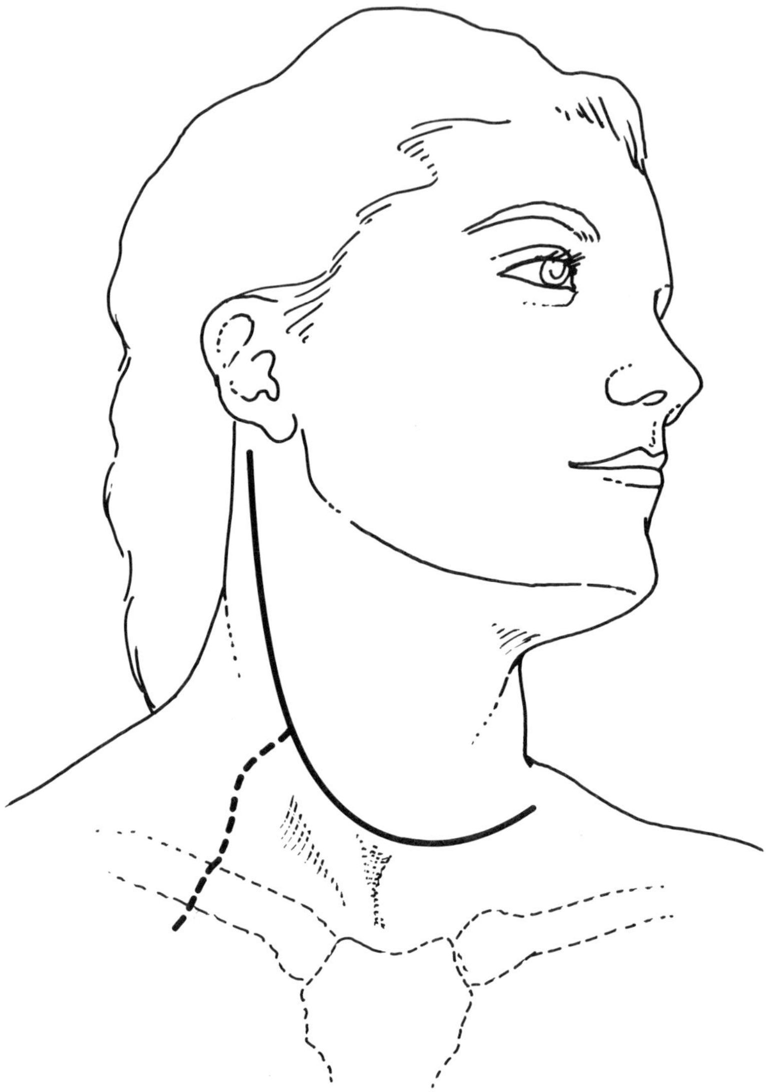

Figure 5.3. The standard thyroid incision has been extended posteriorly and toward the mastoid process to perform a neck dissection. The portion indicated by the dotted line can be added if increased exposure is needed.

forming the hypotenuse of a triangle with the carotid artery as the third leg (Fig. 5.5). The nerve can usually be palpated by running a finger transversely across the trachea just below the inferior thyroid artery. Exploration of the distal branches of this vessel will frequently lead to the lower parathyroid gland. It is essential that the vessels to the gland be carefully isolated and preserved (Fig. 5.6). If the parathyroid gland is located so far anteriorly that its blood supply cannot be preserved, the gland should be removed, minced into 1-mm fragments, and transplanted into the sternomastoid muscle (Fig. 5.7). The location of the inferior parathyroid gland is less consistent than the upper gland. Often it is at some distance from the lobe and, at times, may not be found. In this situation it is good judgment to divide the inferior thyroid artery and its branches as far medially as possible to preserve the blood supply to the parathyroid gland.

Placing a scissors on top of the recurrent nerve and spreading the blades develops a surface that permits the nerve to be dissected

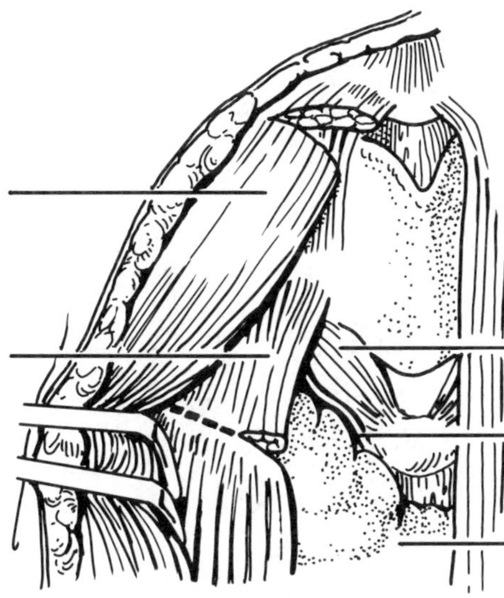

Figure 5.4. The sternohyoid muscle has been divided medially to provide greater access to the thyroid gland, particularly the upper pole. Transection of the sternothyroid muscle, as diagrammed, will further increase the exposure. In this patient, division of the cricothyroid branch of the superior thyroid artery offers increased exposure to the space between the cricothyroideus and the superior pole of the thyroid. Reprinted, by permission, from Schwartz AE, Friedman EW. 1987(32).

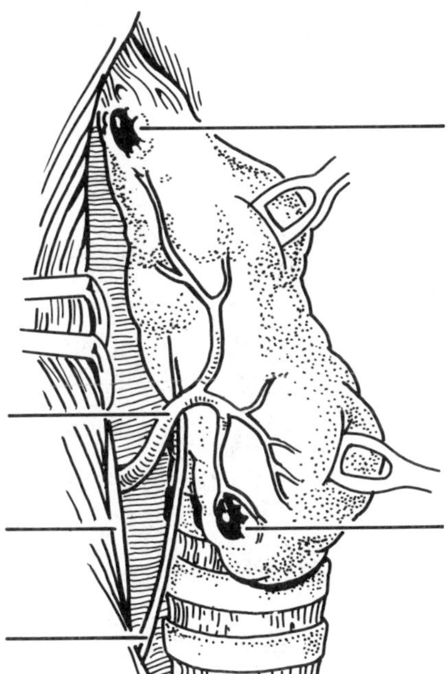

Figure 5.5. The classic position of the parathyroid glands is diagrammed showing the lower gland nourished by a separate branch of the inferior thyroid artery. The artery must be divided distal to this branch to preserve the blood supply of the parathyroid gland. The recurrent laryngeal nerve is seen coursing under the inferior thyroid artery. The upper parathyroid gland is located posteriorly on the upper pole. Although it is also nourished by the inferior thyroid artery, this may be less apparent during the dissection; it may also receive some blood supply from the superior thyroid artery. Reprinted, by permission, from Schwartz AE, Friedman EW. 1987(32).

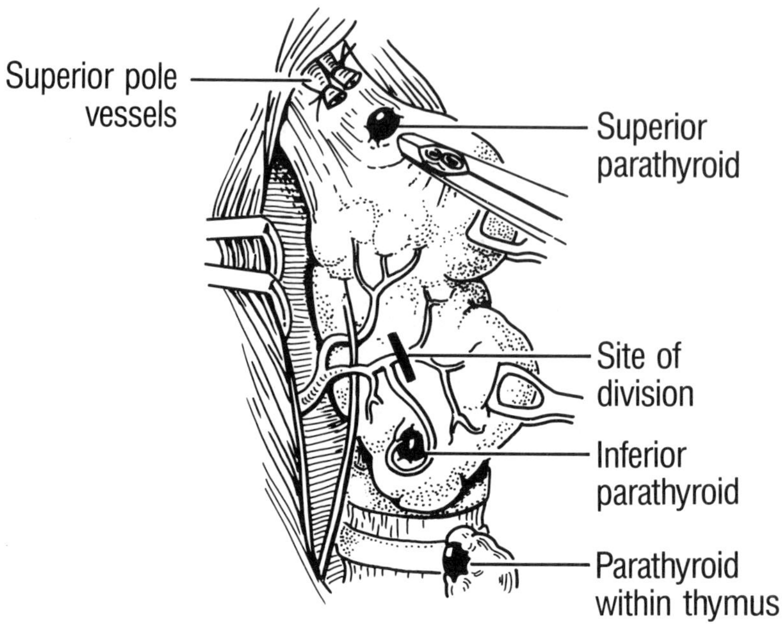

Figure 5.6. The superior parathyroid gland is not found in its classic position but in the areolar tissue adjacent to Berrys' ligament which has not yet been divided. The gland is located only after division of the upper pole vessels. A long segment of the inferior thyroid artery must be preserved to maintain the arterial loop which returns backward to nourish the inferior parathyroid gland. The preferred site for division of the vessel is shown. An additional parathyroid gland present in the thymus will be preserved. Reprinted, by permission, from Schwartz AE, Friedman EW. 1987(32).

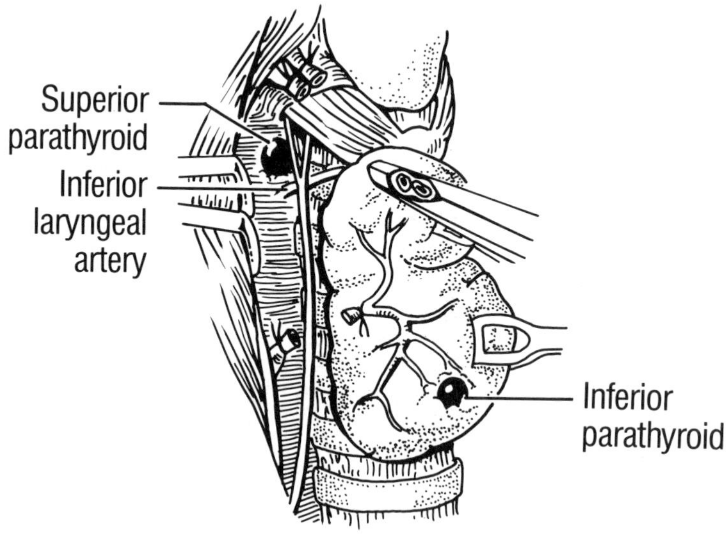

Figure 5.7. The upper pole has been divided, the inferior thyroid artery transected, and the recurrent nerve has been dissected. The superior parathyroid gland has been mobilized, displaced posteriorly, and preserved. The inferior laryngeal artery will be divided as close as possible to the thyroid lobe to avoid injury to the recurrent nerve. The inferior parathyroid gland is located too far from a branch of the inferior thyroid artery to be preserved with its blood supply. It will be necessary to remove the parathyroid gland and implant its fragments into the sternomastoid muscle in order to preserve its function. Reprinted, by permission, from Schwartz AE, Friedman EW. 1987(32).

cephalad to the point where it enters the larynx just below the cricothyroid muscle. The nerve is dissected by separating the tissues that are superior to it, never by disturbing the undersurface. In more than half the cases the nerve splits, often into several strands. All must be preserved. Retracting the thyroid lobe medially and upward straightens the nerve and its branches, facilitating the dissection. If the vocal cord functions preoperatively, every effort is made to preserve the recurrent nerve; if tumor is adherent to the nerve but can be dissected away, the nerve is spared. Berry's ligament is then divided under direct vision, taking care not to injure a parathyroid gland which may be lurking beneath. The upper parathyroid gland has a more consistent location than the lower, and can usually be identified just posterior to the upper lobe of the thyroid gland. It is easily preserved by gently mobilizing it posterior to the recurrent nerve.

After preservation of the parathyroid glands and the recurrent nerve, the thyroid lobe is readily removed from the trachea by sharp dissection. Excision of the pyramidal lobe and thyroid isthmus is an important addition to routine thyroid lobectomy; it clears the midline structures and avoids future anterior nodules that may be clinically confusing. Incomplete removal of the pyramidal lobe is a common cause of failure in total thyroidectomy, as demonstrated by postoperative radioactive scanning of the thyroid.

After removal of a thyroid lobe it is worthwhile to inspect the specimen for a parathyroid gland that may have been inadvertently removed. If it is sufficiently remote from tumor, it should be transplanted.

Near-Total Thyroidectomy

We make the decision to embark on a total thyroidectomy, if it is immediately indicated, on the basis of the status of the parathyroid glands on the side of the initial lobectomy. If they are viable, the opposite lobe can be removed with confidence. If not, it is safer to consider a near-total lobectomy on the opposite side, preserving a posterior rim of tissue to protect the parathyroid glands and the recurrent nerve; the patient will be better off with a bit of residual thyroid gland than with permanent hypoparathyroidism.

Near-total lobectomy is performed by dividing the middle thyroid vein and the superior pole vessels, identifying the recurrent nerve in the area of the lower pole of the thyroid lobe, and placing traction on the lobe medially. The lobe is then transected from its lateral aspect to the trachea, leaving a posterior shell of tissue that protects the parathyroid glands and their blood supply and also shields the underlying recurrent nerve. A small cautery loop is useful to remove additional tissue from within the remaining thyroid capsule without risk to other structures (Fig. 5.8). The capsule of the thyroid is then imbricated into the tracheal fascia (Fig. 5.9). Ninety percent or more of the thyroid lobe can be removed without difficulty by this procedure.

The advantage of near-total lobectomy is that the parathyroid glands and their blood supply are undisturbed and their viability assured. The disadvantage is that the surgeon is unable to visualize the recurrent laryngeal nerve as it completes its upper course without dissecting the parathyroid glands and placing their blood supply in jeopardy. The superior portion of the thyroid lobe is divided without seeing the recurrent nerve beneath. With experience, the nerve can be avoided; however, the surgeon must forego the assurance and confidence of working under direct vision.

Guidelines in the Surgical Management of Well-Differentiated Thyroid Cancer

A determination of the amount of thyroid that should be removed in well-differentiated thyroid cancer can not be made soley on the basis of a formula. It is necessary to balance varying and unresolved degrees of benefit that depend on the age of the patient, extent of the tumor, exact histology, and other features of the cancer, against the risk of permanent hypoparathyroidism and possible nerve injury in an individual patient. We increasingly favor total thyroidectomy as we learn of adverse prognostic factors in a particular case.

No other malignancy shows such a pro-

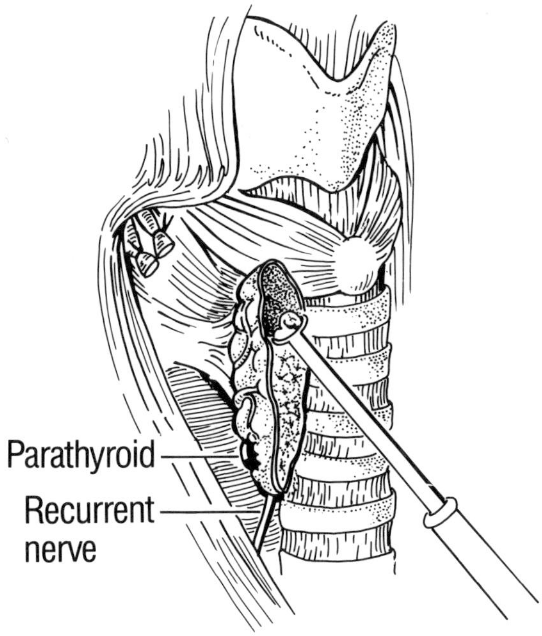

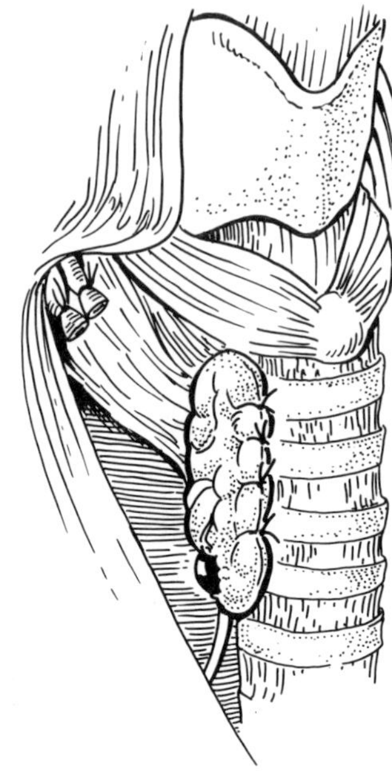

Figures 5.8, 5.9. Near-total thyroidectomy. The superior pole vessels have been divided and ligated. The thyroid lobe is rotated medially and the lower portion of the recurrent nerve is identified. The lower parathyroid gland can be seen in this patient although it is not usually dissected. The recurrent nerve is not visualized at its upper aspect nor is the upper parathyroid gland exposed. These structures are shielded by preserving a posterior rim of thyroid tissue as the thyroid lobe is transected from its lateral to medial side in an oblique direction toward the trachea. Additional thyroid tissue can then be removed from within the capsule with a cautery loop, which also facilitates the inversion of the capsule of the thyroid into the tracheal fascia.

nounced increase in mortality with advancing age as does well-differentiated thyroid cancer. We have never had a death in a patient whose cancer presented below the age of 40; on the contrary, we find that the mortality climbs steeply as the presenting age of the patient advances (Fig. 5.10). In our experience this is the most significant factor in the prognosis of well differentiated thyroid cancer.

Tumors more than 1.5 cm in diameter, particularly those larger than 4 cm, have a more serious outlook in terms of recurrence and mortality for papillary[1] as well as follicular cancer.[33] Penetration beyond the thyroid capsule and into extrathyroidal tissues, without reference to tumor size, is an important prognostic indicator of a decreased rate of survival.[33]

Other factors certainly play a part in the prognosis of well-differentiated thyroid cancer; but in the operating room, we find that the type, size, and extent of the tumor, age of the

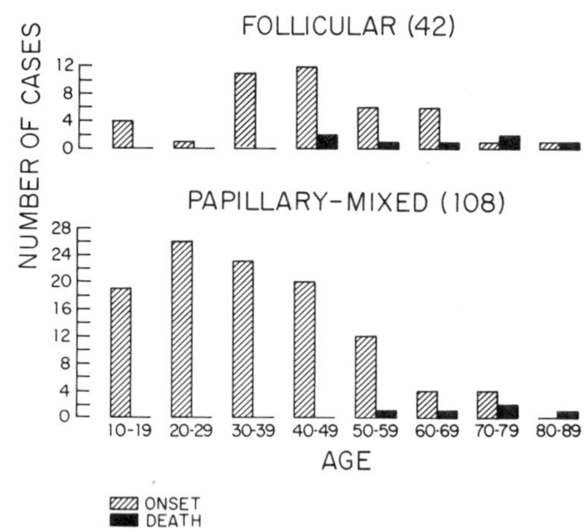

Figure 5.10. Age at onset of disease and at death in 150 patients with well differentiated thyroid cancer followed for more than 15 years. Reprinted, by permission from Friedman EW, Schwartz AE. Well-differentiated thyroid cancer. In: Current Therapy in Endocrinology 1983–1984. Krieger DT, Bardin WD, eds. Toronto: B.C. Decker Publisher.

patient, and history of exposure to radiation, provide the most useful guidance in assessing the outlook of the disease and determining the extent of the procedure. Although a high histologic grade is known to affect survival adversely, it has been difficult to define tumor grade by frozen section examination at our institution.

Our preferences in surgical management are the following:

1. Occult papillary carcinomas (less than 1.5 cm in diameter) confined to one lobe are well managed by lobectomy and excision of the thyroid isthmus in patients below 40 years of age. Subtotal lobectomy (to protect the parathyroid glands) on the opposite side is a valuable addition; if viable parathyroid glands can be preserved on the ipsilateral side, total thyroidectomy is undertaken, particularly in patients over the age of 40.
2. Follicular carcinomas, even those that are small, present a greater threat to the patient. Although we previously managed small lesions by lobectomy, we now prefer to perform a total thyroidectomy. A near-total thyroid lobectomy is an acceptable, and indeed prudent alternative, if it is required to salvage parathyroid glands on the opposite side. Radioactive iodine ablation of any remaining thyroid tissue is routine.
3. Carcinoma in one thyroid lobe and nodularity in the opposite lobe or isthmus requires removal of the contralateral lobe by total thyroidectomy if possible, or near-total lobectomy if necessary to preserve the parathyroid glands.
4. All thyroid malignancies larger than 1.5 cm, and those that penetrate the capsule (even if they are smaller), require more than a lobectomy and excision of the isthmus; a subtotal lobectomy on the opposite side is a reasonable choice if a total lobectomy cannot be safely performed.
5. The presence of carcinoma in one thyroid lobe and a history of radiotherapy to the head and neck mandate a total thyroidectomy if possible, or a near-total lobectomy on the opposite side if the parathyroid glands are endangered.
6. Hürthle cell malignancies, because of their increased aggressiveness, warrant special management. Node metastases are more frequent than in other follicular cancers. Although the incidence of multicentricity within the thyroid gland is the same as in other follicular carcinomas (approximately 15%), Hürthle cell cancer exhibits increased biologic malignancy. These tumors do not trap iodine and do not respond to suppression by thyroid hormone; radioactive iodine is therefore not effective in diagnosing or treating recurrent disease.[34] Total thyroidectomy is the treatment of choice. Neck node metastases are a more significant clinical problem in Hürthle cell cancer; paratracheal and superior mediastinal node dissections are an essential part of the initial surgical procedure. The jugular area is inspected for lymph node metastases at surgery; any that are suspicious are biopsied, but neck dissections are performed only for clinical disease.
7. Dissection of the paratracheal lymph nodes on the side of the lesion and of the superior mediastinal lymph nodes in the neck is a part of our routine management in all thyroid cancers. If lateral jugular lymph nodes are not involved by tumor, no neck dissection is performed. If jugular lymph node metastases are demonstrated, a modified neck dissection is undertaken by extending the original transverse neck incision laterally and toward the mastoid process (Fig. 5.3).
8. Radioactive iodine ablation of residual thyroid tissue following a total or near-total thyroidectomy is a routine part of our management of well-differentiated thyroid cancer. This essentially eliminates any residual thyroid tissue and converts the procedure to a total thyroidectomy. It makes it possible to monitor for recurrence of thyroid cancer by following the level of serum thyroglobulin or by means of radioactive iodine scanning. Should the tumor recur or metastasize, therapy with radioactive iodine becomes a practical treatment modality.

Because medullary thyroid cancer does not concentrate radioactive iodine, it is not useful in the postoperative management of this disease.

Significance and Management of Neck Node Metastases

Neck node metastases are usually present in patients with papillary thyroid cancer, and in most cases are occult. Frazell[35] reported that 61.2% of patients with clinically negative neck nodes had metastatic disease on pathologic examination. Patients under 40 years of age are more likely to present with palpable neck nodes. The significance of these metastases is controversial; many studies show no adverse effect on prognosis.[36,23] Palpable jugular lymph node metastases are rarely life-threatening; if they develop they can usually be readily controlled by neck dissection. Because only 7% to 15% of patients who present with clinically negative necks develop lateral neck metastases,[37] the standard prophylactic radical neck dissections of the past have given way to close observation and modified neck dissection for palpable disease, if it should appear. Often this can be performed with preservation of the sternomastoid muscle, spinal accessory nerve, and jugular vein (Fig. 5.11). Once clinical metastases have developed, limited nodal resections ("berry picking") are inadequate because of frequent recurrence. A block dissection is required.

The frequency of neck node metastases in pure follicular thyroid cancer is considerably lower than in papillary carcinoma: (13.4% is reported by one author[4]) and the same principles of management apply. Hürthle cell cancers, however, have a 50% incidence of neck node involvement and a more aggressive behavior.[5] Prophylactic jugular neck node dissections are not warranted, but the dissection of the paratracheal and superior mediastinal lymph nodes which we advocate in all thyroidectomies for well differentiated thyroid cancer, assumes added importance.

Technique of Neck Dissection

With the realization that lateral neck node disease is not usually life-threatening, and that, if it appears it can be treated at that time, various modifications of neck dissection have been developed. The prophylactic removal of jugular lymph nodes is no longer accepted in most medical centers.

If a neck dissection is to be added to the primary thyroid surgery, the initial transverse incision is made slightly higher than the usual thyroid incision and continued posteriorly and upward toward the mastoid process. This offers a cosmetic incision that provides excellent exposure. If the neck dissection is performed as a secondary procedure, we prefer a curved transverse incision with a short descending limb (Fig. 5.3).

In most neck dissections it is possible to preserve the sternomastoid muscle and spinal accessory nerve; this greatly enhances the cosmetic and functional aspect of the surgery at small cost to the overall effectiveness of the procedure. If there are extensive metastases at the base of the skull or upper jugular lymph nodes, the need to preserve these structures may limit access to this area. In this situation, removing the sternomastoid muscle but preserving the spinal accessory nerve offers excellent exposure, a good cosmetic result, and no loss of shoulder function. If the disease does not infiltrate the jugular vein (and it usually does not), it is possible to preserve this vessel. We do not hesitate to remove the jugular vein if it is involved by, or is adherent to tumor, as its unilateral resection produces no ill effects. We have discarded our previous practice of resecting the contents of the submaxillary triangle because the area is rarely the site of clinical metastases;[35] this eliminates the risk of damage to the mandibular ramus of the facial nerve.

The main sites of metastases to the neck from well-differentiated thyroid carcinoma are the lymph nodes that accompany the internal jugular vein. The primary objective of neck dissection is the excision of these lymph nodes from the level of the subclavian vein upward to the point at which the vessel enters the jugular foramen at the base of the skull. The lymph nodes adjacent to the spinal accessory nerve are less frequently involved but properly should be removed. The nodes overlying the anterior and medial scalene muscles can also be the site of metastases; therefore, this location is cleared of its fatty and nodal tissue, taking care to preserve the phrenic nerve, which

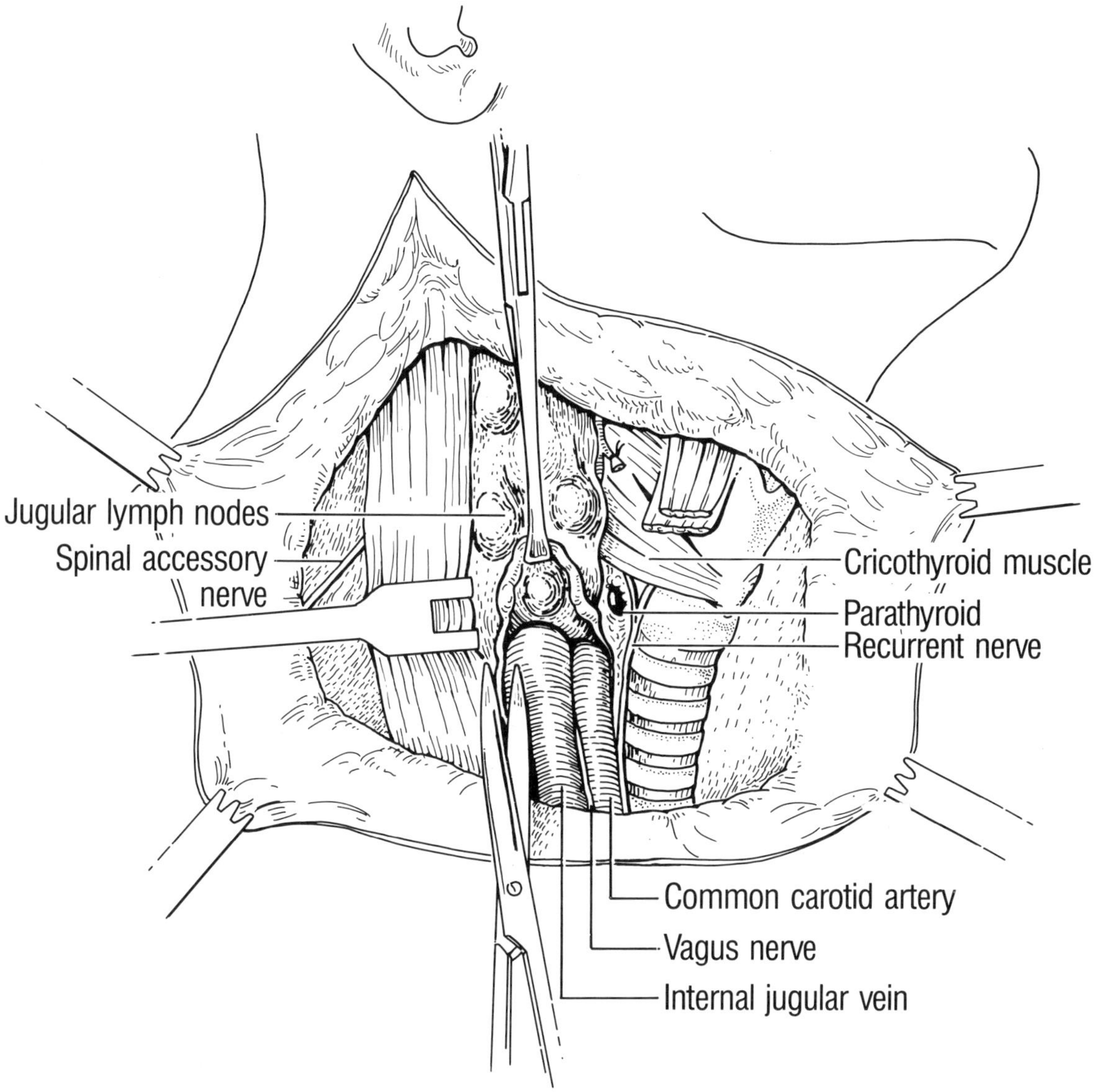

Figure 5.11. Modified neck dissection. The thyroid lobe and strap muscles have been removed. The jugular lymph nodes and accompanying fibrofatty tissue are being dissected from the jugular vein and carotid artery. The vessels will be preserved. The nodal and fibrofatty tissue associated with the spinal accessory nerve are similarly excised, saving the sternomastoid muscle and the spinal accessory nerve.

travels caudad just beneath the fascia of the anterior scalene muscle.

Paratracheal and superior mediastinal lymph nodes are the most frequent sites of metastases in well differentiated thyroid cancer. These are properly dissected as a routine part of the initial thyroidectomy rather than being considered part of a neck dissection.

Midline Recurrence and Dissection

Although death from follicular thyroid cancer is usually the result of metastases to the lungs, bones, or brain, a common terminal event is midline compartment recurrence. This results in the infiltration and obstruction of the airway, or invasion and rupture of the carotid artery. In one study of 56 lethal cases of papillary carcinoma, pulmonary metastases accounted for 37% and local recurrence of midline neck disease accounted for 36% of deaths—an almost equal number.[30] In all thyroid cancer, clearing the midline of thyroid tissue and the resection of the paratracheal and upper mediastinal neck nodes offers an effective means of preventing this catastrophe.

The disastrous consequences of midline recurrence in thyroid cancer make it essential that if the diagnosis is malignant at the time of initial surgery, resection of the thyroid isthmus and the pyramidal lobe and dissection of the paratracheal and superior mediastinal nodes become a routine part of the operative procedure. This is the best opportunity to remove these midline structures and to visualize and preserve the recurrent laryngeal nerves and parathyroid glands. A secondary operation to remove recurrent disease in this area exposes these structure to great risk and is rarely successful. The recurrent laryngeal nerve is exposed and the paratracheal tissues, including the lymph nodes, are dissected free from it under direct vision. The fatty and nodal tissue in the upper mediastinal area is then cleared, leaving a clean trachea. Although the microscopic incidence of lymph node metastases is high, particularly in papillary and medullary cancer, the frequency of local recurrence is minimal in cases in which gross disease does not penetrate into adjacent tissues or into the trachea.

Complications of Surgery

The mortality of thyroid surgery approximates that of general anesthesia. This was reported to be approximately 1.2 per 10,000 in 1982.[38] Since then, the advent of two technologies that are now in general use have produced a quantum leap in safety: the pulse oximeter provides a continuous record of the patient's oxygen saturation; mass spectrometry offers constant monitoring of expired gases (particularly carbon dioxide) ensuring that the airway is intact. The continuing assurance that during the entire procedure the patient's airway and oxygenation is optimal removes the main risk of anesthesia in head and neck surgery.

Postoperative hemorrhage is life threatening. If the closed space in the anterior portion of the neck becomes distended, respiratory obstruction quickly follows. The patient must be closely observed, preferably in a recovery room. Dressings are kept simple so that the underlying wound can be easily examined for bleeding or distention of the neck (Fig 5.12). Drains, even the suction variety, cannot be relied upon to decompress the neck because clotting is frequently associated with bleeding. At the first sign of tracheal compression the wound must immediately be opened at the bedside to relieve the pressure; if possible, the airway must be secured by reintubation or, if necessary, tracheostomy. The patient is returned to the operating room and explored. Occasionally it is discovered that a tie has come off a major vessel; but frequently no definite bleeding site can be identified, and only a generalized ooze is found. This will respond to the removal of all clots, irrigation, and application of a drain or light packing.

Recurrent nerve injury has greatly diminished since dissection and exposure of the nerve has gained acceptance. In experienced hands, nerve injury occurs in less than 2% of patients. If both nerves are divided, stridor may develop and tracheostomy be required. It is our practice and that of most surgeons not to resect the recurrent nerve if it can be grossly dissected free from tumor.

Hypoparathyroidism is not a threat when only one thyroid lobe is resected because only two parathyroid glands are at risk. Nevertheless, every effort is made to preserve the glands, even going to the extent of transplanting those that are nonviable. One never knows if the opposite lobe may require removal in the future. In total thyroidectomy, hypoparathyroidism is the major hazard. The decline in the serum calcium level usually occurs within 24 hours postoperatively. Calcium replacement is usually withheld unless paresthesias or tetany develops, or if the calcium declines to 7.0 mg% or lower. In this event, 1 g of calcium gluconate (10 cm^3 of a 10% solution) is administered

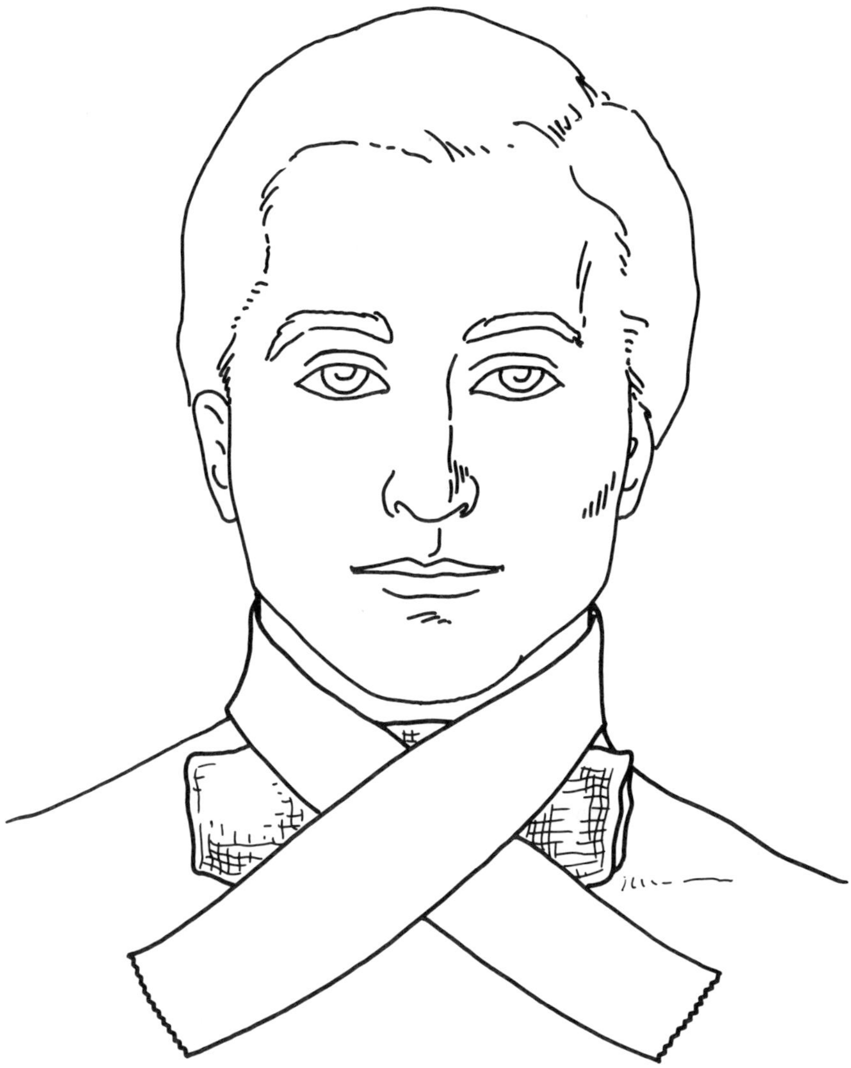

Figure 5.12. The center of a length of 2-in tape is placed on the back of the neck; the ends are brought forward and crossed over the thyroid dressing. Lifting the ends of the tape and removing the dressing provides immediate access to the wound.

intravenously every 6 hours to maintain an adequate serum calcium level while the remaining parathyroid glands recover. Usually the glands reestablish function and the patient can be weaned from medication. If the need for supplemental calcium persists, oral calcium carbonate (which contains the most elemental calcium by weight) and a vitamin D supplement such as dihydrotachysterol or calcitriol is added. The amount is titrated to the need of the patient; the minimum amount necessary to prevent symptoms is prescribed.

Infection can occur after thyroid surgery as it can after any other operation, but it is rare because of the excellent blood supply to the head and neck in general, and to the thyroid gland in particular.

Management of Recurrent Disease

The evaluation of symptoms and physical examination are the most useful tools in patient follow-up. In those patients who have had total thyroidectomies or radioactive ablation of thyroid remnants, monitoring of thyroglobulin levels and sequential uptake scanning can detect recurrence before it becomes evident clinically. Interval chest x-rays are advisable to monitor for pulmonary metastases.

The most commonly accepted adjunct in the management of well-differentiated thyroid cancer is suppression of thyroid stimulating hormone by the administration of thyroid hormone. As a prophylactic measure, and as a therapeutic modality in recurrent disease, we administer levothyroxine to all patients with well differentiated thyroid malignancy. We monitor the levels of thyroid-stimulating hormone (TSH) and try to maintain a level of 0.1 μU/ml or less. However, the usefulness of this classic therapy is challenged by some authors who find no increase in survival from thyroid suppression.[39,40]

Following lobectomy for well-differentiated thyroid cancer confined to one lobe of the thyroid gland, recurrence in the opposite lobe occurs in less than 5% of patients.[11] Surgical resection of the involved lobe is the technique of choice; salvage is achieved in 50% of these patients.[11]

Neck node metastases occur frequently in papillary carcinoma and its variants, less often in pure follicular cancer. Neck dissection is almost always successful in controlling the local disease. Survival has not decreased because therapeutic dissections have essentially replaced those previously performed for prophylaxis. Modifications of the standard neck dissection that spare the accessory nerve, sternomastoid muscle, and even the jugular vein have proved to be cosmetically superior and equally effective in maintaining survival rates.

Recurrent cancer in the local tissues of the neck is a serious threat to life. When well-differentiated thyroid carcinoma penetrates beyond the thyroid capsule into adjacent soft tissues, and when lymph node metastases extend beyond the nodes into adjoining fat and muscle, hopes of controlling the disease locally diminish and the prognosis becomes ominous. These features often characterize the disease in older patients. Wide excisions are indicated, but are often limited by major structures such as vertebrae, the brachial plexus, carotid vessels, and the trachea. The extent to which resection is carried out in these situations must be tempered by judgment. Every effort is justified to maintain the airway; procedures such as tracheal resection, hemilaryngectomy, or even total laryngectomy are justified to accomplish this. Carotid resections with reconstruction may also be considered. Removal of large fungating neck recurrences and resurfacing by myocutaneous flaps may be required for palliation. The limited benefit offered by radiotherapy and chemotherapy in well-differentiated thyroid cancer should not exclude a trial of these modalities. In the late stages of well-differentiated thyroid carcinoma, particularly in older patients, a transition to anaplastic forms sometimes develops. Paradoxically, this may then offer an improved response to chemotherapy and fractionated radiotherapy.

Hematogenous dissemination to lung, bones, or brain is a common feature in pure follicular carcinoma and is the usual cause of death. Although approximately 40% of deaths from papillary thyroid cancer are due to local recurrence, one third succumb to pulmonary metastases,[20] and others die from bone and brain dissemination. This dissemination is often present at the time of initial surgery.

Bone and brain metastases have a very poor prognosis; however, pulmonary lesions are compatible with a prolonged life span. Although cure is rare, many lung lesions of follicular and papillary cancer will concentrate radioactive iodine; palliation may be achieved for many years by this method. Beam radiotherapy is usually more effective than radioactive iodine in the treatment of bone metastases but the result is short-lived.

Surgical Management of Undifferentiated Thyroid Carcinoma

Anaplastic thyroid cancer presents a bleak outlook; it is usually extensive upon presentation and is rarely suitable for curative surgery. In a recent review, the 5-year survival was 3.6% and the median duration of life after diagnosis was 4 months.[41] It is felt by many authors that anaplastic carcinoma develops from transformation of preexisting well-differentiated cancer since they are frequently found together; in one series 89.2% of anaplastic cancers showed areas of differentiated carcinoma[42]—an incentive for the early diagnosis and treatment of well-differentiated carcinoma.

When the disease is extensive, surgery offers no prospect of cure, but considerable palliative benefit can be offered by surgery to clear midline disease and provide an adequate airway; this usually requires a tracheostomy. The recent use of chemotherapy and hyperfractionated radiotherapy offers the hope of restraining the primary lesion so that the patient will not succumb to local recurrence.[43] Sixty percent of anaplastic cancers have hematogenous dissemination.[42]

When the lesion is confined to the thyroid gland, total thyroidectomy with paratracheal and superior mediastinal neck node dissection is warranted to clear the midline structures, prevent local recurrence, and provide a possible cure. The size of the primary tumor appears to be the most important feature determining the prognosis.[41] Once regional lymph nodes are involved, the prospects for a cure are minimal.

Medullary Carcinoma

Medullary thyroid cancer may be a sporadic occurrence or an inherited affliction. All the hereditary forms are preceded by C cell hyperplasia; if the condition can be identified at this stage, cure by total thyroidectomy can be expected. Medullary thyroid cancer and its progenitor, C cell hyperplasia, are unique in that they secrete thyrocalcitonin, a hormone that can be readily identified in the blood stream and accurately quantified. This not only provides an exquisitely sensitive method of diagnosing the tumor in its malignant and premalignant form, but also enables the physician to assay the persistence or recurrence of disease after surgery.

In sporadic medullary thyroid cancer, which constitutes 80% of all cases, the disease is confined to one lobe of the thyroid in four out of five instances.[44] Nevertheless, there are compelling reasons for performing total thyroidectomy. The familial form of the disease, in contrast to the sporadic form, is characterized by multiple foci of malignant cells disseminated throughout both thyroid lobes. It is never possible to know with certainty whether the "sporadic" case is really an index to a kindred with familial disease. Total thyroidectomy resolves this dilemma and also makes it possible to confirm the complete removal of disease by serial sampling of calcitonin levels.

After total thyroidectomy, advisable in all patients with medullary thyroid cancer and C cell hyperplasia, attention must be directed to the most frequent location of early metastatic spread: the central compartment of the neck, including the paratracheal and upper mediastinal lymph nodes. Prophylactic dissection of these lymph nodes from the hyoid bone to the innominate vessels should be routinely performed at the time of initial total thyroidectomy. In patients operated upon at the Mayo Clinic it is reported that extrathyroidal tumor was present in 64% of those with sporadic disease, 60% with MEN 2b, and 26% with MEN 2a.[45] Clark states that 25–75% of patients with medullary thyroid carcinoma have metastases to regional nodes at the time of the original surgical procedure.[46] Involvement of these nodes constitutes a serious threat to life because of the potential for invasion of the trachea and carotid vessels; it is essential that dissection of these lymph nodes be an integral part of the initial surgical management.

Some authors advise routine lateral neck dissection for any palpable medullary thyroid carcinoma.[47] We prefer a more conservative approach; jugular lymph nodes are inspected at the initial exploration. Any that are found to be suspicious are submitted for frozen section. We perform lateral lymph node dissections only for clinical disease, or if sampling of a suspicious lymph node at surgery is reported positive for metastases. If the lymph nodes are minimally involved, we advocate a modified neck dissection sparing the spinal accessory nerve and perhaps the sternomastoid muscle—providing it does not impede an adequate dissection. When lateral neck node disease is substantial, we prefer a standard neck dissection.

References

1. McConahey WM, Hay ID, Woolner LB, VanHeerden JA, Taylor WF. Papillary thyroid cancer treated at the Mayo Clinic, 1946 through 1970: Initial manifestations, pathologic findings, therapy, and outcome. Mayo Clin Proc 1986;61:978–996.
2. Favus MJ, Schneider AB, Stachura ME, Arnold JE. Ryo UY, Pinsky SM, Colman M, Arnold MJ, Frohman LA. Thyroid cancer occurring as a late consequence of head and neck irradiation: Evaluation of 1056 patients. N Eng J Med 1976;294:1019–1025.
3. Schneider AB, Recant W, Pinsky SM, Ryo UY, Bekerman C, Shore-Freedman E. Radiation-induced thyroid carcinoma: clinical course and results of therapy in 296 patients. Ann Intern Med 1986;105:405–412.
4. Young RL, Mazzaferri EL, Rahe AJ, Dorfman SG. Pure follicular thyroid carcinoma; impact of therapy in 214 patients. J Nucl Med 1980;21:733–737.
5. Harness JK, Thompson NW, McLeod MK, Eckhauser FE, LLoyd RV. Follicular carcinoma of the thyroid gland: Trends and treatment. 1984; Surgery 96:972–980.
6. Hawk WA, Hazard JB. The many appearances of papillary carcinoma of the thyroid. Cleve Clin Q 1976;43:207–216.
7. Gosain AK, Clark OH. Hurthle Cell Neoplasms: malignant potential. Arch Surg 1984;119:515–519.
8. Gundry SR, Burney RE, Thompson NW, Lloyd R. Total thyroidectomy for Hurthle cell neoplasm of the thyroid. Arch Surg 1983;118:529–532.
9. Hutter RVP, Frazell EL, Foote FW Jr. Elective radical neck dissection: An assessment of its use in the management of papillary thyroid cancer. Ca 1970;20:87–93.
10. Clark RL, White EC, Russell WO. Total thyroidectomy for cancer of the thyroid: Significance of intraglandular dissemination. Ann Surg 1959;149:858–866.
11. Tollefsen HR, Shah JP, Huvos AG. Papillary carcinoma of the thyroid—recurrence in the thyroid gland after initial surgical treatment. Am J Surg 1972;124:468–472.
12. Attie, JN, Khafif, RA, and Steckler RM. Elective neck dissection in papillary carcinoma of the thyroid. Am. J. Surg 1971;122:464–471.
13. Bloc MA. Surgery of thyroid nodules and malignancy. Current Problems in Surgery. 1983;20:137–203.
14. Hamberger B, Gharib H, Melton LJ III, Goellner JR, Zinsmeister AR. Fine needle aspiration biopsy of thyroid nodules: impact on thyroid practice and cost of care. Am J Med 1982;73:381–384.
15. Schwartz AE, Neiburgs HE, Davies TF, Gilbert PL, Friedman EW. The place of fine needle biopsy in the diagnosis of nodules of the thyroid. Surg Gynec Obstet 1982;155:54–58.
16. Lowhagen T, Granberg P, Lundell G, Skinnari P, Sundblad R, Willems JS. Aspiration biopsy cytology in nodules of the thyroid gland suspected to be malignant. Surg Clin North Am 1979;59:3–18.
17. Evans HL. Follicular neoplasms of the thyroid. A study of 44 cases followed for a minimum of 10 years with emphasis on differential diagnosis. Cancer 1984;54:535–540.
18. Ohman U, Granberg PO, Lindell B. Function of the parathyroid glands after total thyroidectomy. Surg Gynecol Obstet 1978;146:773–778.
19. Ireland AW, Hornbrook, JW Neale FC, Posen S. The crystalline lens in chronic surgical hypoparathyroidism. Arch Intern Med 1968;122:408–411.
20. Smith SA, Hay ID, Goellner JR, Ryan JJ, McConahey WM. Mortality from papillary thyroid carcinoma. A case-control study of 56 lethal cases. Cancer 1988;62:1381–1388.
21. Hubert JP Jr, Kiernan PD, Beahrs OH, McConahey WM, Woolner LB. Occult papillary carcinoma of the thyroid. Arch Surg 1980;115:394–398.
22. Mazzaferri EL, Young RL, Oertel JE, Kemmerer WT, Page CP. Papillary thyroid carcinoma: The Impact of therapy in 576 patients. Medicine 1977;56:171–196.
23. Mazzaferri EL, Young RL. Papillary thyroid carcinoma: A 10-year follow-up report of the impact of therapy in 576 patients. Am J Med 1981;70:511–518.
24. Samaan NA, Schultz PN, Haynie TP and Ordonez NG. Pulmonanary metastasis of differentiated thyroid carcinoma: Treatment results in 101 patients. J Clin Endocrinol Metab 1985;60:376–380.
25. Massin JP, Savoie JC, Garnier H, Guiraudon G, Leger FA, Bacourt F. Pulmonary metastases in differentiated thyroid carcinoma: Study of 58 cases with implication for the primary tumor treatment. Cancer 1984;53:982–992.
26. Starnes HF, Brooks DC, Pinkus GS, Brooks JR. Surgery for thyroid carcinoma. Cancer 1985;55:1376–1381.
27. Cohn KH, Backdahl M, Forsslund G, Auer G, Zetterberg A, Lundell G, Granberg P, Lowhagen T, Willems J, Cady B. Biologic considerations and operative strategy in papillary thyroid carcinoma: Arguments against the routine performance of total thyroidectomy. Surgery 1984;96:957–970.
28. Crile G Jr, Pontius KI, Hawk WA. Factors influencing the survival of patients with follicular carcinoma of the thyroid gland. Surg Gynecol Obstet 1985;160:409–413.
29. Tollefsen HR, Shah JP, Huvos AG. Follicular carcinoma of the thyroid. Am J Surg 1973;126:523–528.
30. Samaan NA, Maheshwari YK, Nader S, Hill CS Jr, Schultz PN, Haynie TP, Hickey RC, Clark RL, Goepfert H, Ibanez ML, Litton CE. Impact of therapy for differentiated carcinoma of the thyroid: An analysis of

706 cases. J Clin Endocrinol Metab 1983;56:1131–1138.
31. Jacobs JK, Aland JW, Ballinger JF. Total Thyroidectomy. Ann Surg 1983;197:542–548.
32. Schwartz AE, Friedman EW. Preservation of the parathyroid glands in total thyroidectomy. Surg Gynecol Obstet 1987;165:327–332.
33. Simpson WJ, McKinney SE, Carruthers JS, Gospodarowicz MK, Sutcliffe SB, Panzarella T. Papillary and follicular thyroid cancer. Prognostic factors in 1,578 patients. 1987;Am J Surg 83:479–488.
34. Gundry SR, Burney RE, Thompson NW, LLoyd R. Total thyroidectomy for Hurthle cell neoplasm of the thyroid. Arch Surg 1983;118:529–32.
35. Frazell EL, and Foote FW. Papillary thyroid carcinoma: pathologic findings in cases with and without clinical evidence of cervical node involvement. Cancer 1955;8:1164–1166.
36. Cady B, Sedgwick CE, Meissner WA, Bookwalter JR, Romagosa V, Werber J. Changing clinical, pathologic, therapeutic and survival patterns in differentiated thyroid carcinoma. Ann Surg 1976;184:541–553.
37. Block MA. Management of carcinoma of the thyroid. Ann Surg 1977;185:133–144.
38. Zeitlin GL. Possible decrease in mortality associated with anaesthesia. A comparison of two time periods in Massachusetts, USA. Closed Claims Study Committee. Anaesthesia 1989;44:432–433.
39. Cady B, Cohn K, Rossi RL, Sedgwick CE, Meissner WA, Werber J, Gelman RS. The effect of thyroid hormone administration upon survival in patients with differentiated thyroid carcinoma. Surgery 1983;94:978–983.
40. Clark RL. Discussion (pp. 417–419) of Harness JK, Thompson NW, Sisson JC and Beierwaltes W.H. Differentiated thyroid carcinomas. Arch Surg 1974;108:410–419.
41. Nel JC, VanHeerden JA, Goellner JR, Gharib H, McConahey WM, Taylor WF, and Grant CS. Anaplastic carcimona of the thyroid: A clinicopathologic study of 82 cases. Mayo Clin Proc 1985;60:51–58.
42. Aldinger KA, Samaan NA, Ibanez M, and Hill CS Jr. Anaplastic carcinoma of the thyroid. A review of 84 cases of spindle and giant cell carcimona of the thyroid. Cancer 1978;41:2267–2275.
43. Kim JH, Leeper RD. Treatment of anaplastic giant and spindle cell carcinoma of the thyroid gland with combination Adriamycin and radiation therapy: a new approach. Cancer 1983;52:954–957.
44. Sizemore GW. Medullary carcinoma of the thyroid gland and the multiple endocrine neoplasia type 2 syndrome. In: Spittell JA Jr, ed. Clinical Medicine, vol 8. Philadelphia: Harper & Row; 1982.
45. Sizemore, GW. Medullary carcinoma of the thyroid. Thyroid Today 1982;5:1–6.
46. Clark OH. Medullary thyroid carcinoma. In: Clark OH, Endocrine Surgery of the Thyroid and Parathyroid Glands. St. Louis: Mosby; 1985:98.
47. Block MA. Surgical treatment of medullary carcinoma of the thyroid. Otolaryngol Clin North Am 1990; 23(3):453–473.

6

Thyroglobulin

ANDREW J. WERNER

Structure and Synthesis

Thyroglobulin, a large glycoprotein molecule measuring 660,000 Kd[1,2] is a product unique to the follicular cells of the thyroid gland. Because of its easy accessibility, it has been the subject of numerous studies since its discovery in 1899. Thyroglobulin functions as the location of thyroid hormone synthesis and storage. Thyroglobulin is formed in the endoplasmic reticulum. Four iodoproteins with sedimentation coefficients of 12S, 17S, 19S, and 27S have been identified in vitro.[3] The 19S variety is the "classic thyroglobulin." Two 12S chains of approximately 330,000 Kd each initially are linked by disulfide bonds; a carbohydrate moiety joins later at the cell apex, forming noniodinated 17S thyroglobulin. As the tyrosyl residues are iodinated, mature 19S classic, thyroglobulin is produced. The 27S protein probably represents two highly iodinated 19S fractions tightly linked together by disulfide bonds.[4]

The oligosaccharide portion of the molecule, roughly 10% by weight, contains sialic acid, galactose, fucose, mannose, *N*-acetylglucosamine and *N*-acetylgalactosamine.[5] Sulfate is also part of the carbohydrate moiety; recently it has been noted that there is differential incorporation of sulfate into the thyroglobulin produced by human thyroid neoplasms.[6] It has been suggested that the structural differences in the thyroglobulin of thyroid cancer and Graves' disease patients may lead to altered immunoreactivity.[7]

The thyroglobulin molecule is stable in the pH range of 5 to 11. In a high alkaline environment, the structure unfolds. causing alteration in iodination. In vitro, low temperature (2°C) causes the formation of 14S and 17S segments. At 25°C, the prevalent type observed is the 19S molecule.[8–13] Of all the thyroid moieties found in thyroglobulin, only 10 to 15% are iodinated; that is, capable of hormone production.[14,15] In vitro, in the presence of excess iodine, 30% of the tyrosyl residues remain deiodinated.[16] Of the 110 tyrosyl residues within a thyroglobulin molecule, only four to eight molecules of thyroid hormone will be formed. Of these, approximately 75% will be thyroxine (T_4) and 25% triiodothyronine (T_3), depending upon the availability of iodine.[17]

Thyroid Hormone Formation

After trapping of iodide, iodination takes place at the apex of the follicular cell (Fig. 6.1). This reaction requires the presence of the enzyme peroxidase, the formation of which is stimulated by thyrotropin (TSH). Monoiodotyrosine (MIT) and diiodotyrosine (DIT) are formed by adding an active iodine to the peptidyl tyrosine molecule at the 3 and 5 positions respectively. DIT is formed preferentially in iodide excess states, while MIT predominates with iodide deprivation. This effect also occurs in the synthesis of 3,5,3′,5′ tetraiodothyronine (thyroxine, T_4) and 3,5,3′ triiodothyronine (T_3) by the coupling reaction. In these cases, two units of DIT, or one of DIT and MIT are each

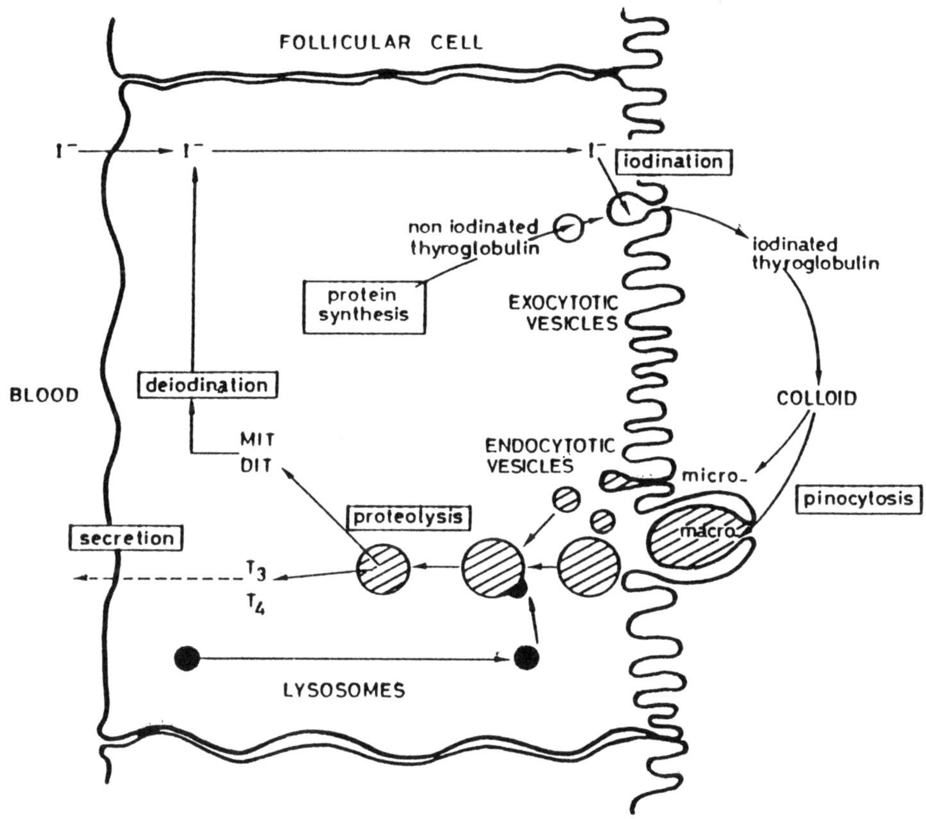

Figure 6.1. Diagrammatic scheme of thyroid hormone secretion.

united to form the active hormones. T_4 and thyroglobulin synthesis, like the coupling reaction itself, cannot take place without the peroxidase enzyme and peroxide, both under the positive influence of TSH.[18]

The newly formed thyroglobulin containing T_4, T_3, MIT, DIT, and dehydroalanine residues, is expelled by exocytosis into the space between the follicular cells and is stored in the form of colloid. Under TSH stimulation, endocytosis of the colloid occurs. Thyroglobulin-containing iodoproteins reenter the cell as droplets that are taken up by lysosomes, forming phagosomes. Near the base of the cell, several enzymes break down the thyroglobulin and liberate T_3 and T_4, which enter the circulation. Some MIT, DIT, and thyroglobulin are also released and can be measured in the blood. While T_3 and reverse T_3 can be found in thyroglobulin, 80% of the former and nearly 100% of the latter are produced by the peripheral monodeiodination of T_4 (Fig. 6.2). The extreme efficiency of the thyroid gland in utilizing iodide is dependent upon the intrathyroidal dehalogenase enzymes that are present in follicular cells. After the enzymatic breakdown of thyroglobulin, these insure the liberation of iodine from iodotyrosines to be reused in new hormone synthesis.

Genetic Abnormalities in the Formation of Thyroglobulin

Due to the complexity of the thyroglobulin molecule, which predisposes to the formation of abnormal protein sequences, it has long been postulated that defects in its synthesis may have a genetic basis.[19] Depending upon the degree of the defect, hypothyroidism or goiter, or both may occur. Theoretically, abnormalities in peroxidase and in the coupling reaction belong to this group of thyroid

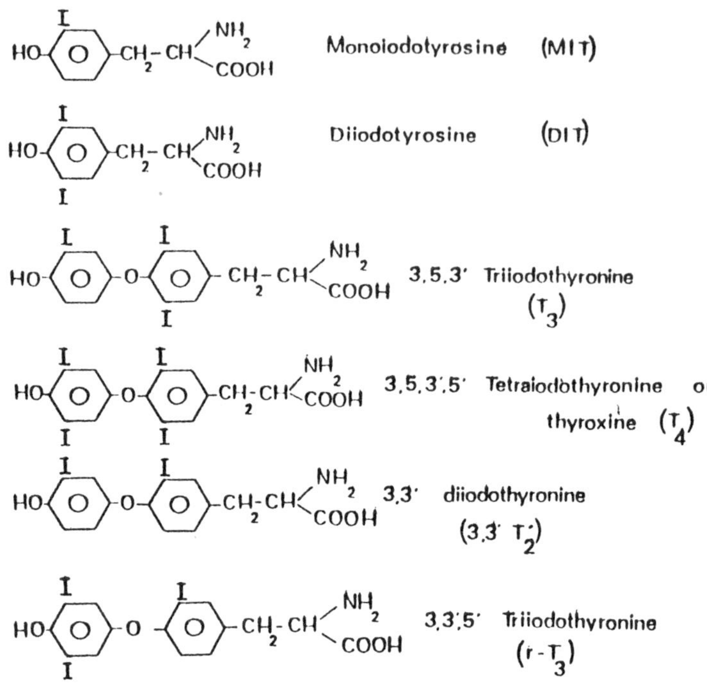

Figure 6.2. The chemical structures of the principal thyroid hormones and related compounds.

dyshormonogenesis.[20,21] Families with thyroglobulin synthesis defects have been identified.[22–24] The clinical characteristics ascribed to these defects are mental retardation and goiter associated with euthyroidism or hypothyroidism. Iodoproteins with a sedimentation constant of 4S, or abnormal 19S subunits, were found in these cases.[24] At least five different types of defects in thyroglobulin formation have been noted.[25–27] No increase in the incidence of thyroid malignancies was found in these kindreds. In rare cases. thyroglobulin is not produced at all.[28] In such patients, iodine is bound to albumin, forming iodoalbumin, which can be found in the gland and in the circulation. MIT and DIT are detected in the blood and urine of these patients. Antithyroglobulin antibodies are not produced.[29]

Physiology

It has been postulated, mostly on the basis of animal studies, that thyroglobulin enters the circulation from intrathyroidal and perithyroidal lymphatic channels.[30] No diurnal variations in thyroglobulin levels have been found. Thyroglobulin's mean half-life is 29.6 ± 2.8 hours.[31] The site of thyroglobulin disposal is in the liver. TRH and TSH stimulation cause temporary elevation in thyroglobulin levels. Thyroglobulin levels may also be elevated after percutaneous needle biopsy, though not after vigorous palpation of the gland.[32]

Thyroglobulin levels are elevated during pregnancy, possibly from an effect of human chorionic gonadotropin (HCG).[33] In the newborn, the formation of thyroglobulin is dependent upon the availability of iodine[34]; it is assumed that thyroglobulin does not cross the placenta.[35,36] In the neonate, levels remain elevated for 2 to 3 months and return to the normal range by the end of the first year.[37] In women, thyroglobulin undergoes age-related changes.[38] It is generally agreed that females have somewhat higher thyroglobulin levels than males. Estrogens cause an elevation of thyroglobulin. There is a slight increase in thyroglobulin toward the second half of the menstrual cycle. In addition, it has been found that smokers have an elevated level of thyroglobulin,[39] and that fasting causes a decrease in normal subjects as an adaptive mechanism.[40]

In pathologic states such as Graves' disease, Hashimoto's thyroiditis, thyroid adenomas, well-differentiated thyroid carcinomas, and multinodular goiter; thyroglobulin levels may be elevated.[41] In subacute thyroiditis, especially in its early stages, thyroglobulin levels can be high. After treatment with radioactive iodine, thyroglobulin is liberated and levels in the blood may be quite elevated.[42]

Thyroglobulin may also be found in the saliva[43,44] pleural fluid of patients with metastatic carcinoma, and may be of diagnostic importance.[45] In such cases, thyroglobulin levels can be markedly elevated, that is, over 1000 ng/ml.[46] By showing an increased thyroglobulin level, one study purported to show that measuring thyroglobulin in patients with childhood neck radiation who later developed thyroid nodules was of prognostic value.[46,47] High thyroglobulin levels, over 40 ng/ml, were found in subjects with metastatic disease with unknown primary sites that later proved to be of thyroid origin.[48,49]

Measurement of Thyroglobulin

The measurement of circulating thyroglobulin in the blood by radioimmunoassay dates back to the late 1960s.[30] Prior to this, other relatively inaccurate methods such as hemagglutination inhibition and electrophoretic immunoretention were used.[50,51] The normal range is quite variable, even among the best laboratories, but in general is between 0 to 30 ng/ml. As many as 6% to 26% of normal controls revealed no detectable thyroglobulin using these assays.[52,53] This phenomenon may be explained either by assay insensitivity or by molecular variability of the intact native molecule.[7] In patients where antithyroglobulin antibodies are present, the test may be invalid. Antithyroglobulin antibody titers, must therefore be determined prior to thyroglobulin measurements in order to assure reliability.

Most radioimmunoassays used today employ a double antibody technique. Newer assays with immunoradiometry (IRMA), or immunoenzymometry (IEMA) are much more sensitive, detecting levels as low as 1 to 2 ng/ml.[54] These assays may be less affected by antithyroglobulin antibody.[55] Some authorities believe that regardless of the presence of circulating antithyroglobulin antibodies, thyroglobulin is of value in detecting recurrent thyroid carcinoma[53] (Fig. 6.3). There is no good correlation between the titer of antithyroglobulin antibodies and its interference with thyroglobulin assay.[54] Thyroglobulin antibodies have been found in 8% to 22% of patients following surgery for differentiated thyroid carcinoma.[56] Monoclonal antibodies against thyroglobulin that differentiate between the products of normal or neoplastic follicular cells may be the definitive diagnostic tool of the future.[57]

Clinical studies utilizing thyroglobulin radioimmunoassay have firmly established its importance in the postsurgical management of thyroid carcinoma. Controversy still exists, however, regarding the absolute sensitivity of thyroglobulin levels as compared with various imaging techniques and as to the proper protocol to employ in order to maximize sensitivity.

In 1975, Van Herle et al. reported that elevated serum thyroglobulin was a useful marker for metastatic thyroid carcinoma.[58] Subsequently, the diagnostic sensitivity of elevated thyroglobulin was found to compare favorably with that of ^{131}I body scanning, even under suppression with thyroxine.[59] In a comparison of thyroglobulin levels and ^{131}I body scans in patients with well-differentiated thyroid carcinoma, thyroglobulin measurements were found to have a specificity of 95% for the dection of recurrence in patients with total thyroidectomy, whereas in patients with subtotal thyroidectomy, 75% sensitivity and 57% specificity were noted.[54]

Collacio et al.[60] found concordance between 2 mCi ^{131}I thyroid scans and thyroglobulin levels in 28 patients with recurrent carcinoma (Table 6.1). Six patients had positive thyroglobulins with negative scans, while three patients had negative thyroglobulins and positive scans. Of the 37 patients with elevated thyroglobulin levels when they were not receiving thyroid

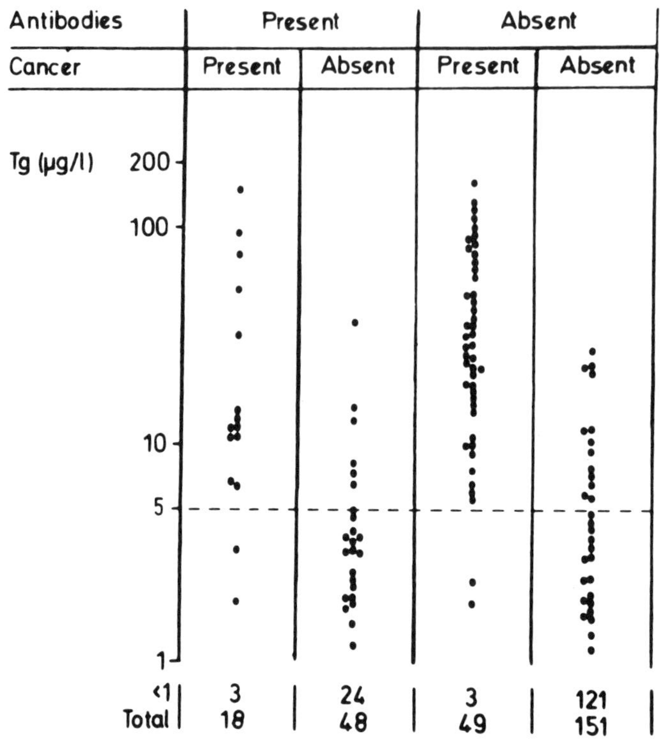

Figure 6.3. Thyroglobulin in patients with or without cancer in the presence or absence of antithyroglobulin antibodies. Reprinted, by permission from Black et al. 1981(53).

Table 6.1. Patients with recurrent thyroid cancer: Total body scand (TBS) versus serum thyroglobulin (Tg)

Positive TBC Positive Tg*	Negative TBS† Positive Tg	Positive TBS Negative Tg	Negative TBS Negative Tg
28	6	3	0

* Serum thyroglobulin ≥ 15 ng/ml.
† No uptake at 48 hours after 2 mCu ^{131}I.
Reprinted, by permission, from Colacchio, TA et al. 1982(60).

replacement, 5 had levels that became normal when thyroxine suppression was resumed (Table 6.2). Collacio et al. recommend that an initial scan and thyroglobulin level be done while the patient is off medication. If both tests are negative, then thyroglobulin on suppression is felt to be adequate follow-up, although periodic discontinuation of suppression and remeasurement was suggested for "young patients at high risk of recurrence."

Pacini[61] noted an incidence of 11/55 "false

Table 6.2. Serum thyroglobulin levels in patients with documented recurrence

On thyroid replacement		Off thyroid replacement*	
Undetectable	8 pts	Undetectable	3 pts
≥15 ng/ml	29 pts	≥15 ng/ml	34 pts†

* TSH equals 26 to 122 μU/ml.
† Twenty-four of these patients had a two- to tenfold increase in Tg.
Reprinted, by permission, from Colacchio, TA et al. 1982(60).

Figure 6.4. Serum hTg concentrations (log scale) and results of scanning in patients with differentiated thyroid carcinoma after surgical thyroidectomy and ^{131}I ablation of residue thyroid issue. In the first column (●) indicates patients with no metastatic thyroid tissue, (○) indicates patients with detectable non-functioning metastases. For each group the mean hTg concentration is indicated (—— for solid circles. ═══ for open circles). The broken horizontal line represents the upper limit of the normal range. ND = not detectable. Reprinted, by permission, from Pacini F, Pinchera A, Giani C, et al. 1980(61).

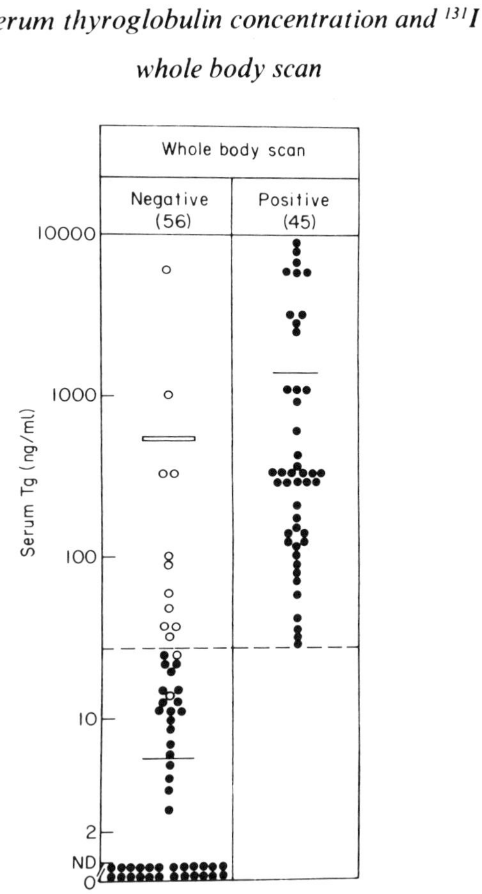

negative" scans of patients with demonstrable thyroglobulin (Fig. 6.4), while Müller-Gärtner[62] found normal thyroglobulin levels in 7 of 321 patients off suppression who were noted to have metastases on high resolution sonography. These patients tended to have very small lesions without palpable adenopathy. Of 30 patients with "certified" metastases and elevated thyroglobulin levels while they were off suppressive therapy, 9 of 22 suppressed their thyroglobulin levels into the normal range when thyroxine was resumed. These patients had papillary carcinoma; subjects with follicular carcinoma did not exhibit the phenomenon of suppression of thyroglobulin levels while they were on thyroxine.

It has been suggested that thyroglobulin levels correlate with the extent of metastases, the bulk of tissue, or the number of functioning thyroglobulin-producing cells. Schneider et al.[63] found no correlation between thyroglobulin level and quantitative 48-hour neck uptake of ^{131}I (Fig. 6.5). Thyroglobulin levels above ten were found in 54 patients, 22 with definite metastases with strongly positive neck scans. Eight patients had proven metastases, negative scans, and thyroglobulin levels greater than 10 ng/ml, suggesting that thyroglobulin was a more sensitive test than scanning (Table 6.3). In contrast, Grant et al.[64] noted that thyroglobulin levels were undetectable in 17 patients with uptake on scan, either on or off thyroxine. Twelve of the metastases were in the thyroid bed. Five further patients had positive scans, and negative thyroglobulin on suppression, but detectable levels of thyroglobulin when thyroxine was withdrawn. In 7 patients, testing positive for thyroglobulin preceded testing positive on a thyroid scan (Table 6.4).

In Schneider's 1981 study, thyroglobulin

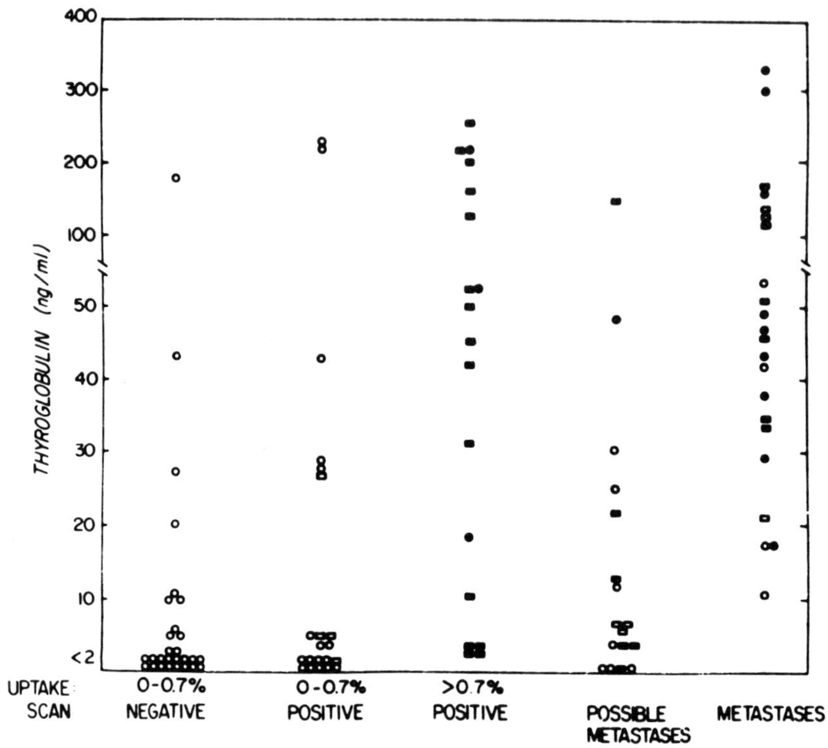

Figure 6.5. Serum TG measurements obtained simultaneously with thyroid scans and 48-h cervical uptake measurements in 44 patients with thyroid cancer. The scans were classified as described in *Materials and Methods*, and the positive category (thyroid remnant) was subdivided according to the 48-h cervical uptake. There were 106 sets of measurements (with antithyroglobulin antibody-positive subjects excluded) divided into the following categories: 28 negative, 21 positive up to 0.7% retention, 18 positive with more than 0.7% retention, 17 possible metastases, and 22 metastases. ○ and ●, Values obtained after previous ^{131}I therapy. □ and ■, Values obtained before any ^{131}I therapy. ● and ■, A 48-h uptake of more than 0.7%. Reprinted, by permission, from Schneider, AB et al. 1981(63). Copyright by The Endocrine Society, 1981.

Figure 6.6. Sequential changes in serum TSH and TG concentrations after cessation of T_3 therapy. T_3 therapy was stopped on day 0. Radioiodine scans were performed on the days indicated by the *vertical arrows*. The 48-h cervical uptakes (or pulmonary uptake in panel 3 are shown *above the arrows*. The patients in panels 5 and 6 resumed T_1 therapy immediately after and 4 days after their scans, respectively. The scans showed cervical metastases for patients 1, 2, and 4, pulmonary metastases for patient 3, residual thyroid tissue for patient 5, and no areas of isotope accumulation for patient 6. All patients had had a total thyroidectomy, except patient 5, who had a lobectomy. Patients 3–6 also who had a lobectomy. Patients 3–6 also had prior ^{131}I therapy (58 to >800 mCi). Reprinted, by permission, from Schneider, AB et al. 1981 (63). Copyright by The Endocrine Society, 1981.

Table 6.3. Patients with negative or weakly positive scans and serum TG levels above 10 ng/ml

TG (ng/ml)[a]	^{131}I therapy (mCi)[b]	Comment
43	1100	Previous pulmonary metastases
172, 28	75	Intraglandular invasive follicular tumor; later positive scan
224, 214	155	Incompletely removed tumor invading trachea; older patient
27, 43	710	Incompletely removed tumor surrounding recurrent laryngeal nerve
20	220	Tumor with extensive intraglandular and lymphatic spread
29	57	
10.4	295	Invasive tumor with bilateral lymph node involvement
27	None	

[a]Measured at least 2 weeks after stopping T_3 therapy.
[b]Total of administered ^{131}I doses.
Reprinted, by permission, from Schneider, AB et al. 1981(63). Copyright by The Endocrine Society, 1981.

Table 6.4. Comparison of serum Tg and ^{131}I radioiodine scans

	Serum thyroglobulin	
	<5 μg/l	≥5 μg/l
^{131}I scan	167	26
−ve	A 17	B 10
+ve		
A:		
Lung metastases	2	
Mediastinal metastases	3	
Thyroid bed	12	
B:		
Lung metastases	3	
Thyroid bed*	7	

*There had biopsy proof of local recurrence (esophagus, trachea, lymph nodes).
Reprinted, by permission, from Grant, S et al. 1984(64).

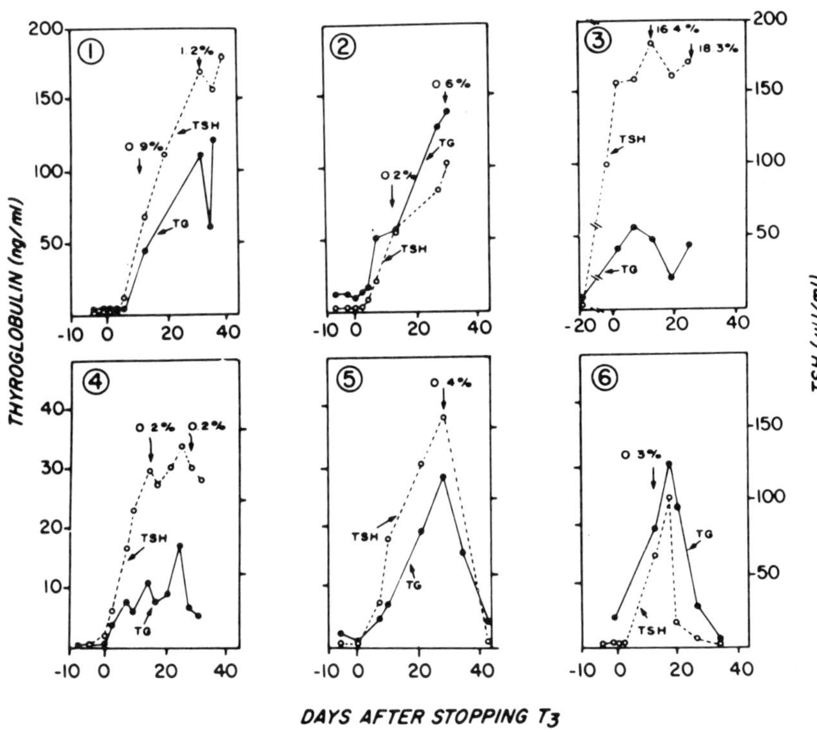

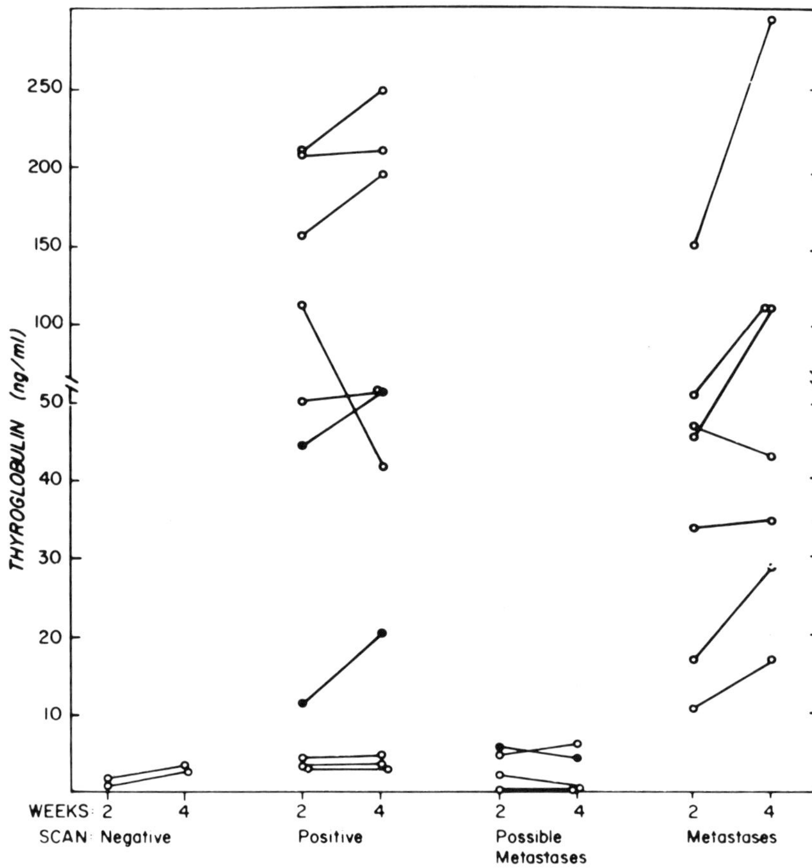

Figure 6.7. Comparison of serum TG measured at 2 and 4 weeks after stopping T_3 ●. Subjects with anti-thyroglobulin antibody levels, through this precluded accurate measurement of TG, the antibody levels did not change appreciably between 2 and 4 weeks. Positive indier thyroid remnant. The four scans showing possible metastases I uptake above the thyroid bed in the midline. Reprinted, by permission, from Schneider, AB et al, 1981(63). Copyright by The Endocrine Society, 1981.

levels were greater than 10 in 5 of 28 patients with negative scans, but less than 2 in 13 of 32 patients with positive scans. While on suppression, 14 of 15 patients had thyroglobulin levels of less than 10. However, after two weeks off triiodothyronine, elevated thyroglobulin levels occurred in all 5 patients with obvious metastases (Fig. 6.6). Four subjects with residual uptake and 2 of 6 patients with no uptake continued to have normal thyroglobulin levels. No significant difference in thyroglobulin levels occurred between the second two and fourth weeks off triiodothyronine (Fig. 6.7). They advised that thyroglobulin on replacement is not a sensitive test, and that the combination of ^{131}I scan and thyroglobulin measurement is "superior to either one alone."

Black et al.[65] followed-up 416 patients for 7 years after thyroidectomy and ^{131}I ablation on thyroid suppression. Initially, 295 patients had thyroglobulin levels of less than 5; of these, only 1.7% revealed evidence of disease after 7 years. Of 121 patients with an initial thyroglobulin greater than five, 19 had no sign of disease at the onset of the study; however, 8 of these 19 later developed an overt recurrence. They noted that the concordance of thyroglobulin levels in the presence of disease improved if they were measured while the patient was on thyroid suppression, which presumably suppressed physiologic but not pathologic thyroglobulin production (Table 6.5).

Pacini et al.[66] reported that 17 patients had elevated thyroglobulin levels and negative 5

Table 6.5. Serum thyroglobulin analysis

		Initial evaluation		Latest evaluation	
		Cancer absent	Cancer present	Cancer absent	Cancer present
Serum Tg					
<5μg/l	Patients (*n*)	288	7	298	7
	%	97.6	2.4	97.7	2.3
>5μg/l	Patients (*n*)	19	102	10	101
	%	15.7	84.3	9.0	91.0
Concordance		93.8%		95.9%	

Reprinted, by permission from Black, EG et al. 1987(65).

Table 6.6. Metastatic Disease Discovered after Therapeutic I^{131}

	First study				Second study*			
Patient no.	Tg ng/ml	5 mCi WBS	^{131}I mCi	Postdose WBS	Tg ng/ml	5 mCi WBS	^{131}I mCi	Postdose WBS
1	15	Neg	80	Residue		Neg		
2	21	Neg	100	Negative	26	Neg		
3	46	Neg	100	Lung Mediastinal nodes	50 (22)†	Lung±	100	Lung
4	153	Neg	90	Lung	84	Neg	100	Negative
5	443	Neg	127	Lung	104 (35)	Neg	100	Negative
6	78	Neg	75	Lung Mediastinal nodes				
7	412	Neg	100	Lung + nodes				
8	53	Neg	100	Residue	51	Neg		
9	61	Neg	111	Mediastinal nodes	48 (28)	Neg		
10	976	Neg	137	Residue, lung, nodes	425	Neg		
11	240	Neg	127	Residue Mediastinal nodes	390	Residue	100	Lung Mediastinal nodes
12	131	Neg	92	Residue Mediastinal nodes	125	Mediastinal nodes	120	Mediastinal nodes
13	22	Neg	95	Residue Mediastinal nodes				
14	60	Neg	127	Residue	52	Neg		
15	51	Neg	140	Lung				
16	120	Neg	80	Lung	80 (10)	Neg	134	Lung
17	72	Neg	112	Lung				

*Second study was performed 8–12 mo after the first study and treatment.
†(n): Number in parenthesis refers to the result of serum Tg for patients who had a third study, 8–12 mo after the second study.
Reprinted, by permission, from Pacini, F et al. 1987(66). Copyright by the Society of Nuclear Medicine, 1987.

mCi ^{131}I scans; after giving 100 mCi ^{131}I therapy doses, uptake was demonstrated in neck residual (7 patients), lung, (9 patients), and mediastinal nodes (8 patients), again illustrating the sensitivity of the thyroglobulin assay (Table 6.6).

It has been suggested that, in the presence of residual normal thyroid, the measurement of thyroglobulin does not discriminate between patients with and without metastatic disease.[67] Recently however, Harvey et al.[68] noted that even in the presence of a residual lobe, a thy-

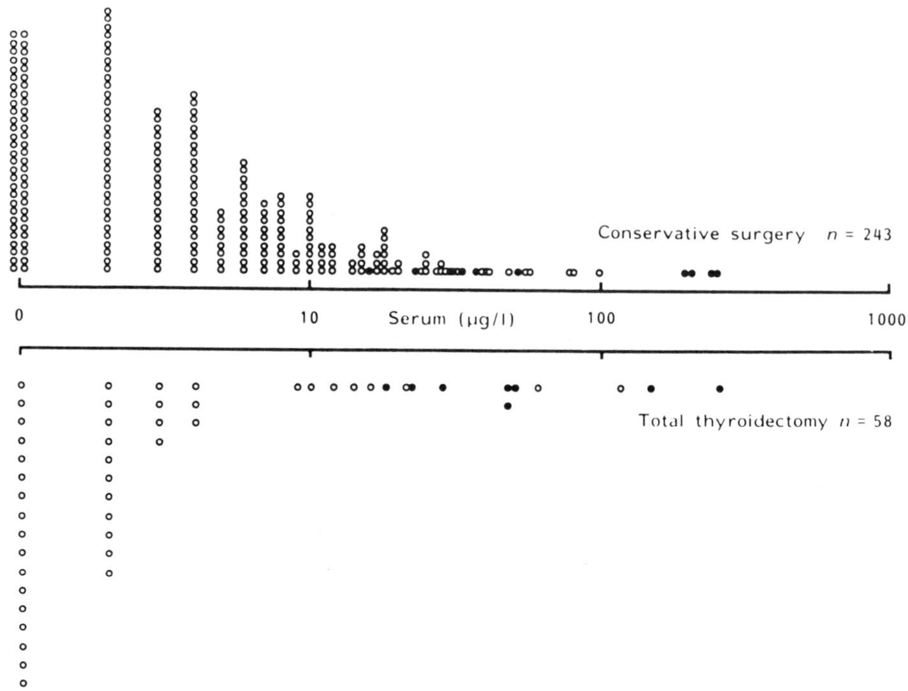

Figure 6.8. Distribution of serum thyroglobulin in all samples according to type of surgery. ● presence and ○ absence of known recurred tumour. Reprinted, by permission, from Harvey, RD et al. 1990(68).

roglobulin level of less than 10 while on suppression "confirms the absence of otherwise known tumor in 100% of cases,"[68] whereas a thyroglobulin level of greater than 10 was diagnostic of recurrence in 92% of 243 samples from 84 patients. In patients without known recurrence, the median serum thyroglobulin level was higher in samples from patients treated by lobectomy compared with those treated with total thyroidectomy; however the overall pattern of distribution was similar since there were unexplained high levels in both groups (Fig. 6.8). Forty-seven samples yielded thyroglobulin levels greater than 10 ng/ml with no known recurrence resulting in a "false positive" rate of 66% in lobectomized patients compared with a false positive rate of 46% for patients who underwent total thyroidectomy. The author states that in the presence of adequate suppression of TSH, an apparently isolated instance of an elevated thyroglobulin level, especially a rising titer, warrants discontinuation of suppression, ^{131}I ablation of the thyroid remnant, and subsequent rescanning to search for occult metastases. In light of the preference of some surgeons to perform conservative therapy (see Chapter 5), this approach appears to be reasonable.

Using sensitive thyroglobulin assays, therefore, may help to formulate a rational approach to the management of thyroid cancer. If a total thyroidectomy or partial thyroidectomy and ^{131}I ablation is performed, a thyroglobulin level and an ^{131}I scan (2 or 5 mCi) while the patient is off medication can be done postoperatively. If both of these are negative then, following Collaccio's suggestion, it seems reasonable to periodically reassess thyroglobulin levels while the patient is on thyroxine suppression. If the level is above ten, and particularly if it is rising, a repeat scan should be done. In the absence of a rising thyroglobulin level, many still recommend rescanning with ^{131}I at an appropriate interval, perhaps every five years, in young patients with low risk. If the thyroglobulin level is elevated and no focus can be found on scan, then high dose ^{131}I may be given with either 100 to 150 mCi of ^{131}I for both scanning and therapeutic purposes.

If a lobectomy and isthmectomy is selected, then thyroxine suppression can be continued; if the thyroglobulin level is greater than 10 and/ or rising, radioiodine ablation and subsequent reevaluation are advised.

References

1. Heidelberger M, Pedersen KO. The molecular weight and isoelectric point of thyroglobulin, J Gen Physiol 1935;19:95–108.
2. Salvatore G, Edelhoch H. Chemistry and biosynthesis of iodoproteins. In: Li CH, ed. Hormonal Proteins and Peptides. vol. 1. New York: Academic Press; 1973:201–241.
3. Salvatore G, Sena L, Viscidi E, Salvatore M. The thyroid iodoproteins, 12S, 19S, 27S in various animal species and their physiological significance. In: Cassano C, Andreoli M, eds. Current Topics in Thyroid Research. New York: Academic Press; 1965:193.
4. Vecchio G, Edelhoch H, Robbino J, Weathers B. Studies on the structure of 27S thyroid iodoproteins. Biochemistry 1966;5:2617.
5. Arima T, Spiro MJ, Spiro RG. Studies on the carbohydrate units. Evaluation of their microheterogeneity in the human and calf proteins. J Biol Chem 1972; 247:1825–1835.
6. Schneider AB, Dudlak D. Differential incorporation of sulfate into the chondroitin chain and complex carbohydrate chains of human thyroglobulin: studies in normal and neoplastic thyroid tissue. Endocrinology 1989;124(1):356–362.
7. Kim PS, Dunn AP, Dunn JT: Altered immunoreactivity of thyroglobulin in thyroid disease. J Clin Endocr and Metabol 1988; 67(1):161–168.
8. Metzger H, Edelhoch H. The properties of thyroglobulin IV. Denaturation kinetics. J Am Chem Soc 1961;83:1423–1427.
9. Seed RW, Goldberg IH. Biosynthesis of thyroglobulin II. Role of subunits iodination and ribonucleic acid synthesis. J Biol Chem 1965;240:764–73.
10. Seed RW, Goldberg IH. Iodination in relation to thyroglobulin maturation and subunit aggregation. Science 1965;149:1380–1382.
11. Vecchio G, Edelhoch H, Robbins J, Weathers B. Studies on the structure of 27S thyroid iodoprotein. Biochemistry 1966;5:2617–2623.
12. Schneider AB, Bornet H, Edelhoch H: Properties of thyroglobulin XX. The biosynthesis of thyroglobulin. Effect of temperature on subunit species. J Biol Chem 1970;245:2672–2678.
13. Schneider AB, Bornet H, Edelhoch H, The effects of low temperature on the conformation of thyroglobulin J Biol Chem 1971;246:2835–2841.
14. Dunn JT. thyroglobulin Structure, function and clinical relevance. Thyroid Today 1985;8:1.
15. DeCrombugghe B, Edelhoch H, Beckers C, DeVisscher M. thyroglobulin from human goiters. Effects of iodination on sedimentation and iodoamino acid synthesis. J Biol Chem 1967;242:5681–5685.
16. Van Zyl A, Edelhoch H. The properties of thyroglobulin XV. The function of the protein in the control of diiodotyrosine residues. J Biol Chem 1967;242:2423–2427.
17. Ingbar SH. The thyroid gland. In: Wilson JD, Foster DW, eds. Textbook of Endocrinology, Philadelphia: W.B. Saunders Co.; 1985.
18. Chirasaveenuprapund P, Rosenberg IN. Effects of hydrogen peroxide-generating systems of the Wolff-Chaikoff effect. Endocrinology 1981;109:2095–2101.
19. Lever EG, Medeiros-Neto GA, DeGroot LJ. Inherited disorders of the thyroid metabolism. Endocr Rev 1983;4:213–239.
20. Stanbury JB, Riccabona G, Janssen MA. Iodotyrosyl coupling defect in congenital hypothyroidism with goiter. Lancet 1963;I:917–920.
21. Morris JH. Defective coupling of iodotyrosine in familial goiters. Arch Int Med 1964;114:417–423.
22. Riddick FA Jr, Desai KB, Stanbury JB, Murison PJ. Familial goiter with diminished synthesis of Tg. Z Ges Exp Med 1969;150:203–212.
23. Mc Kenna TJ, Loughlin T, Ohman M, Schneider A, Towers R. Mild familial goitrous hypothyroidism associated with prolonged 131 iodine retention: possible defect in Tg. synthesis. J Endocr Invest 1989; 12(4):229–234.
24. Dinsart C, Wagar G, Voorthuizen Van F, Vassart G. thyroglobulin complementary DNA as a means to investigate congenital goiters with impaired Tg. synthesis. Ann Endocr Paris 1978;39:133–134.
25. Lissitzky S, Torresani J, Burrow GN, Bouchilloux S, Chabaud O. Defective thyroglobulin export as a cause of congenital goiter. Clin Endocr 1975;4:363–392.
26. DeGroot LJ, Reed Larsen P, Refetoff S, Stanbury JB. Hereditary defects in hormone synthesis, transport and action. In: The thyroid and its Diseases, 5th ed. New York: John Wiley & Sons; 1984:693.
27. Cabret B, Brocas H, Perez-Castillo A, Pohl A, Navas JJ, Targovnik H, Centeneva JA, Vassart G. Normal level of thyroglobulin messenger RNA in a human congenital goiter with Tg. deficiency. J Clin Endocrind Metab 1986;63(4):931–940.
28. Stanbury JB: Inherited metabolic disorders of the thyroid system. In: Ingbar SH and Braverman LE, eds. The Thyroid, 5th ed. Philadelphia: J.B. Lippincott; 1986:690.
29. DeGroot LJ, Reed Larsen P, Refetoff S, Stanbury JB. Hereditary defects in hormone synthesis, transport and action. In: The Thyroid and its Diseases, 5th ed. New York: John Wiley & Sons; 1984:694–695.
30. Daniel PM, Pratt OE, Roitt IM, Torrogiami G. The release of thyroglobulin from the thyroid gland into thyroid lymphatics. The identification of thyroglobulin in the thyroid lymph and in the blood of monkeys by physical and immunological methods and its estima-

tion by radioimmunoassay. Immunology 1967;12:489–504.

31. Izumi M, Kubo I, Taura M, Yamashita S, Morimoto I, Ohtakara S, Okamoto S, Kumagai LF, Nagataki S: Kinetic study of immunoreactive human thyroglobulin J Clin Endo Metab 1986;62(2):410–412.
32. Lever EG, Refetoff S, Scherberg NH, Carr K. The influence of percutaneous fine needle aspiration on serum thyroglobulin J Clin Endocrinol Metab 1983;56:26–29.
33. Rasmussen NG, Hornnes PJ, Hegedus L, Feldt-Rasmussen U. Serum thyroglobulin during the menstrual cycle, during pregnancy and post partum. Acta Endocr 1989;121(2):168–173.
34. Sava L, Tomaselli L, Runello F, Belfiore A, Vigneri R: Serum thyroglobulin levels are elevated in newborns from iodine-deficient areas. J Clin Endocrinol Metab 1986;62(2):429–432.
35. Osotimehin B, Black EG, Hoffenberg R. thyroglobulin concentration in neonatal blood: A possible test for neonatal hypothyroidism. British Med J 1978;2:1467–1468.
36. Pezzino V, Filetti S, Belfiore A, Proto S, Donzelli G, Vigneri R. Serum thyroglobulin levels in the newborn. J Clin Endocr Metab 1981;52:364–366.
37. Ket JL, DeViljder JJM, Bikker H, Gons MH, Tegelaers WHH. Serum thyroglobulin levels: The physiological decrease in infancy and the absence in athyroidism. J. Clin. Endocrinol Metab 1981;53:1301–1303.
38. Feldt-Rasmussen U, Petersen PH, Date J. Sex and age correlated reference values of serum thyroglobulin measured by modified radioimmunoassay. Acta Endocrinol 1979;90:440–450.
39. Christensen SB, Ericsson UB, Janzon L, Tibblin S, Melander A. Influence of cigarette smoking on goiter formation, thyroglobulin and thyroid hormone levels in women. J Clin Endocrinol Metab 1984;58:615–618.
40. Unger J. Fasting induces a decrease in serum thyroglobulin in normal subjects. J Clin Endocrinol Metab 1988;67(6):1309–1311.
41. Van Herle AJ. Serum thyroglobulin measurement in the diagnosis and management of thyroid disease. Thyroid Today 1981;4(2):1.
42. Uller RP, Van Herle AJ. Effect of therapy on serum thyroglobulin levels in patients with Graves' disease. J Clin Endocrinol Metab 1978;46:747–755.
43. Shah D, Dandekar S, Ganatra RD. Thyroglobulin levels in serum and saliva of patients with differentiated thyroid carcinoma. Proc Ind Acad Sci 1978; 87B:169–175.
44. VanHerle AJ, Rosenblit PD, VanHerle TL, VanHerle P, Greipel M, Kellett K. Immunoreactive Tg. in sera and saliva of patients with different thyroid disorders: role of autoantibodies. J Endocrinol Invest 1989; 12(3):177–182.
45. Van Herle AJ, Uller RP, Matthews NL, Brown J: Radioimmunoassay for measurement of Tg. in Human serum. J Clin Invest 1973;52:1320–1327.
46. Schneider AB, Favus MJ, Stachura JE, Arnold JE, Yun Ru, Pinsky S, Colman M, Arnold MJ, Frohman LA. Plasma Tg. detecting thyroid carcinoma after childhood head and neck irradiation. Ann Int Med 1977;86:29–34.
47. Schneider AB, Shore-Freedman E, Ryo UY, Bakerman C, Pinsky SM. Prospective serum thyroglobulin measurements in assessing the risk of developing thyroid nodules in patients exposed to childhood neck irradiation. J Clin Endocrinol Metab 1985;61(3):547–550.
48. Edmonds CJ, Willis CL. Serum thyroglobulin in the investigation of patients with metastases. Br J. Radiol 1988;61(724):317–319.
49. Panza N, Lombardi G, DeRosa M, Pacilio G, Lapenta L, Salvatore M. High serum thyroglobulin levels. Diagnostic indicators in patients with metastases from unknown primary sites. Cancer 1987;60(9):2233–2236.
50. Hjort T. Heamagglutination-inhibition technique with specific antibody (thyroglobulin antibody): A method for the study of the avidity of antisera. Int Arch Allergy Applied Immunol 1968;34:437–454.
51. Assem ESK. Thyroglobulin in the serum of parturient women and newborn infants. Lancet 1964;1:139–141.
52. Pezzino V, Vigneri R, Squatrito S, Filetti S, Camus M, Polosa P. Increased serum thyroglobulin levels in patients with non-toxic goiter. J Clin Endocrinol Metab 1978;46:653–657.
53. Black EG, Gimlette TM, Maisey MN, Casoni A, Harmer CL, Oates GD, Hoffenberg R. Serum thyroglobulin in thyroid cancer. Lancet 1981;2:443–445.
54. Hay ID, Klee GG. Thyroid dysfunction. Endo Metab Clin No Am 1988;17(3)492–494.
55. Wilson R, McKillop JH, Jenkins C, Beastall GH, Thomson JA. Serum thyroglobulin—its measurement and clinical use. Ann Clin Biochem 1989 (pt. 5):401–406.
56. Ross DS. Long term management of differentiated thyroid carcinomas. Endocrinol Metab Clin No Am 1990;3:721–726.
57. Kusakabe K, Mori E, Kano K, Ohta Y, Fujimoto Y, Mori T. Production of monoclonal antibody to thyroglobulin from malignant thyroid carcinoma. Jap J Exp Med 1989;59(1):37–42.
58. Van Herle AJ, Uller RP. Elevated serum thyroglobulin: Marker of metastases in differentiated thyroid carcinomas. J Clin Invest 1975;56:272–277.
59. Reiners C, Reimann J, Schaffer R, Baum K, Becker W, Eilles C, Gerhards W, Schick F, Spiegel W, Wiedemann W, Borner W. Metastasizing differentiated thyroid carcinoma: Diagnostic sensitivity of Tg-RIA in comparison to whole body scintigraphy with I-131. Fortschritte Rontgenstr, 1984;141:306–312.
60. Colacchio TA, LoGerfo P, Colacchio DA, and Feind C. Radioiodine total body scan versus serum thyroglobulin levels in follow-up of patients with thyroid cancer. Surgery 1982;91:42–45.
61. Pacini F, Pinchera A, Giani C, et al, Serum thyroglobulin concentrations and I-131 whole body scans in the diagnosis of metastases from differentiated thyroid carcinoma (after thyroidectomy). Clin Endocrinol (Osv.) 1980;13:107–110.
62. Müller-Gärtner HW, and Schneider C. Clinical eval-

uation of tumor characteristics predisposing thyroglobulin to be undetectable in patients with differentiated thyroid cancer. Cancer 1988;61:976–981.

63. Schneider AB, Line BR, Goldman JM, and Robbins J. Sequential serum thyroglobulin determinations, I-131 scans, and I-131 uptakes after triiodothyronine withdrawal in patients with thyroid cancer. J Clin Endo Metab 1981;53:1199–1206.
64. Grant S, Lultrell B, Reeve T, et al. Thyroglobulin may be undetectable in the serum of patients with metastatic disease secondary to differentiated thyroid carcinoma. Cancer 1984;54:1625–1628.
65. Black EG, Sheppard MC and Hoffenberg. Serial serum thyroglobulin measurements in the management of differentiated thyroid carcinoma. Clin Endocrinol 1987;27:115–120.
66. Pacini F, Lippi F, Formica N, et al, Therapeutic doses of Iodine-131 reveal undiagnosed metastases in thyroid cancer patients with detectable serum thyroglobulin levels. J Nuc Med 1987;28:1888–1891.
67. Schlumberger M, Fragu P, Parmentier C, et al., Thyroglobulin assay in the follow-up of patients with differentiated thyroid carcinoma; comparison of its value in patients with or without normal residue tissue. Acta Endocrinol 1981;98:215.
68. Harvey RD, Matheson NA, Grabonski PS, Rodger AB. Measure of serum thyroglobulin is of value in detecting tumor recurrence following treatment of differentiated thyroid carcinoma by lobectomy. Br J Surg 1990;77:324–326.

7

Radioactive Iodine Treatment of Thyroid Carcinoma

ROBERT LLOYD SEGAL

Introduction

The fact that certain thyroid cancers and their metastases can concentrate iodine and produce biologically effective hormonal products has been known since the classical observation of Von Eiselberg, 1894, who saw the development of myxedema following the radical excision of a cervical thyroid cancer and observed spontaneous cure of the hypothyroid state by a metastatic deposit developed in the sternum.[1]

Malignancies derived from the thyroid gland show a unique ability to concentrate iodine and to form thyroid hormone and its precursors. This physiological fact enabled early investigators to show that localization of radioactive iodine occurred in the metastatic deposits of thyroid tumors.[1]

This capability of some thyroid-derived malignant cells to concentrate iodine is the basis for the diagnostic and therapeutic use of radioactive iodine. Radioactive iodine is utilized diagnostically to determine the location, size, and anatomical limits of thyroid cancer metastases or recurrences. It is used therapeutically for the treatment of differentiated thyroid cancer after primary treatment with surgery.

Therapy with radioactive iodine is the treatment of choice for functioning metastatic or recurrent differentiated thyroid cancer.[2] ^{131}I has distinct advantages over external radiation for the treatment of differentiated thyroid cancer because: (1) the use of ^{131}I in the treatment of metastases or recurrent tumor irradiates the lesion from the inside out, with relative selectivity; (2) assuming a halflife of 4 days, an uptake of 1.0% of the therapy dose of ^{131}I produces 15,000 rads/mCi; and (3) the ionization produced by the 609 kV beta particles (10 rads sec/gm) may be greater than from conventional x-ray therapy and is confined to a smaller area because the beta radiation penetrates only a few millimeters into tissue.[1–3]

There has been a gradual evolution in the evaluation and use of radioactive iodine therapy in the treatment of differentiated thyroid cancer. This change is perhaps best documented by contrasting the relatively gloomy outlook of Silver, who in 1962 stated, "We doubt that the treatment is ever really curative,"[1] with Maxon and Smith's concluding statement: "Radioactive iodine continues to be one of the safest and most effective methods of diagnosis and treating metastatic well-differentiated thyroid cancer."[2]

Evaluation of the efficacy of radioactive iodine therapy for thyroid cancers is difficult because of the unique natural history of these neoplasms. There may be a long latent period between any initial surgical therapy and the occurrence of either metastases or recurrence of the cancer. There may also be marked variations in the biologic activity of these tumors, even among those with similar histology. In addition, radiosensitivity of tumor tissue is not predictable.[2–7]

It is necessary that the groups of patients evaluated have undergone similar therapies. Differing conclusions as to the efficacy of radioactive iodine therapy may be due in part to the heterogeneity of the patients studied. For in-

Table 7.1. Rationale for the use of radioactive iodine ^{131}I in the therapy of differentiated thyroid cancer

Curative

To routinely ablate residual thyroid tissue in order to detect later residual, recurrent, or metastatic disease by means of scanning and/or thyroglobulin determination.
To ablate and "cure" distant metastases present at time of diagnosis following total thyroidectomy sites include:
1. local cervical lesions
2. pulmonary
3. bone
4. liver
5. central nervous system
6. other

To ablate and cure residual thyroid cancer in the neck.

Palliative

To reduce local residual tumors in order to maintain life and prevent local tracheal compression or obliteration.
To relieve pain of distant (bony) metastases.[1,2,7,9,11]

stance, prognosis is influenced significantly by age, which may not be standardized in comparison series.[4,5,7]

Finally, the radioactive iodine may have deleterious side effects, which must be weighed against its therapeutic benefits. Statistical evidence for the advantages of radioactive iodine therapy in differentiated thyroid cancer should ideally include a control group. Such an ideal therapeutic trial has not been performed. Comparison of different protocols for the use of ^{131}I in the diagnosis and treatment of thyroid carcinoma are therefore largely comparisons between different institutions.[2,4,5]

The ideal treatment for differentiated thyroid carcinoma includes the ablation or removal of the primary lesion(s) and prevention, or successful ablation, of local and/or distant metastases, with subsequent significant improvement in both quality and duration of life. Radioactive iodine has a role in both forms of therapy. The present indications for radioactive iodine treatment of thyroid carcinoma are listed in Table 7.1.

The ability of some thyroid cancers to concentrate radioactive iodine is the basis for its therapeutic use. If no radioactive iodine uptake is present, therapy with radioactive iodine is not feasible, and should not be utilized.[1,2,5–7,11] If a sufficient therapeutic dose of radiation is to be delivered by a therapeutic dose of ^{131}I, an uptake of at least 0.1% of the administered dose at 24 hours is necessary.[3] Not all differentiated thyroid cancers concentrate ^{131}I, either in the tumor, local recurrences, or metastases.[11] This unique capacity to concentrate radioactive iodine is initially present in approximately 75% of differentiated thyroid cancer in the young, and in approximately 50% of these cancers in adults.[11–14] After radiation therapy with either radioactive iodine or external radiation, or after chemotherapy, this capacity may disappear.

Isotopic scanning is used to detect the presence of thyroid cancer recurrence or metastases. The usual isotope employed is ^{131}I, which has both beta and gamma energy emissions.[1,2,5] The latter are easily detected by external counting. Thallium 201 has been utilized by one group with some success.[5]

The objectives of scanning include the detection of all tumor sites that may be treatable with radioactive iodine, and the detection of tumor sites that may not be amenable to this therapy due to poor concentration of iodine.[16–18] (Table 7.2).

To enhance the probability of therapeutic success, the concentration of radioactive iodine in thyroid-derived tumor cells may be increased by several preparative methods. The normal thyroid gland competes for ^{131}I so effectively that tumor tissue may not be visualized if any normal tissue is present. Either surgery or ^{131}I ablation will remove this obstacle to the detection of metastases. Complete surgical ablation is recommended in all cases in which the neck is explored and in which subsequent treatment with ^{131}I is being contemplated. This approach saves time because therapy with radioactive iodine can be given soon after the operation; whereas in the case of ^{131}I ablation of residual normal thyroid tissue, an interval of several weeks must elapse before abnormal tissue can be delineated and treated. Total surgical thyroidectomy also spares the patient exposure to unnecessary radiation.[18–20]

Well-differentiated thyroid-derived malignancies retain their dependency on thyroid-stimulating hormone (TSH) for iodine uptake

Table 7.2. Factors affecting the concentration of radioactive iodine in thyroid cancer tissue in scanning and in therapy

Factor	Effect on uptake
Presence of normal thyroid tissue	↓
Hormonal factors	
TSH	↑
Endogenous	↑
Supplemental TSH	↑
Secondary to TRH	↑
Thyroid hormone	
Thyroxine	↓
Triiodothyronine	↓
Inorganic iodine	
Iodine pool	
Medication	↓
Diet	↓
Absorption from skin (iodine preparation of skin in surgery, etc.)	↓
Iodine	
Diuretic therapy	↑
Mannitol therapy	↑
Organic iodine dyes	
CT studies with contrast medium	↓
Vascular studies	↓
Gall Bladder	↓
Myelogram	↓
Medications	
Antithyroid drugs	
Tapazole	↓ (rebound ↑)
Propylthiouracil	↓ (rebound ↑)
Perchlorate	↓
Lithium	↑ ↓
Amiodirone	↓
Dose of ^{131}I administered	
Time of scanning	

↑ indicates increase in uptake, ↓ indicates decrease.

as well as for cell proliferation. If thyroid-stimulating hormone is absent, radioactive iodine uptake is not possible. Increasing the level of TSH will increase the radioactive iodine uptake of thyroid-derived cells.[1-3,10-12]

Since thyroid hormones suppress TSH secretion by the pituitary, when thyroxine is removed by either thyroid ablation or discontinuing the use of supplemental thyroid medication (particularly after total thyroidectomy), the endogenous production of TSH will be stimulated and levels greater than 30 miμ/L will be achieved. This level consistently produces adequate radioactive iodine uptake in susceptible cells. A period of 4 to 6 weeks without replacement therapy is generally sufficient. During this period symptoms of hypothyroidism may occur without thyroid hormone replacement. The duration of these unpleasant symptoms can be shortened by utilizing low dose triiodothyronine (T_3) therapy for the first two weeks of this period. However, since T_3 has a shorter half-life than T_4, a shorter period of withdrawal is sufficient to allow TSH to rise. Some authors have attempted to increase the thyroid-stimulating hormone level by the use of either bovine or human TSH injection. The use of bovine TSH may produce immunological responses of varying severity and may occasionally produce anti-TSH antibodies. For these reasons most institutions have abandoned the use of bovine TSH injection.[22]

Paying adequate attention to increasing the TSH level, decreasing iodine intake, and maximizing iodine uptake will increase the success rate in scanning. A dose of 1 to 2 mCi of ^{131}I is utilized with a rectilinear scan of the neck and with a gamma counter for whole body scanning.[1-3,14,21]

Larger doses of 5 to 15 mCi ^{131}I will increase the yield of information with scanning; however, the larger doses carry the risk of sublethal radiation injury to the metastasis with a subsequent decrease in the percent of uptake after a therapeutic dose of radioactive iodine.[28] TSH is in itself potentially dangerous. Many differentiated thyroid cancers in man are endocrine dependent.[1] Increased growth of such cancers, and conversion from a low-grade differentiated endocrine-dependent tumor to a highly malignant anaplastic non-TSH-dependent cancer has been reported.[2] For this reason, after the use of radioactive iodine therapy, reinstitution of thyroid hormone therapy is mandatory.

The uptake of radioactive iodine is affected by the size of the body iodine pool. The intake of iodine from all sources contributes to the iodine pool. Thus, increased iodine intake from medications including cough mixtures and vitamins, a high iodine diet (e.g., seaweed, kelp, iodized salt, and seafoods), and the absorption of iodine applied to the skin or mucous membranes, all increase this iodine pool and decrease the concentration of radioactive iodine in thyroid-derived cells. Conversely, a low iodine diet used in addition to diuretics to lower the iodine pool will raise the radioactive iodine uptake.[1–3,11]

Organic iodine dyes have a more prolonged depressive effect on radioactive iodine uptake. This effect can last from 2 to 4 weeks for water soluble dyes used in angiography and computerized tomography (CT) scans and for up to 4 to 12 weeks for lipid-soluble dyes such as those used in gall bladder studies. Retained dye in the spinal canal after myelography may be a source of prolonged iodine release and may therefore cause prolonged depression of radioactive iodine uptake.[1–3]

Antithyroid drugs such as tapazole and propylthiouracil inhibit uptake by means of chemical action on the thyroid cells. In the past, these drugs have been utilized to decrease thyroid hormone levels and increase TSH. A high "rebound" radioactive iodine uptake occurs when these medications are discontinued. However, especially in the case of propylthiouracil, a protective effect against radiation, or specifically the action of radioactive iodine in thyrotoxicosis, has been reported; therefore, a similar decrease in radiation efficacy in thyroid carcinoma is implied.[12,24] Perchlorate and similar drugs prevent the trapping of iodine by thyroid-derived cells. Lithium may change uptake for a variable period of time.[25,26] Amiodorone, which has a high iodine content, may depress uptake for months.[27]

Increasing the dose of radioactive iodine that is administered will allow the detection of differentiated thyroid cancer-derived tissue that has low iodine uptake. The percentage of the administered dose of radioactive iodine will remain the same, but a larger amount of radioactivity will be present in tumor sites, enhancing the probability of identifying them.[13,16,23] If scanning is performed at 24 hours, there will be significant blood background radiation due to the distribution of radioactive iodine in tissue and body fluid. If scanning is done after a longer interval of from 48 to 72 hours, the background radiation diminishes and the interference of this background radiation is minimized. False positive scans may occur in certain situations (Table 7.3).

Table 7.3. Factors that contribute to false positives in radioiodine uptake scans

Nasal secretion with the nasal cavity
Contaminates of handkerchief, etc. from nasal secretion
Salivary glands
^{131}I retained in the gastrointestinal tract
Meckel's diverticulum[28]
Urine
Contaminates of bed clothes
Cyst: Renal (or other) with protein content

Protocols for ^{131}I Therapy

Two approaches to the ablation of residual thyroid tissue have evolved. The first involves the administration of a low dose less than 30 mCi of ^{131}I to ablate a thyroid remnant, and assumes that this dose may need to be repeated to be completely effective.[37] In the second approach, an amount of ^{131}I that is sufficient either to ablate all residual thyroid tissue or, if a significant remnant is present, to deliver 50,000 rads is administered in a single high dose of usually 60 to 150 mCi.[2,3,6,9]

Buena and Leeper used dosimetric methods to estimate the largest safe single dose of ^{131}I in therapy of differentiated thyroid cancer metastases.[11,12] Their preparatory protocol includes the ablation of the normal thyroid, discontinuance of thyroxine for 6 weeks, and avoidance of iodine either used as contrast agent or ingested in food and drugs. A dose of 1.0 mCi of ^{131}I is given orally. Body retention is measured at 2 and at 4 hours; thereafter, it is measured once a day for 4 more days. The highest body count measured is considered to represent 100% iodine retention. Urine is collected in daily pools, and heparinized blood is initially drawn at 2 and at 4 hours, and thereafter daily for 4 more days, enabling the radiation dose to the blood to be calculated. A calculated maximum of 200 rads to the blood is a dose-limiting factor.[10–12,30]

In addition, a maximized retained dose of 120 mCi at 24 hours prevented tumor products and iodoprotein containing ^{131}I from increasing the blood radiation above their limits.

One other imposed limitation is that applied when pulmonary metastases are present. A maximum retained dose of 80 mCi at 24 hours has prevented the occurrence of radiation pneumonitis (which had resulted in 2 deaths with a prior protocol without this limit).[29]

Using their dosimetry calculations, the average single dose was 293 mCi and the largest, 694 mCi. They comment that "had an arbitrary fixed dose in the range of 150 to 200 mCi been utilized 92 of the 202 treatment doses would have undertreated the patients and 3 patients would have received doses expected to result in excessive blood radiation."[12] Retesting and retreatment, if necessary, is performed a year later.[11,30]

Beierwaltes usually treats metastases from differentiated thyroid carcinoma that take up radioactive iodine with an empiric dose of 150 to 175 mCi for uptake in regional nodes, 175 to 200 mCi for treatment of pulmonary metastases, and 200 mCi for bony metastases.[3] Retesting and retreatment, if necessary, are performed 1 year after the initial treatment. If recurrence is not present, retesting is done at 3 and 5 years after initial treatment. Late recurrence up to 25 years post-therapy has been documented, necessitating the performance of long-term follow-up studies.

Evaluation of the Effects of Radioactive Iodine on Differentiated Thyroid Carcinoma

The usual course of differentiated thyroid carcinoma is that of a slow growing, rather indolent tumor. The prognosis tends to be more favorable with papillary carcinoma (90% survival at 10 years), than with follicular carcinoma (80% survival at 10 years). Mazzaferi reported that a multivariate analysis of over 1100 patients without distant metastases failed to identify tumor histology as a significant prognostic variable.

There have been many studies of large series of patients with differentiated thyroid cancer. In comparing the effects of treatment on morbidity and mortality from each institution, one must be aware of the possible inherent differences in the populations at risk: the size of the lesion at initial surgery, presence of multicentricity, history of previous radiation, and extent of initial surgical resection; as well as the effects of various doses of radioactive iodine employed for therapy. The incidence of later local recurrence of distant metastases may also vary widely, depending in part upon the duration of follow-up in each series. Some include only those patients who had clinically apparent distant metastases at the time of initial evaluation, while others also include those patients whose metastases were found after residual thyroid ablation by surgery or by ^{131}I followed by total body scans. Still other studies include patients with metastases that developed after many years. Therefore, the percentages of nodal and/or distant metastases as stated in reviews of the literature vary widely. Maxon tabulates and averages these percentages arriving at figures for papillary carcinoma of 35% for initial nodal metastases and 9.4% for later nodal metastases as compared with figures for follicular carcinoma of 12.8% for initial nodal metastases and 6.7% for later nodal metastases. Using the same series, distant metastases were on average more common in follicular carcinoma than in papillary carcinoma, i.e. 16.4% vs 3.8% initially 13% vs 4% later; in some of the series the incidence of distant metastases depended less on histology than on tumor size, grade, and patient age. Later local recurrences occurred in 5.6% of papillary carcinoma and 7.8% of follicular carcinomas.[2]

Residual thyroid cancer that concentrates radioactive iodine after initial surgery may occur because of extra thyroidal tumor invasion or incomplete surgical resection. Reports of successful treatment of residual tumor with ^{131}I are plentiful and indicate that this modality treatment may improve long-term survival. Local recurrent carcinoma is associated with shortened survival, which may also be improved by ^{131}I treatment.[1–7]

The efficacy of ^{131}I treatment for ablation of thyroid remnants continues to be a topic of controversy. In an international survey, 81%

of thyroidologists favored administration of ^{131}I to a thyroid remnant remaining after total or near-total thyroidectomy for papillary carcinoma; 97% recommended such therapy for follicular carcinoma.[36] Mazzaferi has published data indicating that the rate of recurrence is lower when such therapy is given.[4,5] Because local recurrence is associated with shorter survival, such therapy eventually should have long-term impact. In DeGroot's 12-year follow-up of 269 patients with papillary carcinoma, ^{131}I ablation was associated with "decreased risk of death in patients with Class I and Class II tumors greater than 1 cm. in size."[37] He further states that "the data strongly supports the use of more extensive initial surgery in Class I and II patients with tumors greater than 1 cm., as well as postoperative radioactive iodine ablation of thyroid remnant tissue." Among Mt. Sinai Hospital (New York) endocrinologists this practice is nearly universal. De Groot et al report that post thyroidectomy doses of 30 mli of ^{131}I may be expected to ablate all residual normal thyroid tissue in 85% of patients. Doses of 100 to 150 mCi are used if there is suspicion or confirmation of actual residual thyroid tumor, invasion outside of the thyroid bed, or nodal metastases in the immediate postoperative period.

The overall long-term incidence of distant metastases occurring in well-differentiated thyroid carcinoma is somewhat more difficult to calculate because of the relatively small size of most series, as well as the need for a long duration of prospective follow-up required for these relatively indolent tumors. Ruegemer and Hay reported that in the Mayo Clinic series of 988 patients, distant metastases were present in 8.6% of cases,[33] whereas in a series reported by Hoegi, the incidence was 12.4%.[34] In Rasmassen's 1978 series of 158 patients with well-differentiated carcinoma followed up for ten years, 20 initially had distant metastases present, while a further 28 patients with papillary carcinoma, and 22 patients with follicular carcinoma subsequently developed metastases.[32]

Distant metastases are most commonly found in the lungs. In Maxon's tabulation of ten series comprising 810 patients with metastatic well-differentiated carcinoma, 44% of the metastatic sites were pulmonary; 29%, bone; 10%, both bone and pulmonary; 6%, mediastinal; and 8%, other (including brain and liver).[2]

It is estimated that approximately 50% of all metastatic lesions initially concentrate radioactive iodine in quantities significant for therapeutic purposes.[3,4,6,7,33,41]

Pulmonary metastases may be further divided by their pattern of uptake into microfollicular, macrofollicular, and diffuse infiltrative; in some institutions, the pattern of pulmonary metastasis is thought to be a factor influencing response to therapy as well as prognosis.[7,11,32,33] Ordinary chest x-rays will be abnormal in approximately 1/2 of patients with pulmonary metastasis. CT scanning may be positive in patients with micronodular lesions of the lungs.[40] Radioactive iodine scanning may be the only method of diagnosis of the infiltrative variety.[39–41] Hay (Mayo Clinic) reported five deaths among 23 patients with microfollicular disease, compared with 21 deaths among 48 patients with macrofollicular disease after ^{131}I therapy. In Beierwaltes' series, 39 patients with pulmonary metastases were treated with ^{131}I. Of the 22 patients with papillary carcinoma, 8 were alive with disease, while 14 showed no disease. Four patients with follicular carcinoma died of disease while two survived, one with disease, one without. Maheshwari et al. reported on a 28 year follow-up of patients treated with ^{131}I at MD Anderson Hospital (Houston, Texas). Age was a definite factor in prognosis. For all patients who presented initially with pulmonary metastases, the eight who were less than 40 years of age all responded to ^{131}I, while only 60% of those over 40 years old responded. Of patients who developed pulmonary metastases later in the course of their disease, all nine under 40 years of age responded, while only 11 of 26 patients over the age of 40 responded.[7] In all series, survival was better in cases in which pulmonary lesions concentrated radioactive iodine than in cases in which they did not. Survival was also adversely affected by large tumor burden.[7,39–41]

Because the numbers are so small, there are

Table 7.4. Adverse effects of ^{131}I therapy

I. Pregnancy
  A. Fetal hypothyroidism
  B. Teratogenicity

II. Direct effect of radiation resulting in
  A. Salivary gland dysfunction
  B. Hypoparathyroidism
  C. Vocal cord dysfunction secondary to radiation of nerves
  D. Radiation tracheitis

III. Deleterious Effects
  A. Bone marrow
    1. Leukemia
    2. Thrombocytopenia
    3. Pancytopenia
    4. Decreased hemoglobin
    5. Lymphocytes
  B. Lungs
    1. Radiation pneumonitis
  C. Gonads
    1. Sterility, male & female
    2. Chromosomal abnormalities
  D. Bladder
  E. Gastrointestinal

IV. Secondary ^{131}I effects on thyroid tumor & metastases
  A. Anaplastic transformation of well-differentiated thyroid cancer
  B. Thyroid storm (acute hyperthyroxinemia due to release of performed hormone)
  C. Acute neurologic dysfunction

V. Induction of other solid tumors
  A. Bladder
  B. Breast (?)

no series comparing various protocols of ^{131}I dosage administered with survival.

Bony metastases are associated with a less favorable prognosis in both papillary and follicular carcinoma. In the MD Anderson series of 24 patients with bony metastases treated with ^{131}I, only 3 patients were alive without disease after 28 years, 2 were living with disease, and 18 had died of disease (one patient died of unrelated causes without evidence of cancer).[7] In Maxon's review of five other series, only 16 of 233 patients showed complete resolution of bony metastases as evaluated by x-ray or clinical appearance, while 33 of 72 patients showed some improvement.[2] Despite these statistics, most authorities continue to use radioactive iodine, sometimes in combination with external radiation, for palliation of pain from bony metastases, as well as in hopes of tumor regression.[1,2,4,7–9,19,41]

Adverse Effects of ^{131}I Therapy

Table 7.4 outlines the potential deleterious effects of radioactive iodine therapy.

Pregnancy is an absolute contraindication to radioactive iodine therapy. Before any study or treatment with ^{131}I, pregnancy must be ruled out. Most laboratories instruct patients not to become pregnant for a period of 3 to 6 months after radioactive iodine therapy. Strict birth control measures must be employed. We insist upon this agreement before therapy is administered and exclude pregnancy in females by appropriate CG assay.

Several cases of radioactive iodine treatment during pregnancy have resulted in cretinism or chromosomal abnormalities.[43,44] The radiation dose received by the fetus is the sum of the radiation dose to the blood and the radiation received from the radioactive iodine within the bladder, as well as the radiation from ^{131}I within the gastrointestinal tract. After 42 days of fetal life the thyroid anlagen will concentrate iodine and thus raise the fetal radiation burden.[43,44]

The salivary gland secretes iodine. Radioactive iodine may cause acute sialoadenitis. Dry mouth and salivary gland dysfunction may occur following ^{131}I therapy. Stenosis of the salivary ducts and stone formation has been noted.[45,46] The use of atropine in small doses immediately before the use of radioactive iodine will lower the radiation dose to the salivary glands and minimize the risk of these complications of therapy.[47]

The parathyroid glands are sensitive to external radiation in low dose, which may result in hyperparathyroidism due to hyperplasia of the glands as a later complication. This radiation effect has not been reported with radioactive iodine therapy for differentiated thyroid cancer. However, hypoparathyroidism due to radiation damage to the glands following either radioactive iodine ablation of normal thyroid gland or radioactive iodine ablation of recurrent tumor has been reported (personal communication, SB Yohalem).

Vocal cord dysfunction with recurrent laryngeal nerve palsy has been reported with radioactive iodine therapy of recurrent thyroid cancer, although this is a rare complication. Pochin, as quoted by Silver, described one case with such severe symptoms that a tracheotomy was necessary.

Radiation tracheitis following the use of high dose radioactive iodine treatment for thyroid gland ablation has been reported.[1]

The effects of ^{131}I on the bone marrow are the same as those observed after whole-body radiation; they are dependent on the total dose and the time frame in which the radiation is administered. Blood counts should be performed prior to administration of ^{131}I. Bone marrow depression is maximal at approximately 6 weeks; thrombocytopenia, leukopenia, and anemia have been noted following radioactive iodine therapy.[2,18–20] If there is any indication of bone marrow suppression (lymphopenia is an early indicator of change) bone marrow studies are indicated. The deleterious effects of radiation on bone marrow and therefore on blood elements may be the limiting factor in determining treatment dosage. The use of granulocyte stimulating factor and macrophage monocytic stimulating factor in patients with bone marrow depression may obviate this deleterious effect. Leeper noted that 8 of 59 patients had serious bone marrow depression following maximal radioactive iodine therapy.[11,12] The calculated dose to whole blood was 3 Gy or more. After limiting calculated radiation dose to blood to 200 rads and a maximum whole-body retained dose to 120 mCi at 48 hours, no instances of severe or persistent bone marrow depression were noted. Based on whole-body radiation doses, therapy with ^{131}I can be expected to induce leukemia, usually of the acute myelogenous type, if more than 200 rads are received by the bone marrow. In the reported series, except in one instance, leukemia was not reported following radioactive iodine unless total doses exceed 600 mCi. A report by Melvin of 14 cases of leukemia in 2453 treated patients may confirm this complication.[2]

Rall reported radiation pneumonitis lending to death in two patients when large doses of ^{131}I were used to treat pulmonary metastasis. Setting limit of 80 mCi of ^{131}I retained at 24 hours in patients with diffuse lung metastases has prevented this complication.[11,29]

The dose of radiation delivered to the testicles from radioactive iodine therapy is approximately the same as that of radiation to the blood. The testes do not concentrate iodine. Some additional radiation to the testes may occur as a result of radioactive iodine in the bladder. Frequent emptying of the bladder in combination with vigorous hydration will decrease the radiation dose from ^{131}I contained within the bladder. Most studies reported a radiation dose to the testicles of approximately 0.3 rads/mCi after ^{131}I therapy.[1,2] Male infertility and even azospermia has been reported after treatment with ^{131}I.[49] The data suggest that gonadal damage may occur with radioactive iodine therapy, especially at higher levels of administered dose.[50] The report of an elevation of follicle-stimulating hormone (FSH) level peaking at approximately 2 months after radioactive iodine ablation therapy to the thyroid using 50-mCi ^{131}I suggests an effect on spermatogenesis even with relatively small amounts of radioactive iodine therapy. If pelvic or bony metastases are present, the dose to the testicles may be markedly increased. Some radiation to the testicles may occur from the radioactive iodine within the gastrointestinal tract.[48,49] It should be noted that in some cases the radiation changes induced in the gonads may be permanent. Therefore consideration of sperm storage should be considered in appropriate cases.[2]

The ovaries are subject not only to radiation from the blood after therapy with radioactive iodine for differentiated thyroid cancer, but also to significant radiation from radioactive iodine in urine within the bladder.[51] One report of concentration of iodine within the follicular fluid has not been confirmed (personal communication, TF Davies 1990). As in males, ^{131}I treatment for metastases in the bony pelvis will markedly increase the radiation exposure to the ovaries. Any radiation to the ovaries may produce genetic damage either through direct effects on chromosomes or through induced genetic mutations. The naturally occurring rate of mutations is approximately 0.5 per million genes per generation. The doubling dose is that dose which causes the gene mutation rate to double. The doubling dose of ^{131}I would be over 150 mCi. The administration of 150 mCi to females would be expected to produce chromosomal abnormalities in about 50 children per 100,000 live births. The effects of this dose of radiation may cause abnormalities in 0.3% of pregnancies. Given a dose of 500 mCi of ^{131}I, abnormalities would be expected in approximately 1% of pregnancies resulting in a live birth. This would not be clinically apparent and has not been reported to be evident in the small series reported thus far.

There is a theoretical worry concerning genetic effects of radiation on the F_2 generation.[51] Discussion of the statistical probability is beyond the scope of this chapter.

Secondary ^{131}I Effects on Thyroid Cancer and Metastases

The transformation of differentiated thyroid cancer into an anaplastic tumor has been reported to occur spontaneously in the absence of any radiation therapy. Severel cases of this transformation occurred shortly after radioactive iodine therapy, suggesting that there is a greater incidence of the phenomenon after radiation.[52]

Radiation may cause destruction of thyroid tissue and release of preformed thyroid hormones into the circulation. This may lead to a hyperthyroxinemic state or even acute "thyroid storm" if sufficient hormone is released. This sequence of events has been reported after radioactive iodine ablation of the thyroid.[1,2] Acute hyperthyroxinemia has been followed by myocardial infarction.[53] Several cases of thyroid storm have been reported after radioactive iodine therapy, usually in patients with extensive metastatic follicular carcinoma.[54] This complication usually occurs 18 to 96 hours after therapy.

Radioactive iodine therapy for metastatic well-differentiated thyroid cancer to the central nervous system may cause acute neurological syndromes secondary to radiation effects. If cervical cord metastases are present, acute cord compression may result.[54]

Other complications of ^{131}I therapy for thyroid carcinoma include acute symptoms of gastritis. It is important to avoid contamination of the environment if emesis occurs. Excretion of ^{131}I via the urinary tract has not been reported to lead to an increase in renal tumors; however, an increased incidence of bladder cancer has been reported.[21] No increase in gastrointestinal tumors has been reported in patients treated with radioactive iodine.

There are reports of an increased incidence of breast cancer following larger doses of radioactive iodine; however, these data are not statistically significant.[55]

Local radiation control boards dictate when a patient may leave the hospital after treatment with ^{131}I for thyroid carcinoma. In our institution, a patient may return home with a retained dose of 8 mCi of ^{131}I. Children and others may still be at risk for radiation injury if prolonged close contact with treated patients is not prevented.

In the event of death of a patient with a large retained dose of ^{131}I, special arrangements may be necessary for an autopsy to be conducted in order to prevent the danger of personnel being exposed to significant radiation.

Contamination due to emesis or loss of urinary control may be dealt with in accordance with radiation control guidelines.

The amount of radiation exposure to hospital personnel from patients treated with large dose of ^{131}I may be minimized by taking appropriate precautions. Distance is a shield; the patients should be isolated in single rooms. Storage and decay of highly radioactive urine will depend on local plumbing and sewage. If there is sufficient effluent, direct disposal may be permissable. Otherwise, arrangements for storage of waste in order to allow decay of radiation may be required. Personnel should be monitored for radiation exposure. Active rotation of personnel will keep individual radiation doses to a minimum.

The use of ^{131}I in the treatment of anaplastic and medullary carcinoma is covered in Chapters 8 and 9.

Conclusion

Radioactive iodine therapy has been utilized in the treatment of differentiated thyroid cancer recurrences and metastases. Ablation of residual normal thyroid tissue postoperatively, followed by total body scanning is indicated in all patients with unfavorable prognostic factors including large primary cancer, multifocal primary tumors, capsular invasion, vascular invasion, or old age. Treatment of otherwise asymptomatic patients without known or demonstrated metastases is associated with a lower incidence of recurrence or later metastases.[4,5]

Radioactive iodine treatment for local recurrences or pulmonary metastases is associated with a high cure rate. However, treatment of bone, brain, or liver metastases may only be palliative. In the future, prognostic factor analysis and the use of prognostic indicators may result in a delineation of those patients with thyroid carcinoma who will be cured with the initial surgery and those at risks for recurrence and/or metastasis. If these prognostic analysis can be validated then the use of ablative radio iodine will be restricted to those patients with a limited or poor prognosis. The harmful effects of radiation will be avoided in the great majority of patients.

Major deleterious effects of radioactive iodine treatment include bone marrow depression, gonadal dysfunction with azospermia and infertility, induction of anaplastic transformation of differentiated thyroid cancer (although this is questionable), and precipitation of thyroid storm due to acute release of preformed thyroid hormone.

References

1. Silver S. Radioactive isotopes in medicine and biology, 2nd ed. Philadelphia, PA: Lea & Febiger; 1962.
2. Maxon HR III, and Smith HS. Radioiodine-131 in the diagnosis and treatment of metastatic well differentiated thyroid cancer. Endo Metab Clin North America: Thyroid Carcinoma 1990;19:685–718.
3. Beierwaltes WH. The treatment of thyroid carcinoma with radioactive iodine. Seminars in Nucl Med 1978;8:79–94.
4. Mazzaferri E. Controversies in the management of differentiated thyroid carcinoma. In Program Syllabus of the Endocrine Society's 42nd Post-Graduate Assembly 1990;167–189.
5. Mazzaferri EL. Treating differentiated thyroid carcinoma: Where do we draw the line? Mayo Clin Proc 1991;66:105–111.
6. Maxon HR, Thomas SR, Hertzberg VS, Kereiakes JG, Chen I-W, Sperling MI, Saenger EL. Relation between effective radiation dose and outcome of radioiodine therapy for thyroid cancer. N Engl J Med 1983;309:937–941.
7. Maneshwari YK, Hill CS Jr, Haynie TP III, Hickey RC, Samaan NA. 131-I Therapy in differentiated thyroid carcinoma: M.D. Anderson Hospital experience. Cancer 1981;47:664–671.
8. LaQuaglia MP, Corbally MT, Heller G, Exelby PR, Brennan MF. Recurrence and morbidity in differentiated thyroid carcinoma in children. Surgery 1988; 104:1149–1156.
9. Beierwaltes WH, Hishiyama RH, Thompson NW, Copp JE, Kubo A. Survival time and "cure" in papillary and follicular thyroid carcinoma with distant metastases: statistics following University of Michigan therapy. Nucl Med 1982;23:561–568.
10. Medeiros-Neto G, and Gaitan E. A method and rationale for treating metastatic thyroid carcinoma with the largest safe dose of 131-I. Frontiers in Thyroidology 1986;2:1317–1321.
11. Leeper RD, Shimaoka K. Treatment of metastatic thyroid cancer. J Clin Endocrinol Metab 1980; 9(2):383–404.
12. Benua RS, Cicale NR, Sonenberg M, Rawson RW. The relations of radioiodine dosimetry to results and complications in the treatment of metastatic thyroid cancer. 1962;87:171–182.
13. Pacini F, Lippi F, Formica N, Elisei R, Anelli S, Ceccarelli C, Pinchera A. Therapeutic doses of iodine-131 reveal undiagnosed metastases in thyroid cancer patients with detectable serum thyroglobulin levels. J Nucl Med 1987;28:1888–1891.
14. Thomas SR, Maxon HR, Kereiakes JF, Saenger EL. Quantitative external counting techniques enabling improved diagnostic and therapeutic decisions in patients with well-differentiated thyroid cancer. Radiology 1977;122:731–737.
15. Hoefnagel CA, Delpract CC, Marcuse HR and de Vijlder JJM. Role of thallium-201 total body scintigraphy in follow-up of thyroid carcinoma. J Nucl Med 1986;27:1854–1857.
16. Coakley AJ, Page CJ, Croft D. Scanning dose and detection of thyroid metastases. J Nucl Med 1980: 21:803–804.
17. Waxman A, Ramanna L, Chapman N et al. Significance of ^{131}I scan dose in patients with thyroid cancer: determination of ablation: concise communication. J Nucl Med 1981;22:861.
18. Halpern S, Preisman R, Hagan P. Scanning dose and detection of thyroid metastases. J Nucl Med 1980; 8:803–804.
19. Brown AP, Greening WP, McCready CR, Shaw HJ, Harmer CL. Radioiodine treatment of metastatic thy-

roid carcinoma: the Royal Marsden Hospital experience. Br J Radiol 1984;57:323–327.
20. Krishnamurthy GT, Blahd WH. Radioiodine I-131 therapy in the management of thyroid cancer. Cancer 1977;40:195–202.
21. Thomas SR, Maxon HR, Kereiakes JF, Saegger EL. Quantitative external counting techniques improved diagnostic and therapeutic decisions in patienis with well differentiated thyroid carcinoma. J Nucl Med 1971;12:731–737.
22. Hershman JM, Edward CL. Serum thyrotropin: after thyroid ablation compared with TSH levels after exogenous bovine TSH. Implications for 131-1 treatment of thyroid carcinoma. J Clin Endocr 1972;34:814–818.
23. Pacini F, Lippi L, Formica N, Elisei R, Ancilli S, Cacarelli C, Pinchera A. Therapeutic doses of iodine-131 reveal undiagnosed metastases in thyroid cancer patients with detectable serum-thyroglobulin levels. J Nucl Med 1987;28:1888–1891.
24. Connell JMC, Hilditcht E, Rohertson J et al. Radioprotective action of carbimazole radioiodine; therapy for thyrotoxicosis; influence of the drug on iodine kinetics. J Nucl Med 1987;13:358–361.
25. Rifkin N, Quitkin F, Blumberg AG, et al. The effect of lithium on thyroid functioning, a controlled study. J Psych Res 1974;10:115–120.
26. Lazarus JH. Endocrine and metabolic effects of lithium. New York: Plenum Medical Book Co.; 1980:108.
27. Martino E, Saffan M, Aghinihombard F, et al. Environmental iodine intake and thyroid dysfunction during chronic amiodarone therapy. Ann Int Med 1984;101:28–34.
28. Caplan RH, Gunderson GA, Abillcra RM, Kisker WA: Uptake of iodine-131 by a Meckel's diverticular mimicking metastatic thyroid cancer. J Nucl Med 1987;12:760–762.
29. Rall J, Alpers JB, Waller CG, Sonenberg M, Berman M, & Rawson QW. Radiation pneumonitis and fibrosis complications of radioiodine treatment of pulmonary metastases from cancer of the thyroid. J Clin Endocrinol Metab 1957;17:1263–1276.
30. Buena R, Yeh S, Leeper RS. Radioactive iodine in the therapy of thyroid cancer. J Nucl Med 1988, Abstr, p. 88.
31. Blahd WH. Treatment of malignant thyroid disease. Seminars in Nucl Med 1979:9:95–99.
32. Rasmusson B. Carcinoma of the thyroid: a survey of 227 cases. Acta Rad 1978;17:177–188.
33. Ruegemer JJ, Hay ID, Bergstrach EJ, Ryan JJ, Offord KP, Gorman CA. Distant metastases in differentiated thyroid carcinoma: a multivariate analysis of prognostic variables. J Clin Endocrinol Metab 1988;67:501–558.
34. Hoic V Stenwig AE, Kullman G, Limdegaerd M. Distant metastasis in papillary thyroid cancer: A review of 90 patients. Cancer 1988;6:1–6.
35. Beierwaltes WH, Rabbani R, Dmuchowski C, Lloyd RV, Eyre P, and Mallete S. An analysis of "ablation of thyroid remnants" with I-131 in 511 patients from 1947–1984: experience at University of Michigan. J Nucl Med 1984;25:1287–1293.
36. Baldet L, Manderscheid J-C, Glinoer D, Jaffiol C, Coste-Seignovert B Percheron C. The management of differentiated thyroid cancer in Europe in 1988: results of an international survey. Acta Endocr. 1989;120: 547–558.
37. DeGroot LJ, Reilly M. Comparison of 30- and 50 mCi doses of iodine-131 for thyroid ablation. Ann Intern Med 1982;96:52–53.
38. Goolden AM, Davey JB. The ablation of normal thyroid tissues with iodine-131. Br J Radiol 1963;36: 340–345.
39. Massin JP, Savoie JC, Garnier H et al. Pulmonary metastases in differentiated thyroid carcinoma: study of 58 cases with implications for the primary tumor treatment. Cancer 1984;53:982–992.
40. Piekarski JD, Schlumberger M, Leclere J, Couanet D, Masselot J. Parmentier C. Chest computed tomography (CT) in patients with micronodular lung metastases of differentiated thyroid carcinoma. Int J Radiat Oncol Biol Phys 1985;11:1023–1028.
41. Schlumberger M, Tubiana M, de Valthaire F et al. Long-term results of treatment of 283 patients with lung and bone metastases from differentiated thyroid carcinoma. J Clin Endocrinol Metab 1986;62:960–967.
42. Russell KP, Rose H, and Starr P. The effects of radioactive iodine in maternal and fetal thyroid function during pregnancy. Surg Gynecol Obstet 1957;104:560–567.
43. Goh KO. Radioiodine treatment during pregnancy: chronosomal abberations and cretinism associated with maternal iodine-131 treatment. J Am Med Wom Assoc 1981;36:262–265.
44. Becker D. Oral communication presented at satellite meeting VI, International Thyroid Conference. The Hague, Netherlands 1991.
45. Goolden AWB, Mallard JR, Farran HE. Radiation sialitis following radiation therapy. Br J Radiology 1957;30:210–212.
46. Spiegel W, Reiners C, Borner W. Sialadenitis following iodine-131 therapy for thyroid carcinoma. J Nucl Med 1985;26:816.
47. Glazebrook GA. Effect of decicurie doses of radioactive iodine-131 orl parathyroid function. Am J Surg 1987;154–368.
48. Dobyns BM, Maloof F. The study and treatment of 119 cases of carcinoma of the thyroid with radioactive iodine. J Clin Endocrinol 1951;11:1323–1360.
49. Handelsman DJ, Turtle JR. Testicular damage after radioactive iodine (I-131) therapy for thyroid cancer. J Clin Endocrinol 1983;18:465–472.
50. Robertson JS, Gorman CA, Gonadal radiation dose and its genetic significance in radioactive iodine therapy of hyperthyroidism. J Nucl Med 1976;17:826–831.
51. Raymond JP, Izembart M, Marliac V et al. Temporary ovarian failure in thyroid cancer patients after thyroid remnant ablation with radioactive iodine. J Clin Endocrinol Metab 1989;69:186–190.
52. Carcangiu ML, Steeper T, Zampi G et al. Anaplastic

thyroid carcinoma: a study of 70 cases. Am J Clin Pathol 1985;83:135–158.

53. Segal RL, Silver S, Yohalem SB, & Neuberger RA. Use of radioactive iodine in the treatment of angina pectoris. Am J Cardiol 1958;1:671–681.

54. Holmquest DL, and Lake P. Sudden hemorrhage in metastatic thyroid carcinoma of the brain during treatment with iodine-131. J Nucl Med 1975;17:307–309.

55. Edmonds CJ, and Smith T. Long-term hazards of the treatment of thyroid cancer with radioiodine. Br J Radiol 1986;59:45–49.

8

Medullary Carcinoma of the Thyroid

RHODA H. COBIN

Introduction

Medullary carcinoma was first recognized as a distinct clinical entity in 1959 by Hazzard.[1] Since then, information regarding the biology of this tumor, its clinical behavior, and its involvement in multiple endocrine neoplasia type II has rapidly accumulated. Medullary carcinoma comprises only a small fraction of all thyroid carcinomas, but its importance as a model for the study of peptide secretory tumors and as a preventable cause of mortality (in a familial setting) far outweighs its low frequency of occurrence. In addition, recently developed molecular biologic techniques have yielded new insight into the genetic basis of carcinogenicity in inherited neoplasms.

Demographics

In 1973[2] Hill et al. reported the experience at MD Anderson Hospital (Houston, Texas) with medullary carcinoma. Of 777 patients with thyroid cancer, 73 (9%) of the patients had medullary carcinoma, and of these, 43 were female and 31 male (a 1.4:1 ratio, compared with a 2.5:1 ratio seen in other thyroid cancers in their institution). The age range was 15 to 82 years of age and the average was 47 years. There was no predominance by race. This distribution is similar in subsequent series.[3,4] In centers where screening for familial disease has been aggressive, patients are detected at a younger age[5] (*vide infra*). Familial medullary carcinoma of the thyroid is thought to comprise roughly 20% of the total, although as more families of affected individuals are studied, the incidence will surely rise.

Clinical Presentation

While in screening studies for familial disease, patients are now detected chemically, presentation in the sporadic setting is no different from patients with other forms of cancer of the thyroid. All patients present with a neck mass. Only 7% have pressure sensation or dysphagia, and 9% have diarrhea or other symptoms related to distant metastases (although as many as 32% of patients previously diagnosed with medullary carcinoma developed diarrhea, which may be hormonally mediated). Thus, the presence of diarrhea and a neck mass may offer a possible presurgical diagnostic clue.[1]

Radiography

Preoperative clues to the presence of medullary carcinoma of the thyroid may be present in routine x-rays of the neck and chest. Soft tissue films may reveal typical dense homogeneous conglomerate calcifications, generally bilateral, in the thyroid lobes. Metastases to regional nodes may also calcify. The appearance is distinctly different from the faint homogeneous "psammomatous" calcifications seen with other thyroid carcinomas. When medullary carcinoma of the thyroid metastasizes to the liver, the lesions may also develop typically dense conglomerate calcifications. In the lungs an interstitial nodular infiltrate occurs with metastases, sometimes with hilar and mediastinal nodes; calcification does not appear to occur in the chest and mediastinum. Bone lesions of metastatic medullary carcinoma of the thyroid are generally lytic and do not differ from other lytic metastases.[6]

Cytology

Fine needle aspiration biopsy, commonly employed in the evaluation of solitary thyroid nodules, may yield valuable preoperative clues to the presence of a medullary carcinoma (Fig. 8.1). Tumor cells are larger than normal follicular cells. Their size varies; the largest are multinucleated giant cells. Cells may be individual or present in cohesive groups. Spindle shape or triangular cells with dendritic extensions are highly suggestive of medullary carcinoma. The cell cytoplasm is usually amphophilic and structureless, but a distinctive red granulation is seen in up to 5 to 15% of cells. With May-Grunwald-Giemsa staining, they appear azurophilic, do not stain with eosin, and show weak metachromasia with toluidine. The cellular nuclei are eccentrically positioned, dark, sharply outlined, and often binucleate or multinucleate. Distinct nucleoli and mitoses are rarely seen. Amyloid may be recognized in smears as cloudy, amorphous lumps of a substance staining gray-blue or violet with May-Grunwald-Giemsa stain and bright red with hemotoxylin eosin.[7] Although amyloid may be identified presumptively on Papanicolau stains, it is confirmed by restaining with Congo red. With alkaline Congo, the amyloid is bright red in common light and exhibits green birefringence in polarized light. Generally, this material is present outside the cells, but may be present intracellularly as well. Geddie et al.[8] emphasized the importance of spindle cells and note that cytoplasmic granules stain positive for calcitonin by the immunoperoxidase technique. Papanicolau-stained slides may be decolorized for subsequent immunoperoxidase and Congo red stains.

Histopathology

When medullary carcinoma is seen on gross examination, it is firm, solid, grayish, or pale brown, well demarcated from surrounding tissues, or may be infiltrating. Microscopically, the typical appearance is that of polyhedral neoplastic cells arranged in sheets or irregular trabeculae and divided into nests by fibrous connective tissue septae (Fig. 8.2). Spindle cells may comprise anywhere from a small fraction to the predominate portion of the tumor, are generally seen with less amyloid, and may be associated with a relatively poor prognosis.[1,9] Amyloid deposition may be either abundant or scanty (Fig. 8.3); In up to 25% of cases, it may be absent altogether. Amyloid may be seen by Congo red stain under polarized light and is best seen as typical amyloid fibrils on electron miscroscopy. The amyloid in medullary carcinoma is composed of a soluble P component (common to all amyloid) and a unique fibrillar protein of 5700 molecular weight that may have some homology to calcitonin. This is believed to represent a prohormone of calcitonin or a fragment of a precursor.[10] Immunohistochemistry generally reveals dense staining of most tumor cells with calcitonin antiserum.

C-cell hyperplasia[11] is identified by means of immunocytochemistry usually occurring at the junction of the upper and middle half of the thyroid lobes. C-cell hyperplasia begins with a diffuse increase in the number and size of C cells as compared with normal controls. At first the pathology is restricted to the normal parafollicular location; it progressively encircles, displaces, and compresses follicular elements producing solid intrafollicular aggregates of C cells with complete replacement of the follicular epithelium, forming nodular hyperplasia. When C cells break through the basement membrane of the follicle and encircle the interstitium, micromedullary carcinoma of the thyroid is diagnosed.[11] Carcinoembryonic antigen (CEA) immunostaining may be present in either C-cell hyperplasia or micro-medullary carcinoma of the thyroid.[12]

In familial cases there are often microscopic foci of C-cell hyperplasia, or microscopic medullary carcinoma of the thyroid in areas of normal parenchyma, thus demonstrating a multicentric tumor origin.[13]

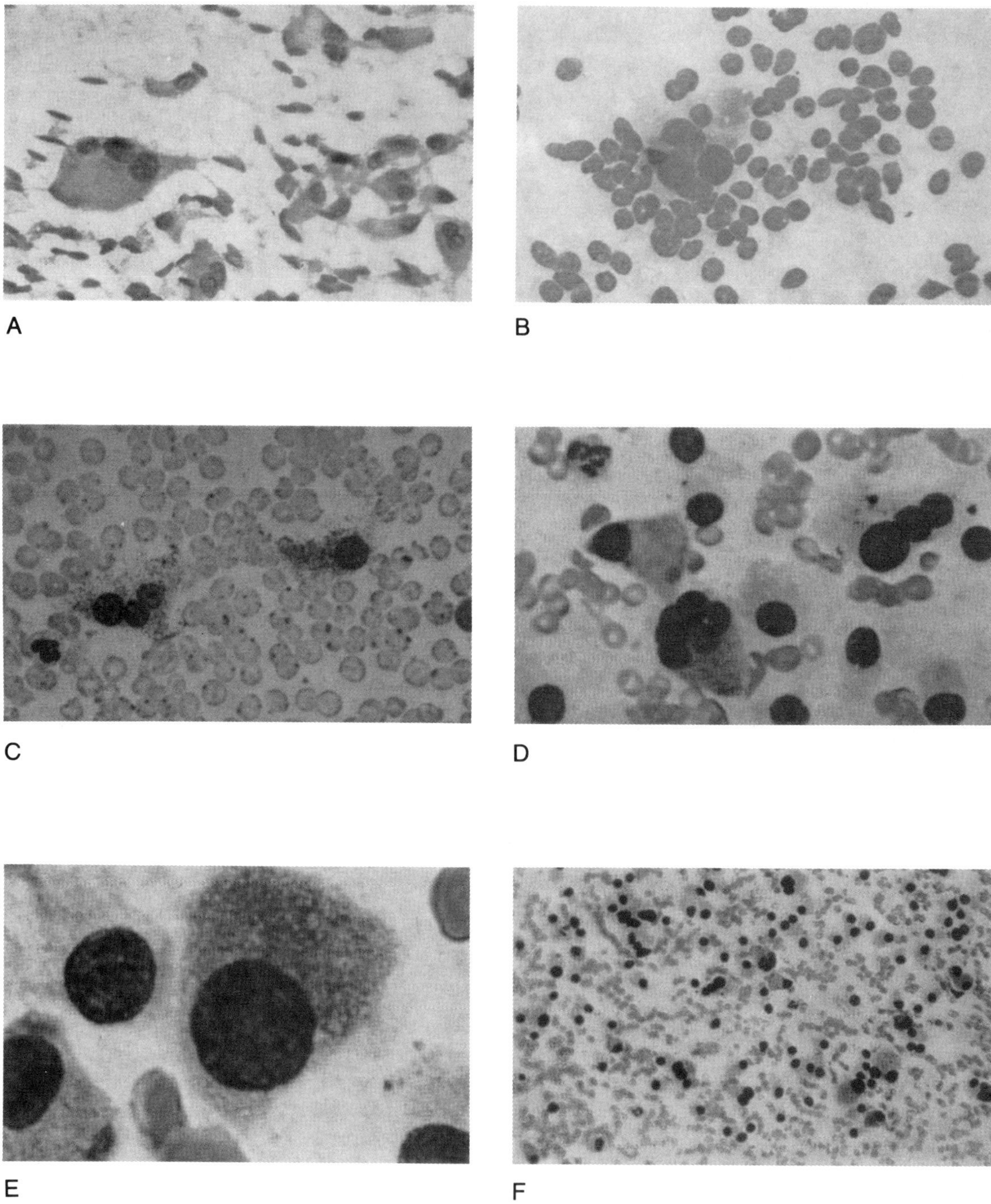

Figure 8.1. Representative samples of cells obtained from fine needle aspirates. In B, nonspecific small tumor cells are seen, along with more diagnostic red-granulated giant cells. C demonstrates angulated dendritic cells with eccentrically placed nuclei, and D shows characteristic triangular cells. In K, the bluish gray cytoplasmic condensations are thought to be amyloid. Aspirates may be stained Congo red for amyloid and viewed with non-polarized light as in G or in polarized light as in F. Reprinted, by permission from Soderstrom N, Telenius-Berg M, Akerman A, 1975. (7)

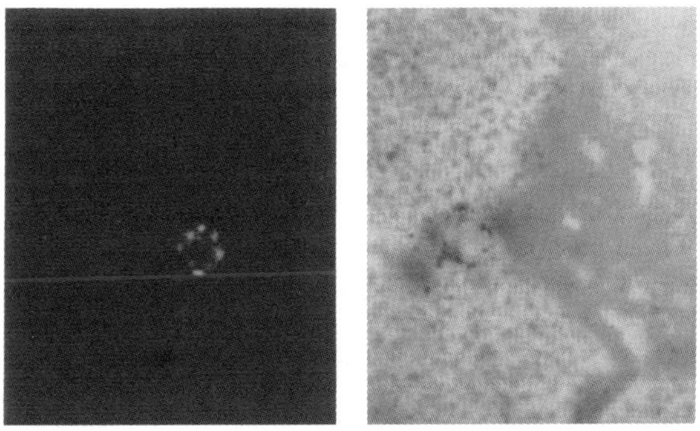
G

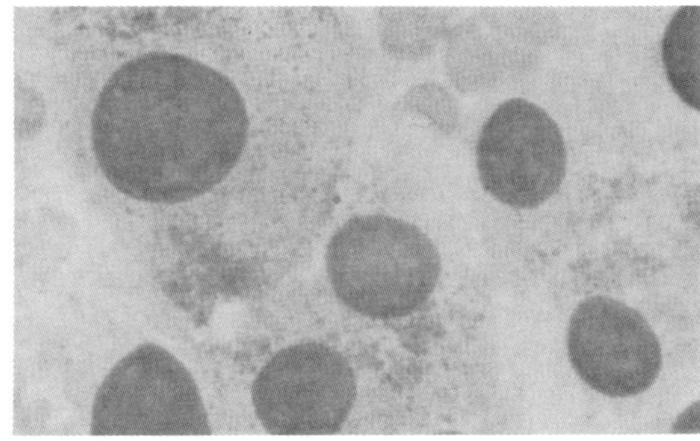
H

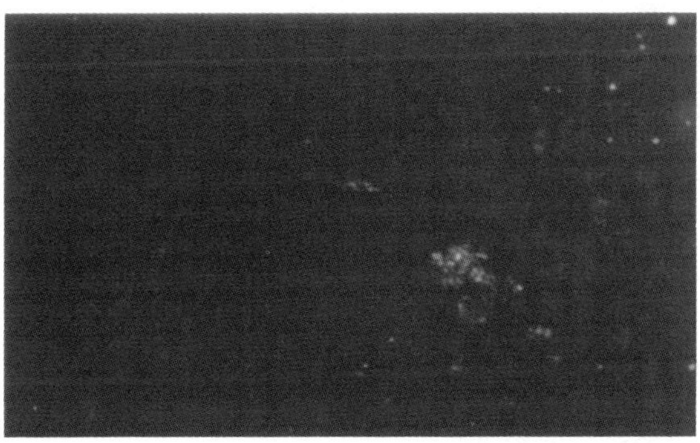
I

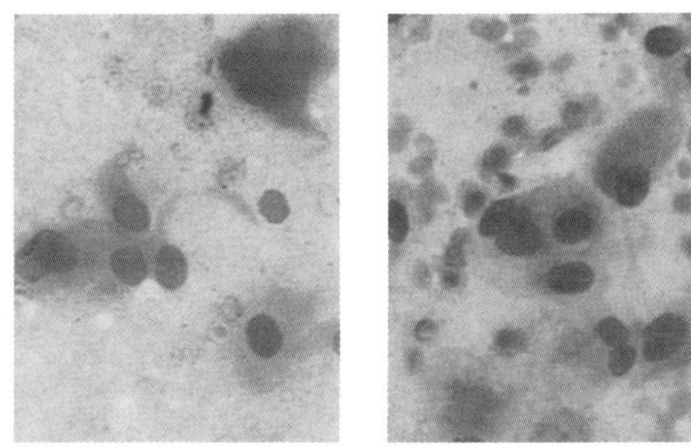
J

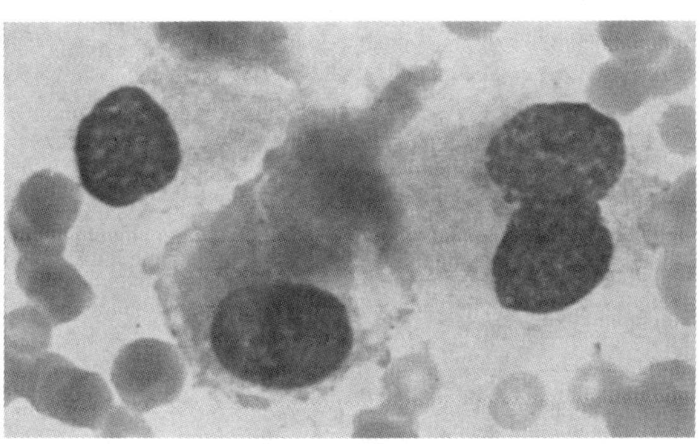
K

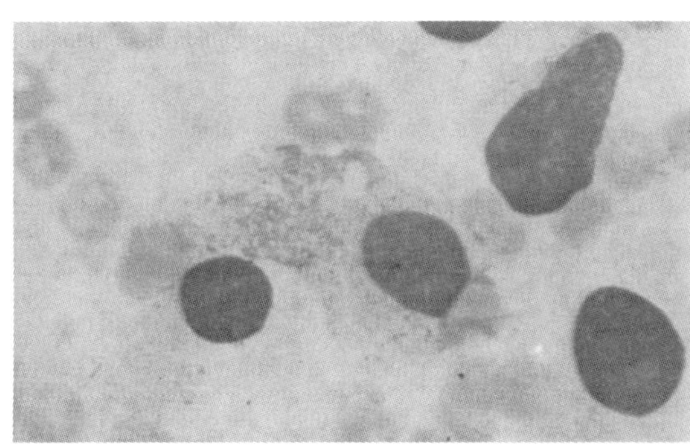
L

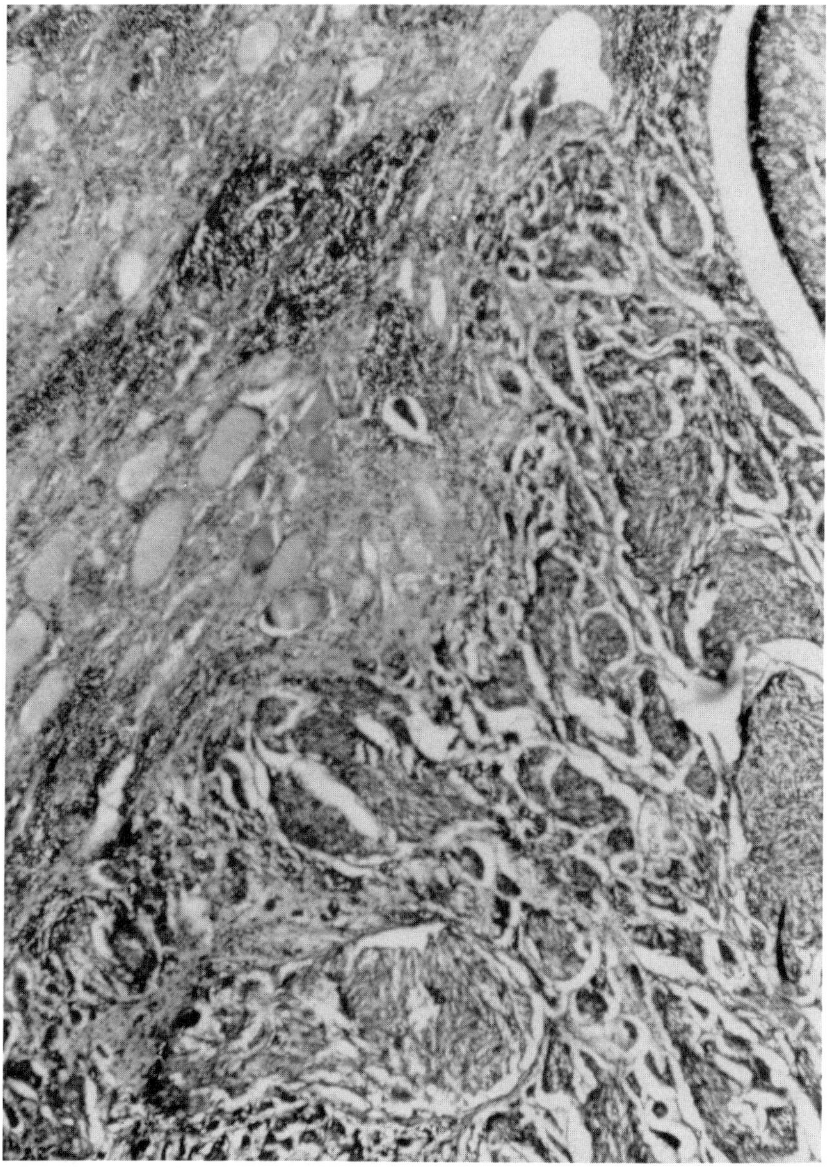

Figure 8.2. Histopathology of medullary carcinoma.

Electron Microscopy

On electron microscopy tumor cells bear a striking resemblance to the thyroid parafollicular cells (C cells) from which they are derived (Fig. 8.4). A well-developed Golgi apparatus is visible, from which small vesicles of 40 to 160 mμ appear to pinch off. These are scattered further throughout the cytoplasm, along with secretory granules and vacuoles containing secretory products. These secretory *vacuoles*, which measure 170 to 530 mμ, are clear and contain only a scanty amount of finely granular material. Secretory *granules* have a single limiting membrane and contain abundant, dense, finely granular material. A narrow, clear halo is sometimes seen just beneath the limiting membrane. Rough endoplasmic reticulum,

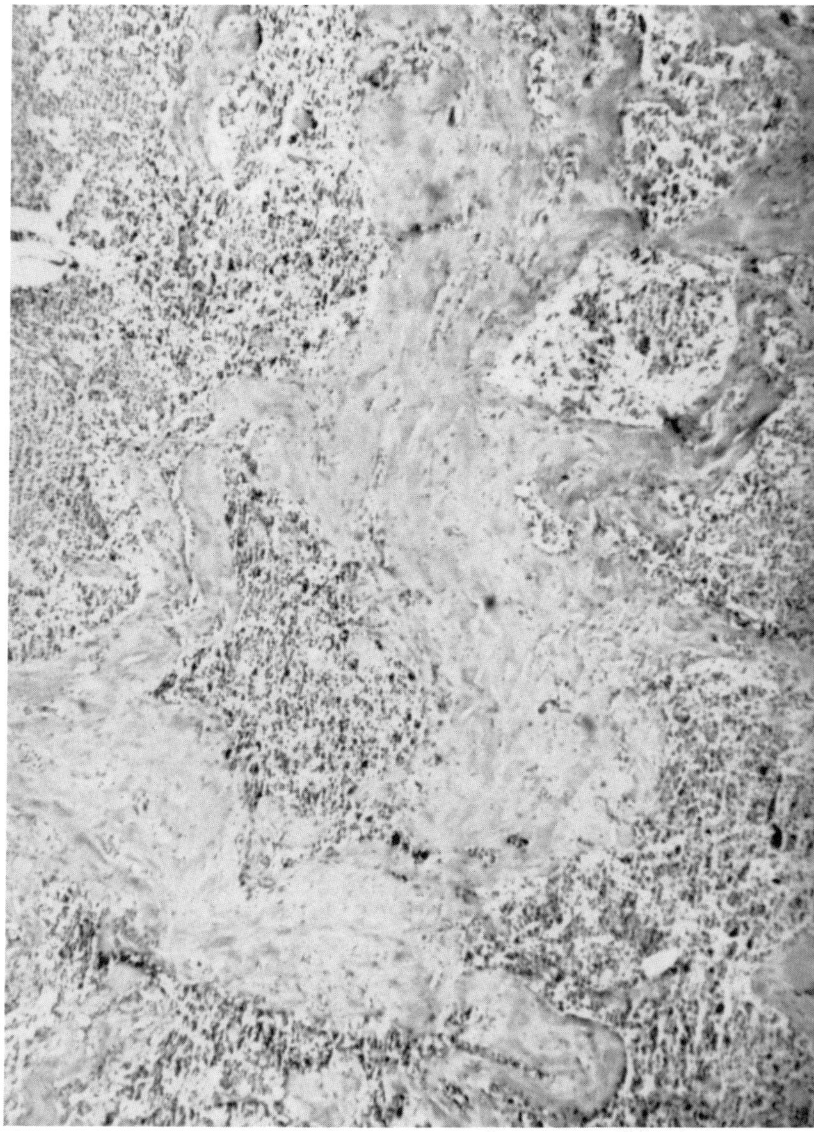

Figure 8.2. (*cont.*)

smooth endoplasmic reticulum, and mitochondria are not numerous. Amyloid fibrils may be identified. By electron miscroscopy, medullary carcinoma often cannot be differentiated from pancreatic islet cell tumors and from carcinoid tumors, lending support to the concept that these cells are all derived from similar primordial, neuroendocrine cells and share a similar oncogenesis.[14,15]

Biogenic Amines

As long ago as 1967, it was recognized that medullary carcinoma stained positive for chromaffin and argentaffin reactions. Formaldehyde vapor-induced fluorescence is able to detect 5-hydroxytryptamine, but epinephrine or norepinephrine in some medullary carcinomas. A similar phenomenon has been found in carci-

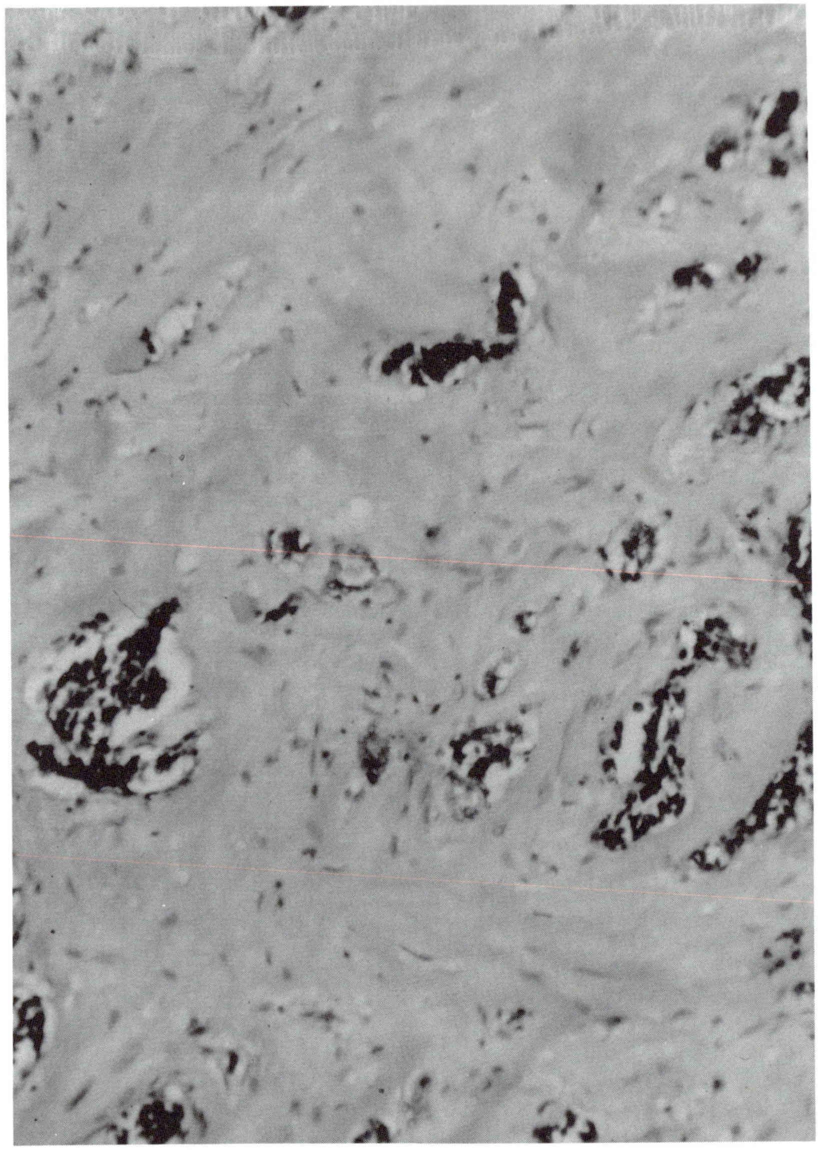

Figure 8.3. Amyloid in medullary carcinoma.

noid tumors.[16,17] The ability of these tumors to pick up amine precursors and decarboxylate them, the demonstration of DOPA-decarboxylase in tissue and the presence of neuron-specific enolase isoenzyme, led to the conclusion that medullary carcinoma, as well as other cells of similar structure, form a series of "APUD-cell" tumors. It was proposed that "neuroendocrine cells migrate into the primitive alimentary tract mucosa and are carried with the developing endocrine glands to their final resting places where they mature in the endocrine cells of the anterior pituitary thyroid, parathyroid, islets of Langerhans, ultimobranchial body and thymus."[18] These cells have the capacity to develop into a wide variety of peptide-producing endocrine tumors, including medullary carcinoma, pheochromocytoma, carcinoid, and islet cell tumors.[19] The similarity in ultrastructural characteristics, as well as the cosecretion of peptides of the gut, both eutopic and ectopic, might be explained

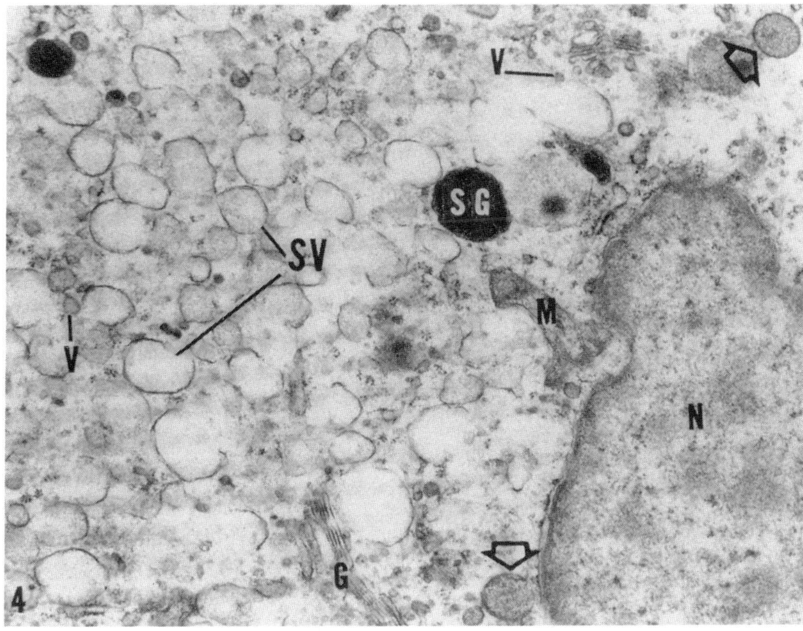

Figure 8.4. Medullary carcinoma of thyroid. There are many secretory vacuoles (**SV**) that appear to be clear and have an incomplete limiting membrane. Some secretory granules (**SG**) are dark and others have a less dense, finely granular content (arrows). Small vesicles (**V**) occur near the Golgi apparatus (**G**) and secretorv bodies. A distorted mitochondrion (**M**) and a portion of the nucleus (**N**) are also shown. Uranyl acetate and lead citrate stain. (original magnification ×22,600) Reprinted by permission, from Gonzalez-Licea A, Hartman WH, Yardley JH, 1968. (14) Copyright by the American Society of Clinical Pathologist 1968.

by the potential of precursor cells to form tumors; hence, the syndrome of multiple endocrine neoplasms could be explained as a "dysplasia of neuroectoderm." This may be genetically determined, at least in familial cases. Although the common neuroectodermal origin of these tumors has been challenged,[20] their ultrastructural and chemical similarities remain.

Pathologic Variants

Variants of medullary carcinoma may present with primarily follicular or papillary architecture.[21] Experienced pathologists differentiate these structures on the basis of their histologic description as being "glandular" rather than truly follicular. Furthermore, these cells stain positive for calcitonin and not thyroglobulin as would be the case if they were truly derived from thyroid follicular epithelium. The papillary structures contain multiple cell layers and small nuclei with condensed chromatin, as contrasted with true papillary carcinoma, in which there is only one cell layer and in which the nuclei show typical ground glass and/or grooved appearance.[22] Since up to 25% of all cases of medullary carcinoma may lack stainable amyloid, this is a poor differential point.

More confusing are the reports of tumors composed of mixed histologic elements,[23] including one tumor that contains elements of medullary, papillary, follicular, and undifferentiated patterns in both primary tumor and metastases. Immunoperoxidase staining localized both calcitonin and thyroglobulin in areas of medullary and follicular elements. The papillary elements fulfilled the classic criteria, including typical nuclei and psammoma bodies. These tumors have been postulated to have an origin from an undifferentiated stem cell derived from primitive pharyngeal pouch tissue.

To further complicate the issue, Holm et al.[24] reported 14 cases of medullary carcinoma with double staining for thyrocalcitonin and thyroglobulin in both primary tumors and metastases, both in solid and follicular areas in otherwise histologically classical-appearing medullary carcinoma. Thyroglobulin and calcitonin were colocalized within the same cell, and in some cases with calcitonin gene-related peptide (CGRP) and bombesin in both the primary and metastatic tumors. Although entrapment of normal thyroid elements and phagocytosis of thyroglobulin have been proposed as a mechanism for the colocalization, it is possible that the tumor derives from primitive stem cells, and then develops characteristics of both follicular and parafollicular cells. In situ hybridization methods to search for RNA for both peptides are necessary to verify this hypothesis.

Finally, C-cell hyperplasia has been found in tissue adjacent to non-medullary carcinomas, both papillary and follicular.[25] In these cases, the primary tumors did not stain positive for calcitonin. In only one case was elevated serum calcitonin measured; the rest of the cases were studied retrospectively, and no correlation was made with serum calcitonin levels. Therefore, the possibility of confusion with a medullary carcinoma in a patient with a thyroid mass and elevated calcitonin was raised. In fact, however, such a patient would come to surgery, and subsequent careful histologic and immunocytochemical staining would resolve any diagnostic dilemmas.

The author has noted occasional cases in which C-cell hyperplasia in a nonfamilial setting has been discovered serendipitously on finding an elevated calcitonin level. In such a situation, when calcitonin can be hyperstimulated with pentagastrin, regardless of the family history, it is still incumbent on the physician to exclude the premalignant variety of C-cell hyperplasia by surgical intervention.

Calcitonin

As early as 1970 it was noted that calcitonin was secreted by medullary carcinoma of the thyroid and could be localized in normal and neoplastic parafollicular C cells; an analogous phenomenon in birds is the secretion of calcitonin in the ultimobranchial bodies, which are derived from the fourth and fifth pharyngeal pouches.[26] Calcitonin is normally present in only low concentration, but in medullary carcinoma of the thyroid, it is increased and usually correlates with the extent of tumor burden.

Using a sensitive radioimmunoassay for calcitonin, Tashjian et al. noted that in normal thyroid glands, tissue calcitonin concentrations correlate well with the presence of C cells stained by the immunoperoxidase technique in the middle third of the lateral lobes, lying deep within the gland, along the hypothetical central axis of each lobe (Fig 8.5). Medullary carcinomas develop at this site. Neonates and children have more C cells. Normal thyroids contain few C cells and less calcitonin, although occasionally small clusters of parafollicular cells have been seen in routine autopsies. The importance of this is unclear, as these subjects were not studied while they were alive.[27]

Calcitonin, a 32 amino acid, 3,500 molecular weight peptide, was first discovered by Copp in 1962.[28] It is initially secreted as a 15,000 molecular weight prohormone, which is then cleaved to form the smaller molecular weight active hormone. Study of the gene encoding the prohormone for thyrocalcitonin predicted that calcitonin gene-related peptide and PDN-21 would also be found, and this has proved to be the case.[29,30] There are species differences in amino acid composition. Radioimmunoassay[26] has resulted in greater ease of measurement, which has significantly affected both the ability to understand normal and pathologic physiology and the practical ease with which medullary carcinoma is detected and managed of. On gel filtration, calcitonin is heterogeneous; it is contained in five or more peaks, particularly in patients with medullary carcinoma and lung tumors.[31,32] Larger molecular weight, biologically inert forms are apparently formed by disulfide linkage and, to a lesser extent, by aggregation and noncovalent protein binding. Monomeric human calcitonin, which is silica extractable, is believed to be the only biologically active hormone; it often comprises 15% or less of the total hormone in patients with tumors, but is the primary calcitonin obtained in stimulated samples. The predomi-

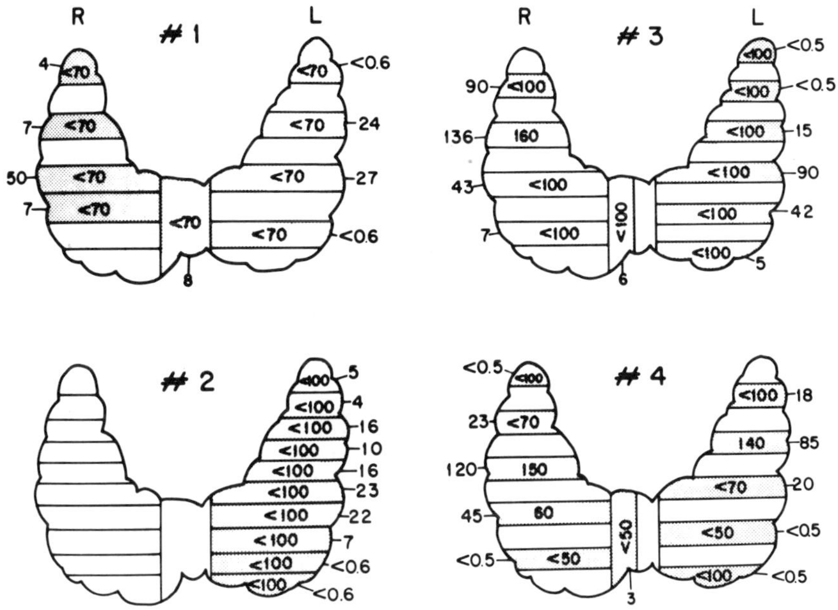

Figure 8.5. Location of C cells and calcitonin content in normal thyroid. Numbers inside refer to calcitonin content while numbers outside refer to C cell population by immunocytochemistry. Reprinted, by permission from Wolfe, Noekel, and Tashjian, cateritonzin-containing all distribution in thyroid. J Clin Endo Metab 1974;38–688. Copyright by The Endocrine Society, 1974.

nance of biologically inactive product may help to explain the relative infrequence of bone mineral abnormalities in affected subjects.[33,34] Radioreceptor assays using bone and renal cell membrane displacement, cyclic AMP production, or both have yielded important physiologic information, but have not yet proven to be practical in the assessment of clinical disease.[31]

Calcitonin is the specific product of the thyroid C cells (parafollicular cells), although immunoperoxidase staining has localized calcitonin in pituitary, lung, thymus, liver, and bladder; and calcium-lowering activity has been found in parathyroid, thymus, and adrenal medulla. Whether or not calcitonin is actually produced in these locations has been the subject of debate, as it could be that simple adsorption may occur. This phenomenon may have some importance when elevated calcitonin is noted postoperatively in patients who have had surgery for medullary carcinoma.[28]

In man, under normal physiologic conditions, calcitonin has been shown to inhibit osteoclastic bone resorption. Bone density may be affected by total thyroidectomy, I-131 ablation of the thyroid, and chronic severe hypercalcitoninemia,[33] although none of these seem to be clinically important. In the kidney, calcitonin increases renal tubular wasting of calcium, phosphate, sodium, potassium, and magnesium. In the bowel, calcitonin decreases gastric and gastric acid secretion and increases small bowel secretion of sodium, chloride, and water. This may contribute to the diarrhea seen in medullary carcinoma. Physiologically, calcitonin secretion is regulated primarily by calcium; it is stimulated by high calcium concentrations and inhibited by low calcium levels (Table 8.1). Secretagogues for calcitonin release of uncertain physiologic importance include gastrin and biogenic amines (alpha-adrenergic stimulatory and beta-adrenergic and dopaminergic inhibitory effect). Somatostatin, which is colocalized in C cells with calcitonin, may play a paracrine inhibitory role. Calcitonin is generally present in higher levels in men, neonates, children, and pregnant and lactating women, and declines slightly with

Table 8.1. Calcitonin responses to calcium and pentagastrin stimulation in normal subjects

	Calcitonin value (pg/ml)					
	Calcium infusion*			Pentagastrin injection†		
Group	Basal	5 min	10 min	Basal	1.5 min	5 min
Men (N = 18)						
Mean‡	7	43	25	7	25	21
Median	7	58	50	6	19	19
Range	3–19	6–190	3–150	<2–19	4–260	2–170
Women (N = 37)						
Mean‡	3	10	8	3	5	4
Median	3	9	9	3	5	4
Range	<2–16	<2–130	<2–130	<2–11	<2–33	<2–24

Reprinted, by permission, from Gharib, H., Kao, P.C. and Heath, H., 1987(92).

advancing age. The marked hyperstimulatability found with synthetic gastrin (pentagastrin) and calcium have formed the basis for stimulation studies that led to the recognition of the premalignant entity C cell hyperplasia and, therefore, to the earlier detection and cure of medullary carcinoma in a familial setting (see below).[36] Calcitonin is elevated in all cases of clinically palpable medullary carcinoma; however, in smaller tumors and C-cell hyperplasia, basal levels may be normal. In these instances, only stimulation will divulge pathology.

Calcitonin levels are also increased in renal failure, in which clearance, especially of the large molecular weight form, is diminished. In pernicious anemia and in Zollinger-Ellison syndrome, calcitonin may be elevated, perhaps in response to chronic elevations of gastrin. In acute gastrointestinal bleeding, acute pancreatitis, regional ileitis, cirrhosis, and hepatocellular carcinoma, calcitonin may also be inexplicably elevated. In acute and chronic pulmonary disease, calcitonin levels are increased, which is possibly being secreted by pulmonary endocrine K (Kulchitsky) cells.[37,38] In hyperparathyroidism, small increases in basal and stimulated calcitonin have been observed,[39] although in most of the other phenomena that cause chronic hypercalcemia this has not usually been noted. In some patients with hypercalcemia of malignancy, calcitonin may be elevated; but it is speculated that calcitonin may in this situation be directly secreted by the tumor itself. Basal calcitonin levels two to three times normal without hyperstimulatability have been seen in patients with hyperthyroidism, as well as in those with hypothyroidism.[40] Body[41] et al. reported the cases of five seemingly normal men with elevated basal and stimulated immunoassayable calcitonin, which did not parallel standard dilution curves, and which was abolished by prior silica extraction of their serum. They speculate that unusual individuals may have circulating high molecular weight, biologically inactive forms of calcitonin that are slowly cleared. These patients, however, were not subject to surgical intervention; hence there was no absolute confirmation that their C cells were indeed normal.

Calcitonin has been shown unequivocally to be produced "ectopically" in non-medullary tumors. Tumors noted to be associated with ectopic secretion of calcitonin include APUD-cell derived tumors, especially small cell carcinoma of the lung, in which elevated calcitonin may be noted in as many as 75% of cases, often with levels as high as those seen in medullary carcinoma. Other tumors in which this phenomenon has been reported include pancreatic islet cell tumors and carcinoid.[42] Non-APUD cell tumors that have been associated with elevated calcitonin include non-islet cell tumors of the pancreas, breast, prostate, colon, stomach, esophageal, uterine, and bladder cancer.[43–45]

In most cases, the serum calcitonin concentration could not be further increased by calcium or pentagastrin stimulation, but in a few cases, notably those of Coombes[46] and Haansen[47], significant increases above baseline did occur. This has caused speculation that, at least in some cases, elevated calcitonin is a manifestation of chronic calcium release from occult bone metastases, and is therefore really of thyroidal origin; that selective venous catheterization reveals a hormone gradient from the thyroid bed strengthens this argument.[48] Calcitonin has been extracted from tumors, and most importantly, calcitonin release from tumor cells has been demonstrated in vitro.[49,50] Becker et al.[37] emphasized that thyrocalcitonin of medullary carcinoma origin may be more heterogeneous in molecular weight than calcitonin produced by other disorders. He and others differentiated the two sources of calcitonin using an antiserum directed at the carboxy terminal of the molecule. Medullary carcinoma calcitonin is universally recognized, whereas the hypercalcitoninemia caused by other nonthyroidal malignancy, especially lung cancer, is better recognized by a midportion antiserum.[51] This differential testing is cumbersome and not practical for most cases, but may have value in the unusual situation in which there is doubt of the origin of calcitonin, especially preoperatively in a nonfamilial case of the disorder.

Additional Secretory Products

Medullary carcinoma, along with other "APUD cell tumors," may secrete a variety of peptide hormones in addition to its normal cell product, calcitonin. DOPA-decarboxylase and histaminase, a diamine oxidase, are frequently detected in both primary tumor and metastases. Histaminase is only detected in carcinoma, not in normal C cells or C-cell hyperplasia.[52] Some studies have suggested that the proportions of the normal product, calcitonin, DOPA-decarboxylase, and histaminase may have prognostic significance,[53] (vide infra). Most of the peptide secretory products are chemically silent, but ectopic production of ACTH has been responsible for Cushing's syndrome;[54,55] and VIP and prostaglandin production in addition to calcitonin excess itself have been implicated in the diarrhea that is often seen, especially with large tumor burdens.[56–59]

Chromogranin, a soluble peptide which is co-stored and co-released by exocytosis with catecholamines from the adrenal medulla, is nearly universally detected in human polypeptide hormone producing tumors, including medullary carcinoma.[60] One case of C cell hyperplasia was positive in the original series, and one case of medullary carcinoma was negative for calcitonin staining, but positive for chromogranin.[61] In vitro, phorbol esters simultaneously stimulate RNA for both chromogranin and calcitonin in medullary carcinoma and lung carcinoma cells.[62] Other peptides detected in medullary carcinoma by immunohistochemical staining include cytokaratin (100% of tumors studied), CGRP (calcitonin gene-related peptide) (92%), CEA (77%), neuron-specific enolase (75%), and Vimentin (53%). Variable smaller numbers of tumors contained neurotensin, somatostatin, neurofilaments, bombesin, alpha human chorionic gonadotropin (hCG), and serotonin.[63]

In rat medullary carcinoma CGRP, an alternate product of the calcitonin gene, is produced. CGRP mRNA is released in vivo because of a defect in transcript processing.[64] Unlike calcitonin, CGRP seems to be unresponsive to calcium stimulation,[65] making it unreliable as a preliminary diagnostic tool, although it may be useful in following up some tumors that have relatively weak calcitonin secretion. Similarly, PDN-21, a 21–amino acid carboxy terminal–adjacent peptide produced from human calcitonin precursor mRNA has also been measured[66] in many normal subjects; its level increases after calcium infusion, with a greater response found in males than in females. No normal subjects, but some subjects genetically at risk for medullary carcinoma, hyperresponed to calcium stimulation.

Gastrin-releasing peptide (GRP), a 27–amino acid mammalian homolog of the amphibian 14–amino acid peptide bombesin is widely distributed in the lung, brain, and GI tract; where it modulates sympathetic and parasympathetic functions in neuronal cells, and stimulates the release of many hormones, including gastrin, glucagon, and growth hormone. It has been implicated as a growth factor and as a factor in the development of neoplasia in pulmonary neuroendocrine cells. Sunday et al.[67] found 20-fold greater levels of this peptide in neonates, with a strong correlation with calcitonin levels. Most neonatal cells are positive for GRP, although only about 5% to 18% of normal adult cells contain this activity. In the cases of C cell hyperplasia and medullary carcinoma, more GRP is identified, lending support to the idea that it may play a role in the growth or neoplastic formation of these cells. The GRP receptor has been shown to be functionally coupled to the P-21 product of the RAS oncogene.[68]

Sikkri et al.[69] studied 25 cases of medullary carcinoma with immunocytochemical and histochemical stains. All tumors reacted to CGRP and PDN 21 stain, sometimes more strongly than to calcitonin antiserum. Somatostatin and bombesin activity were weak or inconsistent markers. As a general marker of neuroendocrine neoplasia, Grumelius argyrophil silver staining and the stain for chromogranin A were more consistent than neuron-specific enolase isoenzyme immunoreactivity.

In vivo however, GI hormones, including vasoactive intestinal peptide (VIP), gastrin, glucagon, insulin and pancreatic polypeptide, bear little relationship to tumor burden or prognosis, nor are they correlated with the presence of diarrhea.[57]

Prognostic Features

It had been hoped that the in vivo biologic virulence of tumor could be predicted by either histologic characteristics of tumor or differential staining of the tumor (perhaps reflecting dedifferentiation) for various products. Baylin's group[53] felt that homogeneous, intense calcitonin staining characterized tumors with an indolent course, while more aggressive tumors had patchy, less diffuse calcitonin staining with more heterogeneity, including more staining for DOPA-decarboxylase and histaminase. Using the density and homogeneity of calcitonin staining as the sole marker, Saad et al.[70] reached a similar conclusion. Markedly elevated or rising CEA levels in both tumor and serum have been associated with a less favorable prognosis than those with low or stable levels of CEA.[71,72] More recently, however, Schroeder et al.[63] demonstrated that prognosis was not found to be related to histologic features such as dominant architectural pattern, cellular shape, presence of amyloid deposits, or immunocytochemical stains for a variety of peptides.

Cytometry

Analysis of DNA content and nuclear cell phase distribution by several methods has been employed in evaluating tumor prognosis in a variety of malignancies. Recently, small numbers of thyroid cancers have been studied, including a very few medullary carcinomas. Although the conclusions have not been consistent, the most recent reports suggest that these exists a definite role for this modality.

In 1983, Tangen[73] studied 10 medullary carcinomas by flow cytometry and concluded that the percentage of cells in S phase was higher than in follicular carcinoma, but lower than in anaplastic carcinoma. DNA histography showed diploid or hyperdiploid patterns that were not correlated with survival rates in five medullary carcinoma of the thyroid tumors subjected to simple cell cytophotometry by Bengtsson et al.[74] The only patient with recurrent or metastatic disease had a hyperdiploid pattern. In Kramer's 1985 report,[75] four patients with medullary carcinoma of the thyroid were included, of whom only one showed aneuploidy; one patient with extensive metastases and a diploid DNA content revealed nonetheless a high proliferative activity. Backdahl[76] analyzed 32 tumors and found that DNA content as determined by cytophotometry correlated to age, tumor size, invasion, or metastases. Knowledge of DNA content yielded a predictive value equivalent to that of postoperative clinical information and, when added to this information, significantly increased prognostic accuracy. In Schroder's 1988 series, 25 patients with medullary carcino-

Feature	Hereditary	Sporadic
Cases	58 in 8 families	24
M-F ratio	22:36	11:13
Others in family affected	Yes	No
Pathologic features	Bilateral in 40/41; associated C cell hyperplasia	All unilateral; no C cell hyperplasia
Other endocrine involvement	Part of MEN-2 syndrome	Not part of MEN syndrome
Parathyroid	9 in 4 families	0
Adrenal medulla	6 in 4 families	0
Ectopic ACTH production	2 in 2 families	0
Associated malignancy	Pancreas in 3	0
Mucosal neuromas	0 in this series	0
Age of onset in cases prior to serum calcitonin assay, yr	36 (average) in 20 cases (20-67)	50 in 24 cases (22-74)
Curability by surgery based on serum calcitonin assay	23/23 nonpalpable (100%); 3/18 palpable (17%)	9/20 (45%), all palpable
Surgical approach	Total thyroidectomy	Total thyroidectomy may not always be necessary
Average life expectancy, yr	50 in 20 cases (44 in those 4 families with pheochromocytomas)	66 in 7 cases
Associated mental illness	14	3

Figure 8.6. Comparison of hereditary and sporadic varieties of medullary thyroid carcinoma. Reprinted, by permission, from Block, MA et al, 1980. (13) Copyright 1980 by the American Medical Association.

ma of the thyroid were analyzed: 20 with flow cytometry, 11 with cytophotometry, and 6 with both. In cases in which both methods were used, the results were similar. A benign course was twice as frequent among patients whose tumors had normal DNA content compared to those patients whose tumors had higher DNA content. Examining cell cycle phase yielded even further information.

The Mayo Clinic[77] retrospectively analyzed 110 familial and sporadic medullary carcinoma of the thyroid tumors resected from 1948 to 1986, with a mean follow-up of 12.3 years. Flow cytometry data revealed that nondiploid DNA was associated with older age, sporadic disease, local invasion, and advanced tumor stage; death from medullary carcinoma of the thyroid occurred in 42% of nondiploid versus only 10% of diploid tumors. Of the fatal diploid tumors, 56% had more than 15% S-phase fraction.

In 1970 McLeod et al.[78] summarized previous series of medullary carcinomas. They believe that flow cytometry might not be as accurate as single nuclei cytophotometry. They calculated that approximately 40% of medullary carcinomas of the thyroid are diploid, with a 22% survival, while 20% to 80% are aneuploid (mean 35%), with 44% patient deaths.

Familial Syndromes

Medullary carcinoma may occur in either a sporadic or familial form (Fig. 8.6). Pathologically, the latter is distinguished by its uniform bilaterality, the consistent association of C cell hyperplasia, and the frequent presence of pheochromocytoma, parathyroid adenoma, or hyperplasia.[13] In about 20% of cases of presumably sporadic disease, there are bilateral tumors.[79] In these cases, it is not clear whether this finding represents undetected familial disease, intrathyroidal spread, or true multicentric origin of the tumor. In hereditary medullary carcinoma of the thyroid, the average age of recognition before calcitonin stimulation was available was 36 years, compared with 50 years for the sporadic type.[13] However, this figure drops dramatically as more frequent screening of families is performed (see below).

Familial medullary carcinoma, which is inherited as an autosomal dominant trait, may present in three distinct forms that are distinguished by the frequency and type of associated lesions. In MEN-2A, medullary carcinoma is 100% expressed and hyperparathyroidism occurs in 34%, and pheochromocytomas in 33% to 50% of cases, depending upon the family (Fig. 8.7). Since the pheochromocytoma

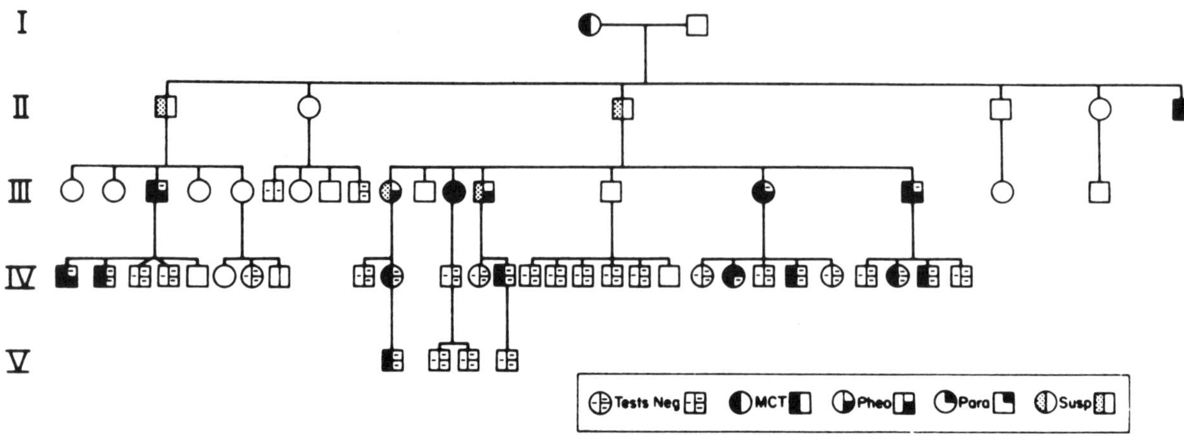

Figure 8.7. A typical kindred of MEN 2A. Reprinted, by permission, from Cance WG and Wells SA Jr, Multiple endocrine neoplasia type IIa. Curr Probl Surg, 1985;22(5):1.

may be clinically silent but potentially fatal during anesthesia, catecholamines should be measured in all patients prior to neck surgery. If pheochromocytoma is found, it must be cured first before surgery is attempted. The medullary carcinoma in this situation is moderately aggressive. In Well's series,[80] 17% of medullary carcinoma patients died of cancer. Clinically palpable lesions may not be present until the second or third decade of life, but C-cell hyperplasia may be found on stimulation in children as young as $1\frac{1}{2}$ years, thus offering the possibility of a cure.

Two families with MEN-2A have recently been described[81] in which cutaneous lichen amyloidosis was described in some but not all affected family members. These raised, firm, papular, pigmented, pruritic lesions occur on the back, leg, arm, or thigh; on pathologic examination they reveal amorphous material that stains positive on Congo red or crystal violet and is located at the dermal–epidermal junction. Keratin stains are positive while stains for calcitonin are negative. No evidence of renal dysfunction or systemic anyloidosis has been found.[81]

Jackson et al.[82] have also reported two unusual consequences of medullary thyroid carcinoma. Endogenous depression, amenable to tricyclic antidepressant therapy, was seen in nineteen patients with hereditary, and seven patients with sporadic medullary thyroid carcinoma. In several, there was improvement after total thyroidectomy, suggesting medication by a tumor-produced biogenic amine. That this was not a reactive depression was suggested by its presence in family members without medullary thyroid carcinoma. In addition, two patients with medullary thyroid carcinoma were reported with nephrotic syndrome secondary to renal amyloidosis; the amyloid deposition stained positive for calcitonin.

MEN-2B is characterized by medullary carcinoma, pheochromocytoma in 90% of cases, and a relatively lower incidence of hyperparathyroidism. Classic findings include multiple mucosal neuromas involving the lids, eyes, tongue, and pharynx (Fig. 8.8), gangleoneuromatosis of the gastrointestinal tract, and a Marfanoid body habitus. Long, thin extremities, decreased body fat, and poor muscle development are all noted. The GI lesions may lead to megacolon. This syndrome may be familial or sporadic, presumably due to new mutation. The medullary carcinoma in this setting is more virulent and may develop before one year of age. Five year disease-free survival is less than 35%, even with relatively early detection. The body habitus and mucosal lesions should alert clinicians to search for early lesions, particularly in childhood.[83]

Farndon et al.[84] reported on two large families in which medullary carcinoma was inherited as an autosomal dominant trait with

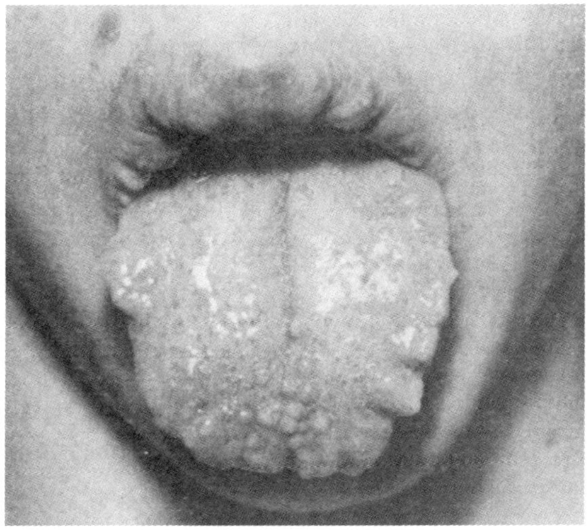

Figure 8.8. Multiple neucrofibromas of the lips and tongue that undoubtedly were a manifestation of von Recklinghausen's disease. Reprinted, by permission, from Carney JA, Sizemore GW, and Hayles AB, 1978. (93)

no associated endocrinopathy. These patients tended to present later in life, even if detected by biochemical stimulation (mean age = 43, compared to age 21 in MEN-2A). The medullary carcinoma seems to be more indolent, with few deaths reported.

By contrast, sporadic medullary carcinoma seems to be more aggressive (though less so than type 2B); it presents later in life with a palpable mass and an 80% frequency of metastases at the time of diagnoses. (see Table 8.2 for a comparison of the characteristics of the variants of famial men.)

As it may be impossible to determine clinically whether an index case is sporadic or whether it represents the propositus of a new family, all of the first degree relatives should be studied with stimulated calcitonin tests.

Screening Studies

Screening studies have assumed an important role in primary prevention in medullary carcinoma. After Sipple first reported the association of medullary carcinoma, pheochromocytoma, and hyperparathyroidism in 1961, many families were discovered,[85] suggesting an autosomal dominant trait with incomplete penetrance. With the availability of a calcitonin radioimmunoassay in 1971, Tashjian et al.[15,86] reported screening the large "J" kindred, uti-

Table 8.2. Authors' experience with medullary thyroid carcinoma, 1972 to 1986

Category of MTC	No. patients	Mean age in years at diagnosis (range)	Ratio of males to females	No. dead from MTC (%)
MEN-IIa	122	27 ± 1.2 (6–71)	62:60	21 (17)
MEN-IIb	10	16 ± 3.5 (7–36)	4:6	5 (50)
Familial non-MEN	41	45 ± 2.4 (15–72)	21:30	0 (0)
Sporadic	27	44 ± 2.8 (19–69)	13:14	8 (30)

Reprinted, by permission, from Wells, S.A., Dilley, W.G., Farndon, J.A., et al, 1985 (110) Copyright 1985, American Medical Association.

Table 8.3. Relationship of method of diagnosis to pathologic staging of MTC

	Group 1	Group 2	Group 3
Number of patients	32	8	50
Mean age at diagnosis	20.5 ± 1.9	32.5 ± 4.7	34.3 ± 2.0
Regional lymph node metastases	2/22 (9%)	3/6 (50%)	17/24 (71%)
Elevated postoperative stimulated CT levels	4/26 (15%)	2/8 (25%)	15/26 (58%)

Reprinted, by permission, from Wells, S.A., Jr., Baylin, S.B., Gann, D.S., et al. Medullary thyroid carcinoma; Relationship of method of diagnosis to pathologic staging. Ann Surg 1978; 188:377–383.

Table 8.4. Plasma calcitonin and prognosis in MTC

Group	Number of patients	Preoperative CT (pg/ml)	Regional lymph node metastases* (%)	Postoperative CT (>300 pg/ml) (%)*	Distant metastases (%)	Death (%)
1	25	250–1,000	1 (4)	1 (4)	0	0
2	36	1,000–5,000	3 (8.3)	6 (16.7)	0	0
3	8	5,000–10,000	1 (25)	1 (12.5)	0	0
4	23	>10,000	13 (57)	14 (61)	4 (17)	2 (8.7)

Reprinted, by permission, from Wells, S.A., Jr., Baylin, S.B., Lineham, W.M., et al, Provocative agents and the diagnosis of medullary carcinoma of the thyroid gland. Ann Surg 1978;188:139–141.

lizing calcium stimulation. These studies again confirmed the autosomal dominant mode of inheritance. Of 12 patients whose mean age was 38 years and whose medullary carcinoma was detected before becoming clinically overt, 7 had already metastasized, emphasizing the need for extremely early detection. C-cell hyperplasia that was felt to be premalignant[87] was found in 3 patients in the initial report. In a follow-up study of the same family published in 1988,[88] it was noted that with the institution of yearly screening, the next 23 cases of the disease were detected at mean age of 11.8 years and at an earlier stage of the disease—13 with C-cell hyperplasia and 9 with C-cell hyperplasia and microscopic medullary carcinoma (one false positive). Of the original 12 subjects, 6 were free of disease at 15 years, including 2 who had originally presented with neck nodes. None of the patients detected by serial testing have died; all are clinically disease-free and none have hyperresponded to secretagogues after total thyroidectomy was performed. When survival curves are reviewed an inverse correlation between mortality and the age of diagnosis (Table 8.3) and concominantly the extent of disease (Table 8.4).

In the Netherlands, Vasen et al.[89] have followed fifteen kindreds since 1975 by using similar screening methods. They note that prior to screening, the average age of death from pheochromocytoma was 34.9 years and for medullary carcinoma, 49.2 years. Since screening has been performed, this has gradually increased, and total cures have become more common. In patients treated after clinical medullary carcinoma was apparent, 72% had metastatic disease at the time of the thyroidectomy and the cure rate as assessed by stimulated calcitonin was 11%. Patients found on initial screening of the family to be without clinically apparent disease had a 33% incidence of metastases and a 57% cure rate, whereas patients who initially had a negative calcitonin response and later converted to positive, had no metastases and a 100% cure rate.

When a new case of medullary carcinoma is detected, all first degree relatives should be screened, since one is never certain if this is an index case to a previously undetected family.

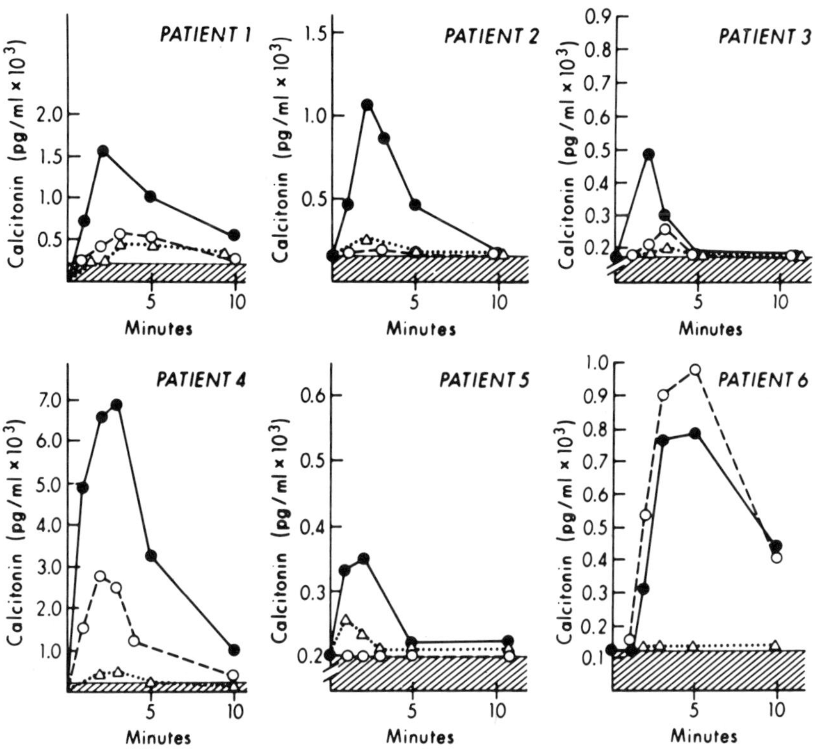

Figure 8.9. ●: pentagastrin, +: Ca gluconate, ○: pentagastrin only, △: Ca gluconate only. Reprinted, by permission, from Wells SA Jr, Baylin SB, Lineham WM, et al., Provocative agents and the diagnosis of medullary carcinoma of the thyroid gland. Ann Surg 1978;188:139–141.

The need for screening is particularly urgent if the propositus has bilateral disease, associated C-cell hyperplasia within the thyroid, or associated endocrinopathy.

Several groups of investigators have compared a variety of secretagogues for use in detection studies, including calcium by infusion[90] or bolus injection,[91] pentagastrin,[92] or a combination of the two,[93] which may produce the lowest incidence of false negative responses (Fig. 8.9). Other secretagogues, including glucagon,[94] ethanol,[95] or thyrotopin-releasing hormone (TRH),[96] also stimulate the C-cells, but not with enough consistency to rely upon them for early detection studies.

Associated Endocrinopathy

Associated endocrinopathy should be sought in all subjects.[97,98] Tashjian and his group[88] emphasized the reliability of 24-hour urine epinephrine secretion (normal = less than 25 μg in 24 hours), and urine epinephrine-to-norepinephrine ratio (normal = less than 0.62) to exclude pheochromocytomas. These assays were more sensitive than other methods of measurement of catecholamine secretion; yet there was one false negative (detected by methyliodobenzlguanidine (MIBG) scan). Adrenal medullary hyperplasia was not uniformly detected. Other authors[99] note that MIBG may reveal functional abnormalities before anatomic changes occur. Magnetic resonance imaging (MRI) reveals ectopic tissue in the paraaortic and caval planes while outlining the adrenals and defining pheochromocytomas with an increased signal on T_2-weighted image. Although this group opts for unilateral adrenalectomy if at surgery only one gland is found to be involved, the 50% to 70% incidence of recurrent contralateral pheochromocytoma in a situation in which it is known that there is preexisting hyperplasia has led others, notably the Mayo Clinic group, toward initial bilateral adrenalectomy, the hazards of Addison's disease notwithstanding.[97] The dangers of untreated pheochromocytoma include arrhythmias, catecholamine crisis, and sudden death. It is fortunate that in the group followed by Tashjian these are not reported to have occurred prior to surgical intervention.

Steinart et al.[85] note that at least one quarter of patients with familial pheochromocytoma have medullary carcinoma. Therefore, in a new case of pheochromocytoma, as in a new case of medullary carcinoma, there should be a search for associated medullary carcinoma and hyperparathyroidism, as well as for familial disease. Parathyroid disease, generally hyperplasia or adenomatous hyperplasia in MEN-2, had been assumed to be a primary part of this syndrome, part of the inherited disease process. It is present in a variable degree in kindred in 2A or 2B, rather than occurring in response to hypercalcitoninemia and possibly minimally lower calcium levels. The fact that no cases of hyperparathyroidism were noted in the cases of 2A or found early in screening studies, challenges this assumption. The authors suggest that the failure to develop parathyroid disease after ten years of follow-up may be ascribed to either the young age of the patients, the practice of removal of one or more inferior parathyroid glands at the time of total thyroidectomy, or the removal of the thyroid (possibly eliminating a source of a parathyroid growth factor or stimulant).[88]

Disease Probability Statistics

With more families being evaluated, Gagel et al.[100] calculated the probability of development of medullary carcinoma in a genetically predisposed individual with a normal stimulated-calcitonin level. Based on 445 members of eleven families, a formula was derived (Figs. 8.10 and 8.11) to predict subsequent risk. It was noted that 50% of the conversions from negative to positive tests occurred before the age of 12, and that 90% of patients had converted before age 25. No conversions were reported after age 40. Amplifying on these statis-

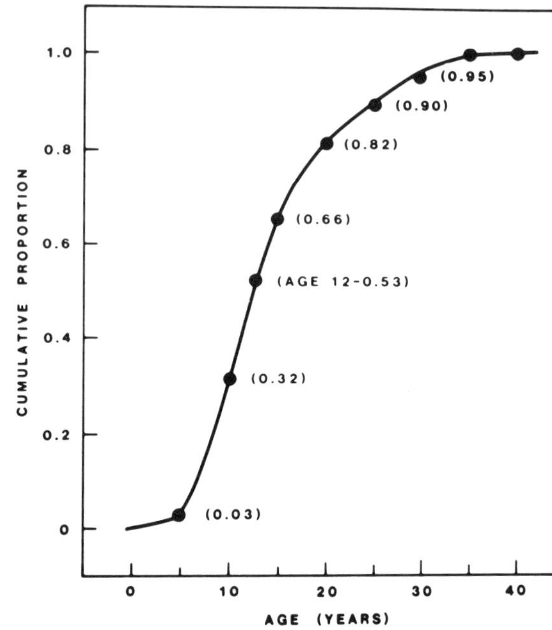

Figure 8.10. Reprinted, by permission, from Gagel RF, Jackson CE, Block MS, et al., 1982. (100).

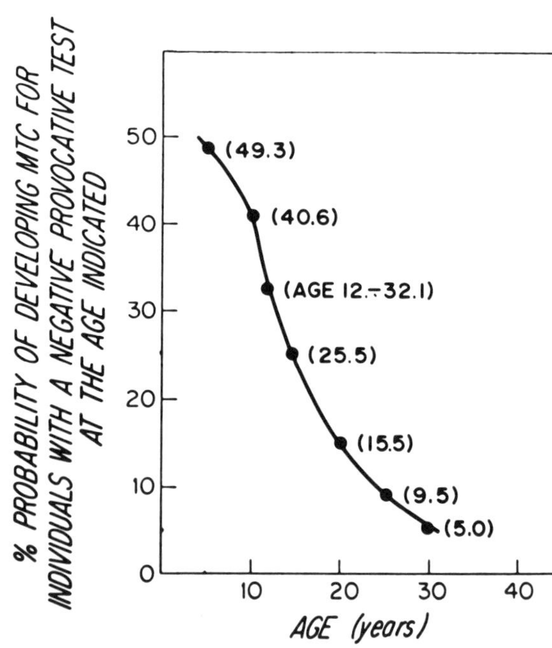

Figure 8.11. The probability of subsequent conversion (development of disease) for an individual at 50% rise who had a negative provocative test result at a given age. Reprinted, by permission, from Gagel RF, Jackson C, Block MS, et al., 1982. (100)

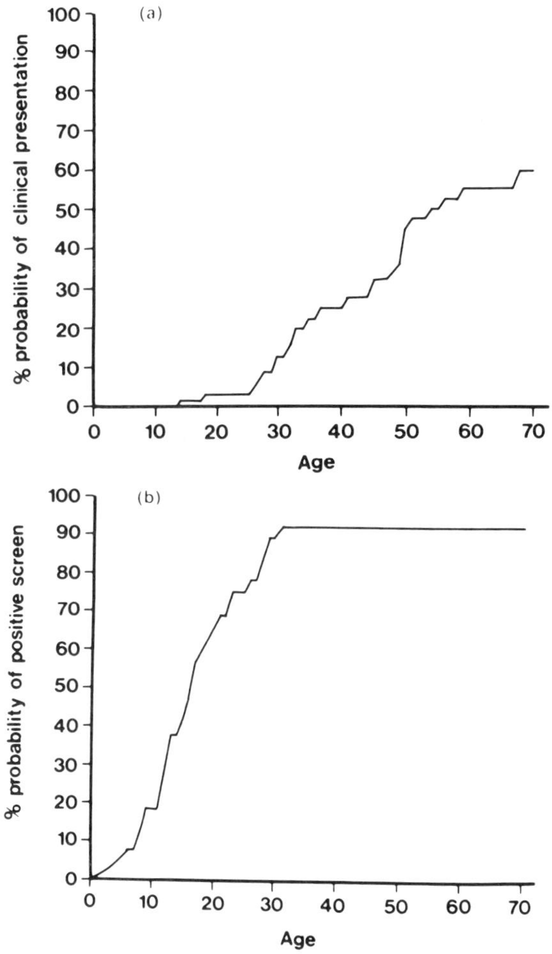

Figure 8.12. Probability of detection of MEN 2a gene carrier with age. Reprinted, by permission, from Ponder BA, Coffey R, Gagel RF, et al., 1988. (101)

tics using the medullary thyroid group registry, Ponder et al.[101] have suggested strategies for the assessment of individual and family risk. They note that only about two thirds of all MEN-2 gene carriers will present clinically by age 70, whereas over 90% could be detected by age 30 on screening studies (Fig. 8.12). Further, they note that in practice, only one half of first degree relatives and only a few second degree relatives of affected individuals are screened. This may lead to incorrect assumptions based on negative clinical assessment. They further emphasize the lack of reliability of basal calcitonin as a measure of involvement. Because clinical disease may not present until patients are older, even in familial cases; it is felt unsafe to assume that transmission of the gene by elderly ancestors who are apparently unaffected is a rare event. Likewise, because of incomplete penetrance, one cannot assume that a particular instance of the disease is sporadic, based on either the advanced age of the patient at diagnosis or the fact that the parents are apparently unaffected. The authors recommend that specimens from all medullary carcinoma patients be searched carefully for C-cell hyperplasia by immunocytochemical stain. They further recommend that the parents of all cases be screened, and if they are not available, that all siblings be screened. If neither parent (over the age of 40) is positive, the probability of familial disease is only 1.7%. If only siblings are available for testing and all are negative, then the risk of familial disease is 4.8%. Thus, the children of the new case in question would be at minimal risk. The possibility that the index case is a new mutation for familial disease, however, suggests that children should be screened, particularly if the proband presented at a young age (since the proportion of familial to truly sporadic cases declines with age), and certainly if there is associated C-cell hyperplasia pathologically.

Therapeutic Modalities

Surgery

The treatment of medullary carcinoma of the thyroid should consist of a total thyroidectomy in all cases, since a presumed sporadic case may be an index case in a new family. Since local recurrences may ultimately prove fatal, aggressive and meticulous surgery is required. Central neck node dissection should be performed with removal of all nodal tissue from the hyoid bone superiorly, to the innominate vessels inferiorly, and to the internal jugular veins laterally. This procedure may yield up to 50% positive nodes. New jugular nodes should be sampled, and modified neck dissection should be performed if positive nodes are found.[80]

In patients with residual or recurrent disease manifested with elevated calcitonin levels, careful reoperation may result in normalization of calcitonin levels and presumably longer survival or cure. Tissel[102] reported that in 11 patients who were reoperated on a mean of 3.3 years after initial thyroidectomy, microdissection lasting 8 to 12 hours was performed with the goal of removing residual lateral and superior anterior mediastinal lymph node metastases. Four cases had normal calcitonin results, even after pentagastrin testing postoperatively. Patients with unilateral disease did well, while patients with large infiltrating tumors and large nodal metastases did not generally normalize their calcitonin levels. Although in many centers, surgical procedures are performed repeatedly when there is evidence of residual disease, there is no proof that this approach ultimately prolongs survival.[103] Certainly, relief of obstructive symptoms should always be sought, and palpable or easily visible tumors may be resected again. In some situations, surgical debulking may effectively improve symptoms caused by hormone production; for example, diarrhea and ectopic Cushing's syndrome.

Detection of Residual Disease

When hypercalcitoninemia persists after aggressive surgery, there is the presumption that residual disease is present, generally with the calcitonin level reflecting the mass of tumor burden. In a few patients, postoperative hypercalcitoninemia gradually declines, suggesting either autonecrosis of tumor, delayed clearance of large molecular weight calcitonin, or in some cases, more virulent, less well differentiated tumor.[104] When elevated calcitonin levels persist, localization studies may have implications for further therapy and for prognosis.

In 1985, thallium/technetium scans were found to localize residual disease in the neck, superior mediastinum, liver and lungs in 5 of 10 patients with elevated calcitonin postoperatively[105] in one study, but in only 1 of 6 patients in another series.[106] Uptake of radiolabeled, monoclonal antibodies against CEA, combined with transaxial tomoscintigraphy gave positive results in a few patients.[107] MIBG scanning in patients with relatively high levels of calcitonin in MEN-II localized residual tumor in seven of fifteen cases.[108] The other cases suggest that positive results depend upon volume and/or secretory activity. Therapy with ^{131}I MIBG has also been suggested in cases where uptake is substantial.

In a 1988 study, Clarke et al.[109] compared DMSA, MIBG, and technetium diphosphonate scanning in nine patients with persistent elevation of calcitonin postoperatively. Eight of these patients had metastases visible on computed tomography (CT) scan. This group noted that all patients with metastases demonstrated by CT scanning showed positive DMSA uptake in both bone and soft tissue metastases, with 88% of patients detected (94% bone, and 100% soft tissue). One patient with elevated calcitonin levels failed to show uptake with DMSA, or localization with CT. MIBG uptake occurred in only 39% of soft tissue and 10% of bone metastases, while technetium 99m localized all known bone metastases but no soft tissue metastases (see Table 8.5).

Wells and others suggest selective venous sampling in all patients with elevated calcitonin levels in whom localization is not otherwise demonstrated.[110] After administering 0.6 μg of pentagastrin per kilogram intravenously, simultaneous samples are obtained from multiple sites. This modality is costly and invasive, but offers the advantage of being independent of the need for large tumor masses to produce adequate radionuclide for visibility. Certainly, when reoperation of the neck or mediastinum is under consideration, the presence of distant metastases particularly in the viscera, may temper the surgeon's judgement. MRI scanning has not been systematically applied to the study of medullary carcinoma, but undoubtedly will be utilized in the future.

After failures of complete neck and mediastinal dissection to completely eradicate either clinical disease or persistent calcitonin elevation, adjuvant therapy has been sought. The goal of this therapy may be considered either complete cure, prevention of rapid growth of clinically important tumor, or palliation once residual tumor produces either locally obstructive symptoms or distant paraneoplastic symptoms secondary to hormone production. A

Table 8.5. Percent metastases identified

	[131]MIBG			[99mTc]MDP			[99mTc](V)DMSA		
		Soft tissue			Soft tissue			Soft-tissue	
	Bone	Local	Distant	Bone	Local	Distant	Bone	Local	Distant
Lesion sensitivity	5/52(10%)	0/10(20%)	3/23(13%)	52/52(100%)	2/10 (0%)	0/23(0%)	49/52(94%)	10/10(100%)	23/23(100%)
Overall sensitivity		10/85(12%)			52/85(61%)			82/85 (95%)	

Reprinted, by permission, from Clarke, S.E.M., Lazarus, C.R., Wraight, P., et al, 1988(109). Copyright by The Society of Nuclear Medicine, 1988.

variety of measures have been attempted, none with particular success.

Radiation Therapy

Because medullary carcinoma of the thyroid is not of follicular origin, it does not concentrate radioiodine; rather, some groups have speculated that significant doses of beta radiation may be delivered to residual radiosensitive medullary carcinoma cells if adjacent normal thyroid traps sufficient ^{131}I, particularly when it is stimulated by high levels of TSH. In 1979, Hellman et al.[111] reported a single case of medullary carcinoma of the thyroid with residual ^{131}I neck uptake who received 150 mCi of ^{131}I, amounting to 34,000 rads to the thyroid bed. Postoperatively and before receiving ^{131}I, calcitonin levels were 800 pg/ml basally, rising to 1200 pg/ml after calcium infusion, while three and ten months after ^{131}I administration, calcitonin levels were less than 100 pg/ml and could not be further stimulated by calcium or pentagastrin. Deftos and Stein[112] reported a second case with residual ^{131}I uptake in a thyroglossal duct remnant; here, 2 courses of ^{131}I 30 mCi (four months postoperatively) and 150 mCi (two years postoperatively) reduced thyrocalcitonin levels from over 500 pg/ml unstimulated, rising to more than 5000 pg/ml after pentagastrin stimulation to undetectable levels before and after stimulation.

In contrast, Samaan's group at MD Anderson (Houston, Texas) reported in 1983[113] their results with ^{131}I in 84 patients treated with surgery alone, as compared to 15 patients with positive ^{131}I scans treated with surgery and ^{131}I in doses of 52 to 200 mCi. When patients with tumors localized to the thyroid were compared with these patients, there was no significant difference between groups in terms of course of disease, increase of recurrence, or survival rates.

External radiation was reported to result in local control of tumor in three of four patients treated by Steinfeld[114] who initially presented with enlarging neck masses and cervical adenopathy. These patients were followed from three to six years until their deaths of metastatic disease. They were considered to be resistant to low doses of radiation therapy.

Tubiana[115] reporting on the experience at Villejuif, France, noted that of 72 patients treated for medullary carcinoma, 26 were treated with surgery alone, 29 received radiotherapy which was considered to be prophylactic in 15 and necessary because of incomplete excision in 14. He noted that while the "most unfavorable" tumors received radiation therapy, their 20-year survival was 50% compared to 25% for patients treated with surgery alone. Eight patients whose tumors were inoperable were treated with radiation therapy, and lived 6 to 10 years after therapy. Three had incomplete tumor regression; one is alive and well with elevated calcitonin levels postoperatively; in two, radiation therapy was considered ineffective. Eight patients were also treated for bone metastases; one had a complete remission and four experienced "significant palliation."

Once again, the MD Anderson group[116] found no difference in survival rates when patients treated with surgery alone or a combination of surgery and radiation therapy were matched for age and involvement of the thyroid gland and cervical nodes, neck soft tissue, and distant metastases. Fifty-seven patients had received 2500 to 600 rads over five weeks because the surgeon thought there was a possibility of microscopic residual disease in the neck. Because patients with sporadic disease were found to have more extensive disease at the time of diagnoses as compared with patients with familial disease, more were included in the group that was treated with radiation therapy (52 vs. 5). Again, because of the younger age and earlier stage of disease at diagnosis, MEN II patients (A & B) survived longer than sporadic cases (see Fig. 8.1). Yet when subgroups of comparable disease extent were compared, there was no improvement, and in fact a worsening in survival rates in those patients given radiation therapy as compared with those treated with surgery alone. Thus, the recommendation for ^{131}I or external beam radiotherapy in postoperative medullary carcinoma is certainly not standardized at this time. Attempts may be made to relieve locally obstructive symptoms that are not amenable to surgery, but routine radiation therapy is not considered necessary or useful.

Chemotherapy

Until recently, chemotherapy for medullary carcinoma has been considered ineffective, but many patients have been treated with a variety of agents in attempts to palliate advanced disease. Adriamycin and CIS-platinum used separately were reported[117] to be ineffective in 13 patients treated at Duke. In a 1985[118] series from Mt. Sinai (New York), one patient with medullary carcinoma of the thyroid treated with a combination of both agents showed a brief partial remission.

Using a cell line derived from human medullary thyroid carcinoma cells in vitro, Goretzki et al.[119] noted that the addition of Nerve Growth Factor enhanced cell proliferation and caused an increased sensitivity to doxorubicin in vitro. This agent has not yet been included in current in vivo therapeutic trials.

The somatostatin analogue octreatide[120] was reported to cause partial improvement in three patients with medullary carcinoma of the thyroid. Symptoms of diarrhea, weight loss, and malaise improved; calcitonin and CEA levels decreased by 40% to 80% for as long as 17 months of treatment; however, size could not be evaluated and eventually all the patients relapsed.

Molecular Biology

The availability of molecular biology techniques has yielded a quantum leap in our understanding of the neoplasia present in Multiple Endocrine Neoplasia type II, as well as offering the incipient theoretical possibility that genetic markers might be useful for clinical detection of family members at risk.

Using DNA restriction fragment length polymorphism studies of lymphocyte DNA, the mutant allele for multiple endocrine neoplasia type 2A has been linked to the centromeric region of chromosome 10.[121–123] This finding has been confirmed in several studies involving many families of varied genetic background. The largest cooperative study performed by the members of a French group studying medullary carcinoma was reported by Sobol and Rod in the *New England Journal of Medicine* in 1989.[124] Three genetic probes were used to study 11 MEN-2A families. The results of linkage analysis were compared with conventional pentagastrin stimulation. In some families, linkage studies may not be informative using presently available probes; secretagogues will continue to be required. In other families, restriction fragment length polymorphism (RFLP) information has identified the carrier state even before the pentagastrin test became positive. Theoretically, patients at extremely high risk genetically could be screened intensely when very young, thus allowing surgical interventions to be performed detecting the most minimal C-cell hyperplasia, as well as permitting those family members who have not inherited the carrier alleles to be spared yearly provocative tests.[125,126]

Interestingly, in this study two obligate carriers were identified who had reached old age (80 and 86 years) without manifesting either clinical or chemical evidence for the carrier state of medullary carcinoma. This fact alone underlines the importance of further genetic information to the offspring of such patients.

Linkage analysis in the French study in 18 families with probes specific for the pericentromeric region of chromosome 10 disclosed that the genetic mutation for medullary carcinoma was in genetic disequilibrium with the marker alleles of the two closely linked probes, IRBPH4 and MCK2. Families with and without pheochromocytoma exhibited genetic homogeneity among groups, suggesting that the different mutant alleles of the same gene or closely linked mutations account for the variation in penetrance of pheochromocytoma.[127] Thus, there appear to be two subgroups of families with medullary carcinoma: those with either high (62%) or low (4%) penetrance of pheochromocytoma. The latter group, previously reported by Fardon et al., seem to present at a later age, have less aggressive tumors and a more favorable prognosis.[84] DNA screening of patients with multiple endocrine neoplasia type 2B is not yet possible due to the limited number of families, the small amount of genetic information available, and the presence of a number of seemingly new mutations with this clinical syndrome.

Molecular biologic techniques have also provided data that elucidates the molecular abnormalities underlying the initiation of the growth of neoplasia and subsequent cellular changes during tumor progression. Matthew et al.[128] reported that there was a loss or marked reduction in intensity in one of two alleles in a hypervariable "mini-satellite" region in chromosome 1 in tumor DNA using a lambda MSI probe in 7 of 14 informative pairs. Because in some cases the derivation was not from the affected parent, it was felt that this deletion did not reflect the site of inherited mutation. As previously noted, chromosome 10 seems to be inherited in linkage disequilibrium with medullary carcinoma in MEN-2A. Expounding upon this information, Baylin and his group suggest that the classical "two hit series" of Knudson,[129] as in retinoblastoma, may not be operant in the case of medullary carcinoma. Here it is felt that the first hit might not be silent, as in the retinoblastoma model, but rather may "confer a growth stimulus on the target thyroid C cells and adrenal chromaffin cells."[130] This would then result in generalized hyperplasia of the entire thyroid C cell and adrenal chromaffin cell population. The tumors, medullary carcinoma and pheochromocytoma, then evolve as multifocal clonal tumors, each tumor coming from a different cell clone.[130] Thus, the original chromosome 10 abnormality would confer it a loss of suppression of stimulus for hyperplasia. In the final phase tumorogenesis would result from an abnormality elsewhere, for example, the chromosome 1 abnormalities found by Matthew. In genetic terms, the "second hit" frequently occurs through "gross structural changes" such as extensive chromosomal deletions or loss of the entire chromosome, that are detectable as a "reduction to homozygosity" for polymorphic DNA markers in the region involved. Failure to detect a reduction to homozygosity might be due to a mechanism of inactivation of the normal allele function that does not involve the loss of a large segment of the chromosome involved, such as point mutations, or due to smaller interstitial deletions. Such a reduction to homozygosity in chromosome 10, or loss of chromosome 10, has been reported to occur in extremely low incidence by Nelkin et al.[131]

Finally, Baylin and his group[132] have also studied the molecular events that control transcription and RNA processing in medullary carcinoma cells. The biology of calcitonin gene expression is at least partially related to the dedifferentiation of the tumor; the expression of calcitonin gene-related peptide and relative loss of calcitonin expression from differential RNA processing is associated with more poorly differentiated tumors which have in turn been associated with more aggressive biologic characteristics.[132] Since it is known that cell signal processing may be affected by exogenous stimuli, Baylin and his group attempted stimulation with protein kinase C and A. Both of these produced a partial differentiation of the cells that was characterized by slowing of cell growth and increased transcription of the calcitonin gene; however, the splicing events for the gene did not revert to a more normal pattern.

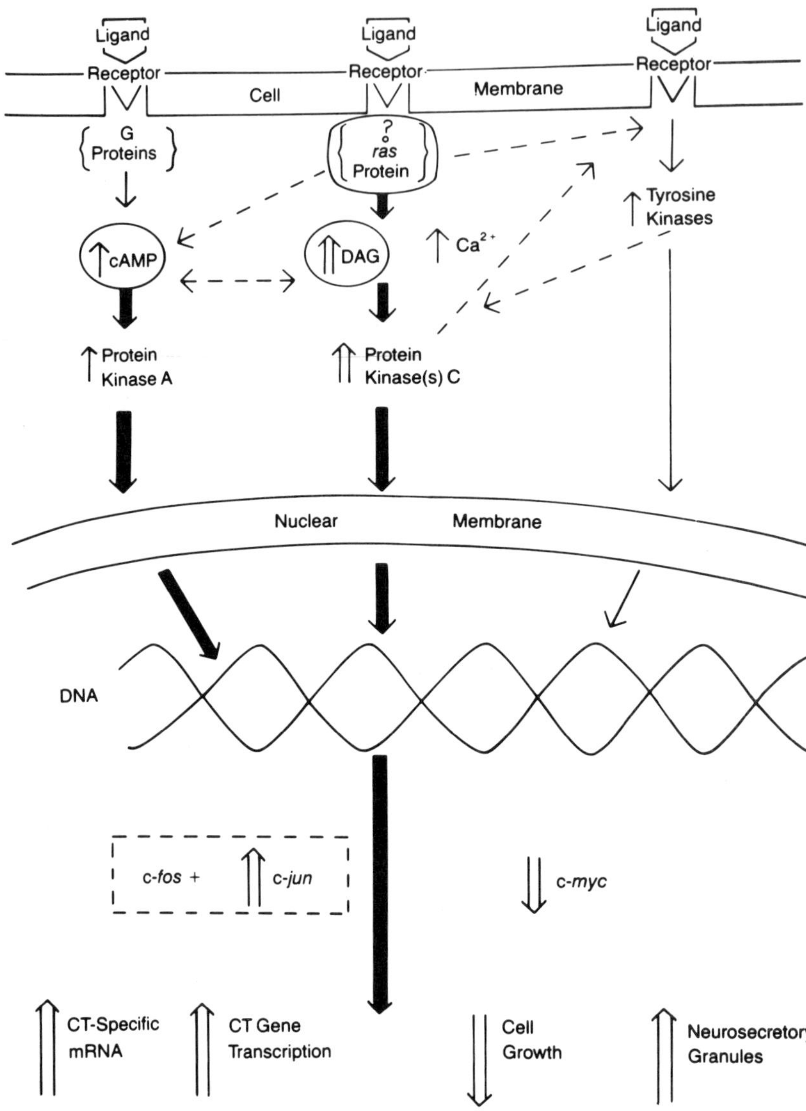

Figure 8.13. Reprinted, by permission, from Nelkin BD, DeBustras AC, Mabry M, and Baylin SG. 1989. (132) Copyright 1989, American Medical Association.

Conservation of cells by mutated *ras* genes that appear to depend upon the activation of the signal transduction pathway, including protein kinase C, are known to cause differentiation of rodent pheochromocytoma and, according to Baylin, insertion and expression of the v-*ras* gene, alteration of the *CT* gene, RNA splicing events that are more characteristic of mature C cells, and the appearance of abundant mature cytoplasmic neurosecretory granules. In these cells, these events were associated with stimulation of protein kinase C pathway and with increased expression of the nuclear oncogene c-*gun*, which may act as a transcription factor for some genes responsive to protein kinase C–mediated signal transduction events (Fig. 8.13). Baylin postulated that the *ras* oncogene may stimulate a pathway of differentiation not otherwise available for the tumor cell, thus bypassing a more proximal defect in the normal signal transduction pathway in the membrane of the tumor cells, such as a defect in a receptor coupled to a *ras* gene protein. They further speculate that such manipulation in vitro may ultimately have therapeutic usefulness for modifying the biologic behavior of tumors in vivo.[132]

Medullary carcinoma represents a fascinating entity for molecular biologists. In its familial form it can be detected chemically before clinically apparent disease is present; in the near future, genetic markers may allow detection in utero or at birth and genetic engineering may allow modification of its virulence once its presence is detected.

References

1. Hazard JB, Hawk WA, Crile G Jr. Medullary (Solid) carcinoma of the thyroid–A clinicopathologic entity. J Clin Endo 1959;19:152–161.
2. Hill CS Jr, Ibanez ML, Samaan N, Ahearn MJ, Clark, RL. Medullary (Solid) carcinoma of the thyroid gland: An analysis of the M.D. Anderson Hospital experience with patients with the tumor, its special features and its histogenesis. Medicine 1973;52:141–171.
3. Chong GC, Bearhrs OH, Sizemore GW, Medullary carcinoma of the thyroid gland. Cancer 1975;35:695–704.
4. Saad MF, Ordonez NG, Rashid RK, Medullary carcinoma of the thyroid. A study of the clinical features and prognostic factors in 161 patients. Medicine 1984;63:319–342.
5. Melvin KE, Miller HH, Tashjian AH. Early diagnosis of medullary carcinoma of the thyroid gland by means of calcitonin assay. New Engl J Med 1971; 285:1115–1120.
6. Kaiser HR, Beaven MA, Doppman J, Wells S Jr, Buja LM. Sipples Syndrome: Medul lary thyroid carcinoma, pheochromocytoma, and parathyroid disease, studies in a large family. Ann Int Med 1973;78:551–579.
7. Soderstrom N, Telenius-Berg M, Akerman A. Diagnosis of medullary carcinoma of the thyroid by fine needle aspiration biopsy. Acta Med Scan 1975; 197:71–75.
8. Geddie WR, Bedard YC, Strauobridge HT. Medullary carcinoma of the thyroid in fine-needle aspiration biopsies. Am J Clin Path 1984;82:552–558.
9. La Volsi VA. Medullary carcinoma in surgical pathology of the thyroid. Philadelphia: W.B. Saunders, pp. 213–252.
10. Sletten K, Westermak P, Natvig JB. Characterization of amyloid fibril proteins from medullary carcinoma of the thyroid. J Exper Med 1976;143:993–998.
11. DeLellis RA, Nunnemacher G and Wolfe HJ. C-cell hyperplaisia: an ultrastructural analysis. Lab Invest 1977;36:237–248.
12. Cox CE, Van Vickle J, Froome LC et al. Carcinoembryonic antigen and calcitonin as markers of malignancy in medullary thyroid carcinoma. Surgical Forum, 1979;30:120–121.
13. Block MA, Jackson CE, Greenawald KA, Yott JB, Tashjian AH. Clinical characteristics distinguishing hereditary from sporadic medullary carcinoma. Treatment implications. Arch Surg 1980;115:142–148.
14. Gonzalez-Licea A, Hartman WH, Yardley JH. Medullary carcinoma of the thyroid. Ultrastructural evidence of its origin from the parafollicular cell and its possible relation to carcinoid tumors. Am J Clin Path 1968;49:512–520.
15. Braunstein H, Stephens CL, Gibson RL. Secretory granules in medullary carcinoma of the thyroid. Arch Path 1958;85:306–313.
16. Falck B, Ljungberg O, Rosengren E. On the occurrence of Monoamines and related substances in familial medullary carcinoma with pheochromocytoma. Acta Path Microbiol Scandinav 1968;74: 1–10.
17. DeLellis RA. Formaldehyde induced fluorescence technique for the demonstration of biogenic amines in diagnostic histopathology. Cancer 1971;28:1704–1710.
18. Weichert RF. The neural ectodermal origin of the peptide secretory endocrine glands–a unifying concept for the etiology of multiple endocrine adenomatosis and the inappropriate secretion of peptide hormones by non-endocrine tumors. Am J Med 1970;49:232–239.
19. Pearse AGE. The APUD concept and hormone production. Clinics in Endo and Metab 1980; Vol. 9, number 2 (July), pp. 211–221.
20. Stevens RE, Moore GL. Inadequacy of the APUD concept in explaining production of peptide hormones by tumors. Lancet, 1983;1:118–119.
21. Sambade C, Baldaque-Fana A, Cardoso-Oliveira, Sohrinho-Simoes M. Follicular and papillary variants of medullary carcinoma of the thyroid. Path Res Pract 1989;184:98–103.
22. Franssila KO. Letter to the case. Path Res Pract 1989;184:104–105.
23. Parker LN, Kollin J, Wu SL, Rypins EB, Juler JL. Carcinoma of the thyroid with a mixed medullary, papillary, follicular and undifferentiated pattern. Arch Int Med 1985;1507–1509.
24. Holm R, Sobrinho-Simoes M, Nesland JM, Sambade C, Johannessen JV. Medullary thyroid carcinoma with thyroglobulin immunoreactivity; a soecial entity. Lab Invest 1987;57:258–268.
25. Albores-Saavedra J, Monforte H, Nadji M, Morales A. C-cell hyperplaisia in thyroid tissue adjacent to follicular cell tumors. Human Path 1988;19:795–799.
26. Tashjian AH, Wolfe HJ, Voelkel EF. Human calcitonin; immunologic assay, cytologic localization and studies on medullary carcinoma. Am J Med 1974;56–848.
27. Gibson WCH, Pensitic, Croker BP. C cell nodules in

adult human thyroid: a common autopsy finding. Am J Clin Pathol 1980;73:347–351.
28. Austin LA, Heath H. Calcitonin, Physiology and pathophysiology. New Engl J Med 1981;304:269–278.
29. Poston GL, Seitz PK, Townsend CM et al. Calcitonin gene-related peptide: possible tumor marker for medullary thyroid cancer. Surgery 1987;102:1049–1054.
30. Ittner J, Dambacher MA, Born W, Ketelslegers JM et al. Diagnostic evaluation of measurements of carboxyl-terminal flanking peptide (PDN-21) of the human calcitonin gene in human serum. J Clin Endo Metab 1985;61:1133–1137.
31. Goltzman D, Tischler AS. Characterization of the immunochemical forms of calcitonin released by a medullary carcinoma in tissue culture. J Clin Invest 1978;61:449–458.
32. Body JJ, Heath H. Estimates of circulating monomeric calcitonin: Physiologic studies in normal and thyroidectomized man. J Clin Endo Metab 1983;57:897–903.
33. Hurley DL, Tiegs RD, Wahner HW, Heath H. Axial and appendicular bone mineral density in patients with long term deficiency or excess of calcitonin. N Eng J Med 1987;317:537–541.
34. Chen JJS, La France ND. Bone mineral density in medullary thyroid cancer (letter to the editor). N Engl J Med 1988;318:517–518.
35. Heath H, Sizemore G. Plasma calcitonin in normal man, differences between men and women. J Clin Invest 1977;60:1135–1140.
36. McLean GW, Rabin D, Moore L, Deftos L, Loberber D, McKenna J. Evaluation of provocative tests in suspected medullary carcinoma of the thyroid: heterogeneity of calcitonin responses to calcium and pentagastrin. Metabolism 1984;33:790–796.
37. Becker KL, Silva OL, Snider RH, Moore GF, Geelhoed. The surgical implications of hypercalcitonemia. Surg Gyn Obs 1982;154:897–908.
38. Conte N, Ceccehelting M, Manente R et al. Calcitonin in hepatoma and cirrhosis. Acta Endocrin 1984;106:109–111.
39. Parthemore JE, Deftos LJ. Calcitonin secretion in primary hyperparathyroidism. J Clin Endocrinol Metab 1979;49:223–226.
40. Oishi S, Shimada T, Tajiri J, Inove J, Sato T. Elevated serum calcitonin levels in patients with thyroid disorders. Acta Endocrin 1984;107:476–481.
41. Body JJ, Heath H. "Non-specific" increases in plasma immunoreactive calcitonin in healthy individuals: discrimination from medullary carcinoma by a new extraction technique. Clin Chem 1984;3014:511–514.
42. Schwartz K, Woffsen A, Forster A, Odell W. Calcitonin in nonthyroidal cancer. J Clin Endo Metab 1979;49:438–443.
43. Mulder H, Hackeng WHL. Ectopic secretion of calcitonin. Acta Med Scand 1978;204:253–256.
44. Hillyard CJ, Coombes RC, Greenberg PB, Galante LS, MacIntyre Calcitonin in breast and lung cancer. Clin Endo 1976;5:1–8.
45. Milhaud G, Calmette C, Taboulet J, Julienne A, Moukhtar MS. Hypersecretion of calcitonin in neoplastic conditions. Lancet 1974;1:452.
46. Coombes RC, Greenberg P, Hillyard C, MacIntyre I. Plasma immunoreactive calcitonin in patients with non-thyroid tumors. Lancet, 1974;1:1080–1083.
47. Hansen M, Hansen H, Tryding N. Small cell carcinoma of the lung: serum calcitonin and serum histaminase (diamine oxidase) at basal levels and stimulated by pentagastrin. Acta Med Scand 1978;204:257–261.
48. Silva OL, Becker KL, Primack A, Doppman JL, Snider RH. Hypercalcitonemia in bronchogenic cancer, evidence for thyroid origin of the hormone. JAMA 1975;234:183–185.
49. Ellison M, Woodhouse D, Hillyard C, Dousett M, Coombes RC et al. Immunoreactive calcitonin production by human lung carcinoma cells in culture. Br J Cancer, 1975;32:373–379.
50. Bertagna XY, Nicholson WE, Pettengill OS, Sorenson GD, Mount CD, Orth DN. Ectopic production of high molecular weight calcitonin and corticotropin by small cell carcinoma cells in tissue culture: evidence for separate precursors. J Clin Endo Metab 1978; 47:1390–1393.
51. Becker KL, Snider RH, Silva OL et al. Calcitonin Heterogeneity in lung cancer and medullary thyroid cancer. Acta Endocrinol 1978;89:89–93.
52. Baylin SB, Bearen MA, Bujal LM, Keiser HR. Histaminase Activity: a biochemical marker for medullary carcinoma of the thyroid. Am J Med 1972; 53:723–733.
53. Lippman SM, Mendelsohn G, Trump DL, Wells SA, Jr, Baylin SB. The prognostic and biologic significance of cellular heterogeneity in medullary thyroid carcinoma: a study of calcitonin, L-DOPA decarboxylase, and histaminase. J Clin Endocrinol Metab 1982;54:233–240.
54. Goltzman D, Huang SN et al. Adrenocorticotropin and calcitonin in medullary thyroid carcinoma: frequency of occurrence and localization in the same cell type by immunocytochemistry. J Clin Endo Metab 1979;49:364–370.
55. Melvin KEW, Tashjian AH et al. Cushing's Syndrome caused by ACTH and calcitonin secreting medullary carcinoma of the thyroid. Metabolism 1972;19:831–832.
56. Said SJ. Evidence for secretion of vasoactive intestinal peptide by tumors of pancreas, adrenal medulla, thyroid and lung: support for the unifying APUD concept. Clin Endocrincol (OXF) 1976 suppl. 5:201–204.
57. Rasmusson B. Gastrointestinal polypeptides in patients treated for medullary carcinoma of the thyroid. Acta Endocrinol 1984;106:112–115.
58. Williams ED, Karim SM, Sandler M. Prostaglandin secretion by medullary carcinoma of the thyroid: a possible cause of the associated diarrhea. Lancet 1968;1:22–123.
59. Roberts LJ, Hubbard WC, Bloomgarden ZT et al.

Prostaglandins: role in the humoral manifestations of medullary carcinoma of the thyroid and inhibition by somatostatin. Trans Assoc Am Physicians 1979; 92:286–291.
60. O'Connor DT, Burton D, Deltos LJ. Immunoreactive human chromogranin A in diverse polypeptide hormone producing human tumors and normal endocrine tissues. J Clin Endocrinol Metab 1983; 57:1084–1086.
61. Sobol RE, Memoli B, Deltos L. Hormone-negative, chromogranin A-positive endocrine tumors. N Engl J Med 1989;320:444–447.
62. Murray SS, Burton DW, Deftos LJ. The coregulation of secretion and cytoplasmic ribonucleic acid of chromogranin-A and calcitonin by phorbol ester in cells that produce both substances. Endocrinology 1988;122:495–499.
63. Schroder S, Bocker W, Baisch H et al. Prognostic factors in medullary thyroid carcinomas; survival in relation to age, sex, stage, histology, immunocytochemistry and DNA content. Cancer 1988;61:806–816.
64. Boultwood J, Wynford-Thomas D, Richards GP, Craig RK, Williams ED. In-site analysis of calcitonin and CGRP expression in medullary thyroid carcinoma. Clin Endo 1990;33:381–390.
65. Poston GJ, Seitz PK, Townsend CM et al. Calcitonin gene-related peptide: possible tumor marker for medullary thyroid cancer. Surgery 1987;102:1049–1054.
66. Ittner J, Dambacher MA, Born W, Ketelslegers JM et al. Diagnostic evaluation of measurements of carboxyl-terminal flanking peptide (PDN-21) of the human calcitonin gene in human serum. J Clin Endocrinol Metab 1985;61:1133–1137.
67. Sunday ME, Waffe HJ, Roos A, Chin WW, Spindel ER. Gastrin-releasing peptide gene expression in developing hyperplastic and neoplastic human thyroid C-cells. Endocrinology 1988;122:1551–1558.
68. Wakelam MJO, Davies SA, Houslay MD, McKay I, Marshall CJ, Hall A. Normal p21N-ras couples bombesin and other growth factor receptors to inositol phosphate production. Nature 1986;323:173–177.
69. Sikri KL, Varndell IM, Qutayba A et al. Medullary carcinoma of the thyroid, an immunocytochemical study of 25 cases using eight separate markers. Cancer 1985;56:2481–2491.
70. Soad MF, Ordonez NG, Girdo, JJ, Samaan N. The prognostic value of calcitonin immunostaining in medullary carcinoma of the thyroid. J Clin Endocrinol Metab 1984;59:850–856.
71. Rougier PH, Calmettes C, Laplanche A, Travagli JP, Lefeure M. The value of calcitonin and carcinoembryonic antigen in the treatment and management of non-familial medullary thyroid carcinoma. Cancer 1983;51:855–860.
72. Saad MF, Fritsche HA, Samaan NA. Diagnostic and prognostic values of carcinoembryonic antigen in medullary carcinoma of the thyroid. J Clin Endocrinol Metab 58:889–891.
73. Tangen KO, Lindmo T, Sobrinho-Simoes M, Johannessen JC. A flow cytometric DNA analysis of medullary thyroid carcinoma. Am J Clin Path 1983;79:172–177.
74. Bengtsson A, Malmaeus J, Grimelius L et al. Measurement of nuclear DNA content in thyroid diagnosis. World J Surg 1948;8:481–486.
75. Kramer BB, Srigley JR, Batsakis JG, Silva EG, Goepfert H. DNA flow cytometry of thyroid neoplasms. Arch Otolaryngol 1985;111:34–38.
76. Backdahl M, Carstensen J, Aver G, Tallroth E. Statistical evaluation of the prognostic value of nuclear DNA content in papillary, follicular, and medullary thyroid tumors. World J Surg 1986;10:974–980.
77. Hay ID, Ryan JJ, Grant CS et al. Flow cytometric nuclear DNA ploidy determination: A significant predictor of outcome in sporadic and familial medullary carcinoma, (abstr.). Proc. 64th Ann Meeting Am Thyroid Assoc, San Francisco. 1989, abstract 8, p. T4.
78. McLeod MK. The measurement of DNA content and ploidy analysis in thyroid neoplasms, otolaryngol. Clinics of N Am 1990;23:271–290.
79. Sizemore GW. Medullary carcinoma of the thyroid gland. Seminars in oncology 1987;14:306–314.
80. Brunt LM, Wells SA. Advances in the diagnosis and treatment of medullary thyroid carcinoma. Surg Clin North Am 1987;67:263–278.
81. Gagel RF, Levy MD, Donvan DT et al. Multiple endocrine neoplaisia Type 2A associated with cutaneous lichen amyloidosis. Ann Int Med 1989;111:802–806.
82. Jackson CE, Talpos GB, Kambouris A et al. The clinical course after definitive operation for medullary thyroid carcinoma. Surgery 1983;94:995–1001.
83. Carney JA, Sizemore GW, Hayles AB. Multiple endocrine neoplaisia, Type 2b. Pathobiol Am 1978;8:105–149.
84. Farndon JR, Leight GS, Dilley WG et al. Familial medullary carcinoma without associated endocrinopathies: A distinct clinical entity, Br J Surg 1986;73:278–281.
85. Steiner AL, Goodman AD, Powers SR. Study of a kindred with pheochromocytoma, medullary thyroid carcinoma, hyperparathyroidism and Cushing's Disease: Multiple endocrine neoplaisia Type 2. Medicine 1968;47:371–409.
86. Melvin KEW, Tashjian AH, Miller HH. Studies in familial medullary carcinoma. Rec Prog Horm Res 1972;28:399–407.
87. Wolfe HJ, Melvin KEW, Cervi-Skinner S et al. C-cell hyperplaisia preceding medullary carcinoma. N Engl J Med 1973;289:437–441.
88. Gagel RF, Tashjian AH, Cummings T et al. The clinical outcome of prospective screenings for multiple endocrine neoplaisia Type 2a—An eighteen year experience. N Engl J Med 1988;318:478–484.
89. Vasen HFA, Nieuwenhuijzen-Kruseman AC et al. Multiple endocrine neoplaisia syndrome, Type 2: The value of screening and central registration. Am J Med

1987;83:847–857.
90. Sizemore GW, Go V. Stimulation tests for diagnosis of medullary thyroid carcinoma. Mayo Clin Proc 1975;50:53–56.
91. Rude RK, Singer FR. Comparison of serum calcitonin levels after a one minute calcium injection and after pentagastrin injection in the diagnosis of medullary thyroid carcinoma. J Clin Endocrinol Metab 1977;44:980–982.
92. Gharib H, Kao PC, Heath H. Determination of silica-purified plasma calcitonin for the detection and management of medullary carcinoma: comparison of two provocative tests. Mayo Clin Proc 1987;62:373–378.
93. Linehan WM, Farrell RE, Cooper CW, Wells SA, Jr. Analysis of pentagastrin and calcium as thyrocalcitonin secretagogues in the early diagnosis of medullary carcinoma of the thyroid gland. Surgical Forum 111–112.
94. Tashjian AH, Howland BG, Melvin KEW et al. Immunoassay of human calcitonin; clinical measurement, relation to serum calcium and studies in patients with medullary carcinoma. N Engl J Med 1970;283:890–895.
95. Dymling JF, Whisky: A new provccative test for calcitonin secretion. Acta Endocrin (Copen H) 1976, July 82(3):500–509.
96. O'Connell JE, Dominiczak AK, Isler CG et al. A comparison of calcium pentagastrin and TRH tests in screening for medullary carcinoma in MEN IIA. Clin Endocrinol 1990;32:417–421.
97. Carney JA, Sizemore GW, Sheps SG. Adrenal medullary disease in multiple endocrine neoplaisia, Type 2 pheochromocytoma and its precursors. Am J Clin Path 1976;66:279–290.
98. Ponder BAJ. Screening for familial medullary carcinoma, a review. J Royal Soc Med 1984;77:585–594.
99. Mathieu E, Despres E, Delepine N, Taieb A. MR Imaging of the adrenal gland in Sipple Disease. J Comp Asst Tomo 1987;11(5):790–794.
100. Gagel RF, Jackson CE, Block MS et al. Age-related probability of development of hereditary medullary carcinoma. J Pediatr 1982;101:941–946.
101. Ponder BAJ, Coffey R, Gagel et al. Risk estimation and screening in families of patients with medullary thyroid carcinoma. Lancet 1988;1:397–400.
102. Tissell LE, Hansson G, Jansson S, Salander H. Reoperation in the treatment of asymptomatic metastasizing medullary thyroid carcinoma. Surgery, 1986; 90:60–66.
103. Block MA, Jackson CE, Tashjian AH. Management of occult medullary thyroid carcinoma. Arch Surg 1978;113:368–372.
104. Normann TV, Tautvik KM, Johanessen JV, Brennhord ID. Medullary carcinoma of the thyroid in Norway, clinical course and endocrinologic aspects. Acta Endocrinol (kbh) 1976;83:71–75.
105. Talpos GB, Jackson GE, Froelich JW et al. Localization of residual medullary thyroid cancer by thallium/technetium scintigraphy. Surgery 1985;98:1189–1196.
106. Poston GJ, Thomas AMK, MacDonald DWR et al. ^{131}I-MIBG Uptake by medullary carcinoma of the thyroid (letter). Lancet 1985;2:560.
107. Goldenberg DM. Tumor imaging with monoclonal antibodies. J Nucl Med 1983;24:350–362.
108. Baulieu JL, Gilloteau P, Delisle MJ et al. Radioiodinated Metaiodobenzylguanidine uptake in medullary thyroid cancer; a French cooperative study. Cancer 1987;60:2189–2194.
109. Clarke SEM, Lazarus CR, Wraight P et al. Pentavalent [99mTc] DMSA, [^{131}I] MIBG, and [99mTc] MDP—An evaluation of three imaging techniques in patients with medullary carcinoma of the thyroid. J Nucl Med 1988;29:33–38.
110. Wells SA, Dilley WG, Farndon JA et al. Early diagnosis and treatment of medullary thyroid carcinoma. Arch Int Med 1985;145:1248–1252.
111. Hellman DE, Kartchner M, Van Antwerp JD et al. Radioiodine in the treatment of medullary carcinoma of the thyroid. J Clin Endocrinol Metab 1979;48:451–455.
112. Deftos LJ, Stein MF. Radioiodine as an adjunct to the surgical treatment of medullary thyroid carcinoma. J Clin Endocrinol Metab 1980;50:967–968.
113. Saad MF, Guido JJ, Samaan NA. Radioactive iodine in the treatment of medullary carcinoma of the thyroid. J Clin Endocrinol Metab 1983;57:124–128
114. Steinfeld AD. The role of radiation therapy in medullary carcinoma of the thyroid. Radiology 1977;123: 745–745.
115. Tubiana M. External radiotherapy and radioiodine in the treatment of thyroid cancer. World J Surg 1981;5:75–84.
116. Samaan NA, Schultz PN, Hickey RC. Medullary thyroid carcinoma: Prognosis of familial versus sporadic disease and the role of radiotherapy. J Clin Endocrinol Metab 1988;67:801–805.
117. Leight GS, Farrell RE, Wells SA, Falletta JM. Effect of chemotherapy on calcitonin levels in patients with metastatic medullary thyroid carcinoma. 1980; AACR Abstracts, 622.
118. Sridhar KS, Holland JF, Brown JC et al. Doxorubicin plus asplatin in the treatment of apudomas. Cancer 1985;55:2634–2637.
119. Goretzki PE, Wahl RA, Becker R et al. Nerve growth factor sensitizes human medullary carcinoma cells for cytostatic therapy in vitro. Surgery 1987; 102:1035–1042.
120. Mahler C, Verhelst J, DeLongueville M, Harris A. Long-term treatment of metastatic medullary thyroid carcinoma with the somatostatin analogue octreotide. Clin Endo 1990;33:261–269.
121. Mathew CGP, Chin KS, Easton DF et al. A linked genetic marker for multiple endocrine neoplaisia type 2A on chromosome 10. Nature 1987;328:527–528.
122. Simpson NE, Kidd KK, Goodfellow PJ et al. Assignment of multiple endocrine neoplaisia Type 2A to chromosome 10 by linkage. Nature 1987; 328:528–530.
123. Nakamura Y, Mathew CGP, Sobol H et al. Linked

by markers flanking the gene for multiple endocrine neoplaisia type 2A. Genomics 1989;5:199–203.

124. Sobol H, Narod S, Nakamura Y et al. Screening for multiple endocrine neoplaisia type 2A with DNA-polymorphism analysis. N Engl J Med 1989;321:996–1001.

125. Sobol H, Narod S, Assouline D et al. Genetic screening of endocrine tumor syndromes with DNA probes: the example of medullary thyroid carcinoma. Horm Reg 1989;32:34–40.

126. Jackson CE, Norum RA. The molecular biology of Laron dwarfism and medullary thyroid cancer. N Engl J Med 1989;321:1039–1040.

127. Narod SA, Sobol H, Nakamura et al. Linkage analysis of hereditary thyroid carcinoma with and without pheochromocytoma. Hum Genet 1989;83:353–358.

128. Mathew CGP, Smith BA, Thorpe K et al. Deletion of genes on chromosome one in endocrine neoplaisia. Nature 1987;328:524–526.

129. Knudson AG. Mutation and cancer: statistical study of retinoblastoma. Proc Natl Acad Sci USA 1971;68820–823.

130. Baylin SB, Gann DS, Hsu SH. Clonal origin of inherited medullary thyroid carcinoma and pheochromocytoma. Science 1976;193:321–323.

131. Nelkin BD, Nakamura Y, White RN et al. Low incidence of loss of chromosome 10 in sporadic and hereditary human medullary carcinoma. Cancer Res 1989;49:4114–4119.

132. Nelkin BD, DeBustras AC, Mabry M, Baylin SB. The molecular biology of medullary thyroid carcinoma—a model for cancer development and progression. JAMA 1989;261:3130–3135.

9

Anaplastic Thyroid Carcinoma

MARVIN W. SINKOFF

Introduction

In any discussion concerning anaplastic thyroid carcinoma (ATC), one is struck by the rapid growth and fulminating quality of this malignancy, which results quite frequently in a fatal outcome. This most malignant of all thyroid carcinomas is also one of the less frequent malignancies encountered in practice, despite the estimate that there must be about 200 million goiters in worldwide incidence.[1] Indeed, goiter is most likely the most common endocrine condition throughout the world, probably because of dietary, environmental, and genetic factors.[2] The concept of anaplastic thyroid carcinoma has undergone changes in interpretation and diagnostic criteria during the past several decades. The terminology also has changed so that "anaplastic carcinoma of the thyroid" is synonymous with the term "undifferentiated thyroid carcinoma" or "undifferentiated thyroid tumor." It does not include other aggressive forms of thyroid malignancy, which have now been delineated and categorized as not originating from epithelial cells.

Livolsi has estimated that carcinoma of the thyroid is diagnosed in 25 patients per million each year in the United States,[1] and represents 1.3% of all malignancies. Thyroid carcinomas produce 0.4% of all carcinoma deaths in the United States. Of all the thyroid carcinomas, the most frequently encountered is papillary carcinoma, followed in order of frequency by follicular carcinoma, mixed papillary–follicular carcinoma, and medullary carcinoma (which still is more frequent than anaplastic thyroid carcinoma.) In Aldinger's series from the M.D. Anderson Hospital in Texas, the incidence was about 7% of 1174 cases of thyroid carcinoma.[2] Histologically proven ATC was demonstrated in 84 cases. Shields has demonstrated an incidence in his series of 12%, with 156 thyroid malignancies reported, of which 20 had anaplastic thyroid carcinoma.[3] Other authors report on series in which ATC is present in an incidence of about 11% to 16%. Jereb found this to be true in 79 cases studied for thyroid malignancy.[4] Woolner found an incidence of 14% of all thyroid carcinomas,[5] and Schneider in the *Acta Cytologica*, in 1980, indicated that the rate of incidence is probably around 12%.[6] The overall incidence in the literature ranges from 7% to 12% to 14%. The incidence seems to be higher in areas of endemic goiter such as Switzerland; this higher incidence seems to be attested to in the European literature, especially in the early decades of this century. This has been attributed to a less clearly defined interpretation and definition of anaplastic thyroid carcinoma, and to the fact that the term included a number of small cell carcinomas that were eventually characterized as lymphoma. It is also conceivable that there may have been a higher incidence of well-differentiated carcinomas in these areas, which then provided the tissue "soil" for transformation and dedifferentiation into the anaplastic form of thyroid carcinoma to take root.

Incidence

Age

Older patients are afflicted with anaplastic carcinoma. The age dividing line used in the literature is below and above fifty. Livolsi reported 29 cases of anaplastic carcinoma with an average age of 67, a range of 60 to 80, and only 2 patients under 50 years of age.[7] Nishayama reported the average age as more than 63 years.[8] Woolner's average age was more than 57 years,[5] and Shvero reported that the mean age was 66 years.[9] In Iceland, the literature reveals the mean age to be 73 among women and 69 among men.[10] Spires indicates that the carcinoma is found most often in the sixth and seventh decades of life.[11] Ekman reports a mean age of 72 years with a range of 41 to 89 years.[12] The Mayo Clinic report, over a 25-year period covering 1161 thyroid carcinomas of which 82 (7.1%) were anaplastic, revealed a mean age of 65 years.[13] Carcangiu found the mean age to be 66 years with only three patients under 50, the range being from 37 to 90 years of age.[14] Aldinger reported that 70% of patients were above the age of 60 and 8% under the age of fifty.[2]

Sex

As in most thyroid cancers, there is a preponderance of females among patients with ATC. The female-to-male ratio is 3:1.2 in Ekman's group,[12] and 3:1 in Shvero's group.[9] Livolsi reports a 4.1:2.1 ratio.[7] Nishayama had 43 cases of female ATC and 10 of male ATC.[8] Spires' female-to-male[11] ratio based on a very small number of cases (14) was 1.3:1; Aldinger reported a 1.5:1 ratio in 1100 cases of cancer, of which 84 were ATC.[2] Carcangiu reported a 3.1:1 female-to-male ratio.[14] Chang from Taiwan reports a female-to-male ratio of 1.4:1 in a small series of 28 cases.[15]

Clinical Picture

The most common symptoms reported in anaplastic thyroid carcinoma are due to the effects of the tumor on the structures of the neck; namely, dysphonia, dysphagia, and dyspnea. In Thomas' series of 84 patients, hoarseness was present 31% of the time, dyspnea, 19%; and dysphagia, 30%. Roughly one third of all patients had these symptoms.[16] These symptoms rarely occur with well-differentiated carcinoma, so that once they present, the physician should suspect the existence of a most malignant process. Fulminating tumors, namely, sarcoma, hemangioendothelioma, osteoclastic sarcoma, and even medullary carcinoma may present in the same way. The patient is very aware of an enlarging mass; in the Mayo series, this was present 59% of the time in 71 patients.[13] Again, dyspnea, dysphonia and dysphagia were very prevalent; however, most of the patients suffered from neck pain, 25 had a cough, and 20 showed profound weight loss. Aldinger reports that there were cervical nodes present in 20 cases and distant metastases in 11.[2] In more than 70 cases, 42 patients were totally unresectable, 17 received radiotherapy, and 13 received chemotherapy. A recent increase in size was reported by Nishayama in 27 of 53 cases,[8] and 15 of the 53 cases had new masses in the neck without previous enlargement of the thyroid. These masses showed no uptake. Nineteen of the cases had lung metastases and eight had vocal cord paralysis.

Silverberg reported that of 23 cases, 20 had pulmonary metastases and other lesions.[17] The cause of death in 11 of these cases was by direct extension. The sites and numbers of metastases were as follows: lung, 12; lymph nodes, 4; pleural, 6; adrenal involvement, 6; liver, 2; kidney, 4; pancreas, 4; heart, 4; bowel, 2; brain, 0; spleen, 2; ovaries, 0 and dura, 0. The tumor is so aggressive that it easily spreads through the capsule of the gland, beyond the lymph nodes into the muscles and soft tissues of the neck, thereby producing its symptomatology and its physical signs. Shvero[9] reported that 34.5% of his patients had a cervical mass, 46% had enlarged thyroid, 15% had metastases to the cervical nodes and 12% to the lungs; and that there was one case of metathesis each to the brain, esophagus, and ribs. There were 11 cases of vocal cord paralyses and 5 cases in which the trachea was invaded. These tissues were all fixed by tumor. The mass could not be delineated and was adherent to trachea, esophagus, and neck muscles. It is believed that neither age nor sex greatly affect survival rates. It is well known that patients with follicular and papillary forms of the disease have greater survival and that those with medullary carcinoma, unless it has metastasized, have a better survival rate than patients with any of the anaplastic thyroid carcinomas.[10] Simpson,[18] in the *Canadian Medical Association Journal*, indicated that prognostic factors could only provide limited means of predicting survival greater than a few months; the factors he listed were age of the individual (the younger patients succumbing more quickly than the older), the size of the tumor, nodal involvement, and the presence of distant metastases with extrathyroidal invasion. Size as a predictor of prognosis was evaluated by the Mayo group.[13] Of 82 cases, 17 were less than 5 cm and 75 were greater than 5 cm. It was believed that the size of the lesion as well as the extent and nodal involvement might have some effect upon prognosis. Forty-two patients of the 82 required tracheostomies to survive, some of which were performed prophylactically prior to radiation therapy.[13] Aldinger believes that the only clinical factor affecting survival, if any, is the amount and size of the anaplastic focus in the initial lesion, especially if it is within a well-differentiated carcinoma.[2] Carcangiu's study of 57 cases revealed that one half were already beyond the thyroid at the time of diagnosis, with cervical node involvement in 20 cases and 11 distant metastases.[14] Forty-two of the 57 cases were unresectable.

Aldinger provides a fairly well defined staging schema of thyroid carcinoma.[2] In 1174 cases, he defined the staging as follows: stage I, confined to the gland; stage II, extension to the regional lymph nodes; stage III, extension to lymph nodes and soft tissues of the neck; and stage IV, distant metastases. Thomas has varied this staging[16]: stage I, limited to the thyroid gland; stage II, regional nodes; and stage III, beyond the regional nodes. There is no differentiation made between extension to regional nodes and extension to the soft tissues of the neck and direct contiguity beyond that.

The staging of the tumor is of some value in describing the extent of disease. Inasmuch as we are dealing with a most malignant tumor, the therapeutic objective is palliation and the prevention of respiratory distress. Knowing the degree to which a tumor has extended from its base within the gland into the regional lymph nodes and from there into the soft tissues of the neck or to distant locations by metastasis is helpful. Surgical intervention may be needed in any case to prevent respiratory death, but should not be employed in cases in which there is evidence for massive extension into other organ systems and fixation of neck tissue. In these cases, radiation and chemotherapy and combined therapeutic techniques are now employed. The clinical extent of the disease process facilitates and enhances the staging. Once tissues involved in the tumor process are identified and localized, one can stage the tumor and proceed with an attempt at appropriate therapy.

Pathology

In 1969 Sidney Werner chaired a committee that devised a classification of thyroid tumors.[19] This classification has been more stringently defined with time; small cell undifferentiated carcinoma no longer is part of the anaplastic thyroid category. The small cell category will be discussed in other sections on lymphoma, medullary carcinoma and sarcoma in this chapter. In the 1970s, classification was more specific in differentiating epithelial cell origin from nonepithelial cell. Anaplastic carcinoma usually represents 5% to 14% of all thyroid malignancies.[2–6] The term ATC has also been used interchangeably with undifferentiated carcinoma of the thyroid, specifically that of epithelial origin. The techniques of electron microscopy have been most helpful in delineating the epithelial origin of anaplastic thyroid carcinoma and excluding the sarcomas and the lymphomas from this origin. On gross examination, all undifferentiated carcinomas share an appearance of high mitotic activity with large foci of necrosis and a marked degree

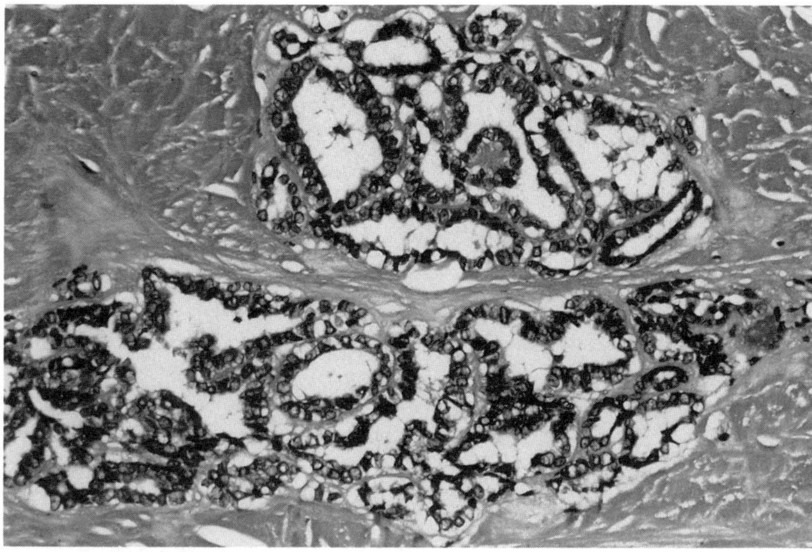

Figure 9.1. Patient with thyroid cancer showing an area of well-differentiated papillary adenocarcinoma. Note papillations, optically clear nuclei, and follicles.

of invasion of the muscle walls in veins with tumor emboli.[20] Indeed, there is replacement of muscle walls of veins and arteries by tumor. Skin ulcerations can occur. Occasionally, because of the fibrous nature of these tumors, the term *sarcomatoid change* has been used interchangeably with "undifferentiated" and "anaplastic" in the literature. In his article, Spires indicated that the term be used exclusively for giant cell and/or spindle cell patterns, thus reflecting a very high grade carcinoma with solid epithelial patterns without evidence of follicle formation.[11]

Cell Types

Giant Cell

By the use of both light and electron microscopic techniques and tissue culture techniques, there has been an intensive study of the giant cell and spindle cell types of anaplastic carcinoma (see Figs. 9.1–4). The undifferentiated epithelial neoplasm at times is so fibrous or spindled that it mimics fibrosarcoma. There are multinucleated giant cells with marked eosinophilic cytoplasm resembling rhabdomyoblasts or malignant histiocytes. There are numerous abnormal mitoses.[1] Indeed, at times the giant cells may resemble osteoclasts. The examination of the ultrastructure on electron microscopy will reveal many cytoplasmic organelles and dense bodies similar to thyroid follicular epithelium. In addition, desmosomes and poorly developed filaments are seen as well. Nishayama reported that large amounts of cytoplasm at times resemble fusiform shapes similar to those seen in fibrosarcoma. Mature connective tissue is seen in some cases with the previously aforementioned eosinophilic-like cytoplasm.[8] All observers agree that the giant cells often have bizarre shapes and that there are acidophilic cells that sometimes resemble Hürthle cells. Occasionally, some follicular carcinoma elements with well encapsulated follicles are detected. Further description of this tissue reveals the presence of intracellular junctions. Follicular remnants may be identified in the tumor. There are occasionally nonneoplastic epithelial cells that resemble thyroid follicles.[21] There are also transitional forms found that can mimic mesenchymal tissue and resemble cells seen in mesenchymal tumors and granulomatous lesions. The cytoplasm has been described as being similar to spindle cells, with prominent ribosomes. There is no linking of ribosomes by well-defined attachment com-

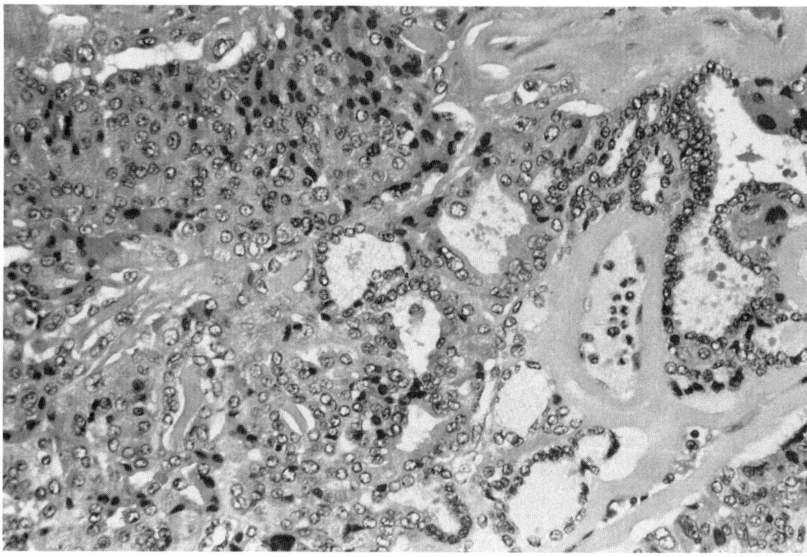

Figure 9.2. This is a specimen from the same patient as Figure 9.1 demonstrating areas of thyroid tumor with both well differentiated and poorly differentiated papillary-thyroid carcinoma.

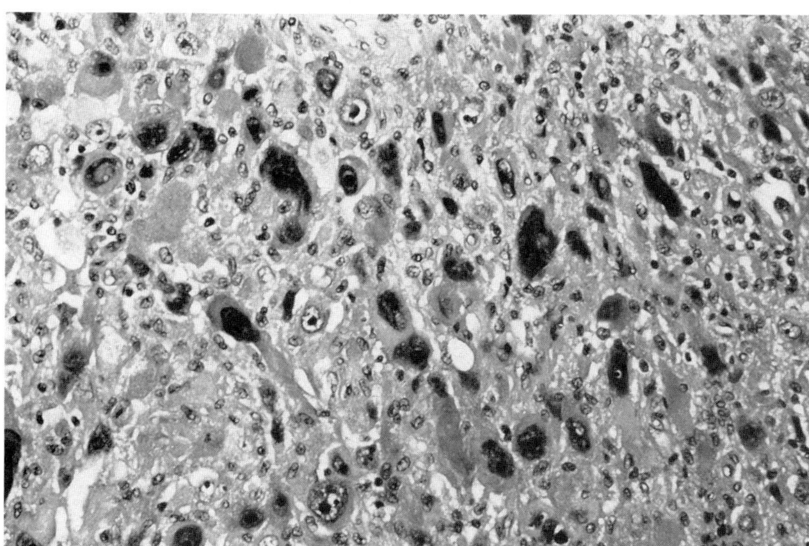

Figure 9.3. In the same patient there is a demonstration of areas of thyroid carcinoma with anaplastic features, namely giant cells and spindle cells.

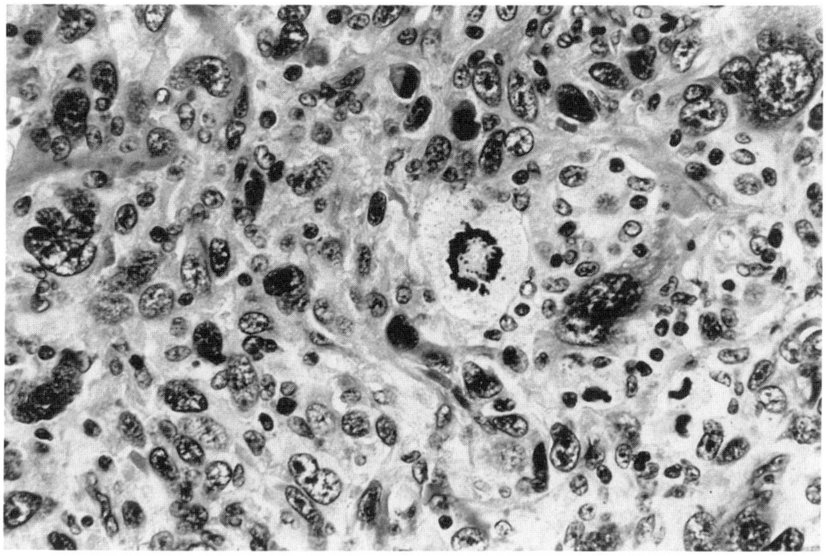

Figure 9.4. Anaplastic thyroid carcinoma exhibiting characteristic spindle and giant cell forms.

plexes, and they are not surrounded by basal laminae. The stroma reveals a moderate amount of collagen fibrils, and abundant microvilli can be found.

Spindle Cell

In many anaplastic thyroid carcinomas both giant and spindle cells are present in tissue specimens; the presence of one of these two cell types does not determine an exclusive tissue category. Nevertheless, the spindle cell anaplastic carcinoma has certain features which are of unique interest. Here again, electron microscopy has been much more valuable than light microscopy. The importance of the electron microscopy technique lies in its ability to differentiate mesenchymal tissue from epithelial tissue, and sarcoma from carcinoma.[22] Desmosomal attachment plates are seen with microvilli. There are transitional forms between the acinar and neoplastic cellular elements. A conversion of round and giant cells into a spindle form is demonstrated. Ultrastructure features demonstrated in tissue culture resemble the cells seen from a primary tumor. On the other hand, if the ultrastructure on electron microscopy reveals an origin in fiberblasts, the tumor must then be categorized as fibrosarcoma. Jao reported that in follicular carcinoma, prominent mitochondria would be seen together with rough endoplasmic reticulum and evidence of secretory activity.[23] Desmosomes were seen to have complex cellular attachments, and basal laminae were present. However, in the spindle cell carcinoma, desmosomes were rare and there were no basal laminae. Gaal reports that the presence of junctional complexes are characteristic of epithelial tissue and can be demonstrated in electron microscopic studies.[21] Gaal also described the spindle cells as having elongated nuclei, and deep indentations containing nuclear bodies. The cytoplasm showed moderately large amounts of rough cytoplasmic reticulum, Golgi complexes, fine filaments, liposomes, and relatively large mitochondria. Tumor cells sometimes include microvilli and rare cilia. Occasionally, the presence of abortive follicular forms have been demonstrated, surrounded by basal laminae.[21]

Squamous Cell

Primary squamous cell carcinoma may be confused with spindle and giant cell carcinoma. Squamous cell carcinoma is a rare lesion. The process of squamous metaplasia has been implicated in the formation of squamous cell carcinoma. It is well known that squamous cell metaplasia occurs in many epithelial tissues in the body, including the thyroid.[24] The squamous cell carcinoma can be as aggressive and fulminating as anaplastic thyroid carcinoma. Squamous cells may be present in spindle and giant cell sections. The thesis that squamous metaplasia occurs is facilitated by the fact that histologically the thyroid gland contains no squamous cell tissue. The term "squamoid pattern" has been attributed to anaplastic carcinoma in combination with spindle and/or giant cells; however, the entity of squamous cell carcinoma still is considered distinct from anaplastic carcinoma although clinically it behaves like anaplastic carcinoma. The squamous component may be seen in the spindle and giant cell tumor, but is not a predominanting pattern. The consensus of the literature is that this entity, squamous cell carcinoma, in terms of its aggressiveness, its fulminating course, and its dismal and fatal outlook behaves like anaplastic thyroid carcinoma. Therapy has been found wanting in this particularly aggressive tumor as it is in the classic giant and spindle cell carcinomas.[24]

Confusion with Lymphoma, Medullary Carcinoma and Sarcoma, and So-called "Small Cell" Carcinoma

The pathologic differential diagnosis of giant cells and spindle cells must consider soft tissue sarcomas; namely, fibrosarcoma, malignant fibrous histiocytoma, malignant hemangiopericytoma, and angiosarcoma. Occasionally, metastasis of the spindle and giant cell carcinoma leads to formation of mature cartilage and bone. True sarcomas of the thyroid constitute 0.6% of all thyroid tumors. Aldinger reported 3 sarcomas in 1174 malignant thyroid cancers.[2]

In addition, a large literature has developed that separates and excludes small cell carcinoma, which is now considered to be malignant lymphoma of the thyroid gland. Occasionally, aggressive and quickly growing medullary carcinoma may mimic an anaplastic carcinoma in its clinical outcome. The only anaplastic neoplasms of epithelial origin are spindle cell and/or giant cell tumors.[2] Thomas,[16] in 1973, indicated that it was rare for small cell carcinoma to coexist with well-differentiated carcinoma, whereas well differentiated and anaplastic carcinoma could coexist in from 5% to 10% of patients. Pathologically, the absence of follicles in the lymphomatous tissue or acini formation by neoplastic cells are the criteria for establishing the diagnosis of lymphoma.[24] It is also known that small cell carcinoma responds better to radiation—an additional reason to separate this category from anaplastic carcinoma, which has different clinical implications and requires different therapeutic approaches.[25] In the past, with the use of light microscopy, it was difficult to differentiate the small cell from anaplastic carcinoma, but with the advent of electron microscopy, ultrastructure studies proved useful in separating the two.

There is also an entity known as poorly differentiated insular carcinoma,[20] which is a separate pathologic entity. It is composed of solid nodes or nodules. There are some small follicles with a monotonous growth of small cells of follicular derivation. There is necrosis; mitoses are also noted. These tumors are negative for calcitonin and positive for thyroglobulin. They metastasize aggressively to regional and distal organs, but they are not giant or spindle cell carcinomas. As mentioned, leiomyosarcomata have been reported together with various other forms of sarcomata. In anaplastic carcinoma of the thyroid, sarcomatous malignant changes have been seen; these changes may very well represent the spindle cell form of the anaplastic carcinoma. A note should be made about osteoclastic-like giant cell thyroid carcinoma. Vizel-Schwartz reported such a case in 1981 in which there was osteoclastoma-like material seen in giant cell carcinoma.[26] He stated this was a rare variant of anaplastic thyroid carcinoma.

Another rare variety of undifferentiated carcinoma is an adenosquamous carcinoma of the thyroid reported by Nicolaides in 1989.[27] This is characterized as a rare, aggressive tumor, similar to anaplastic carcinoma in its prognosis and course. Histologically, there is a blending of glandular and squamous elements. It is important to identify the malignant nature of the squamous epithelium as opposed to benign squamous metaplasia, which as indicated can be found in papillary carcinoma. Once again, it must be emphasised that squamous metaplasia occurs in most epithelial tissues in the body, including the thyroid; one must not confuse this phenomenon with the rare squamous cell or adenosquamous cell carcinoma of the thyroid gland.

Immunopathology (Immunohistology)

Hormonal Tumor Markers

Shvero in 1988[9] studied 26 cases in which thyroid-associated antigens were sought using immunoperoxidase techniques. He categorized thyroglobulin as being an excellent marker for follicular cells, calcitonin for medullary cells, factor-8–related antigen for hemangioendothelioma, and leukocyte common antigen for lymphoma. Of interest was that 10 cases of the 26 were negative for all antigens, indicating the lack of differentiation and primitive nature of the anaplastic cells. Livolsi[7] reported that 27% of the thyroid carcinomas stained for thyroglobulin and 0% for calcitonin. In that series, 30% showed no markers of any expression, thus indicating a total lack of differentiation. Of 29 cases in which calcitonin was not present, thyroglobulin was demonstrated in 8, but not in metastases. There was no evidence of medullary or parafollicular cell differentiation. 70% of the tumors that had epithelial characteristics expressed epithelial membrane antigen (EMA), keratin, or both. 40% with epithelial characteristics expressed vimentin.[7] Böcker, in 1980,[28] analyzed 72 cases of malignant neoplasms of the thyroid, of which 37 were papillary, 9 follicular, 10 anaplastic, and 9 medullary; there were 7 other neoplasms of various types. Thyroglobulin analysis was helpful in distinguishing the anaplastic thyroid carcinoma from follicular carcinoma and papillary carcinoma. The use of thyroglobulin was considered to be adjunctive to light microscopy. Thyroglobulin as a hormonal marker has been found to be localized in the cytoplasm of tumor cells. It is found to a far less degree in the interpapillary spaces and in the glandular laminae. It is apparently not secreted by tumor cells. Most observers report that tests for thyroglobulin in anaplastic thyroid carcinoma are negative. If they are positive,[20] it is assumed that the thyroglobulin detected is a product of nonneoplastic follicles entrapped within the anaplastic carcinoma and composed of fairly normal follicular cells, or that there is a preexisting area of better-differentiated tumor cells.[29] It is known that in differentiated medullary carcinoma, there is a failure of calcitonin to be a specific marker. This has evoked controversy in the literature. Carcangiu,[14] in 70 cases of which 54 were followed up, found no evidence for the expression of thyroglobulin or calcitonin.

Epithelial and Sarcomatous Markers

Beitrami studied 12 cases of anaplastic thyroid carcinoma with antibody studies[29] and found a coexpression of cytokeratin and vimentin in 66% of these cases. He felt that the antidesmoplastic antibody could be used to differentiate sarcomatous changes from carcinoma of the thyroid. Livolsi[7] indicates that monoclonal keratin studies are specific for the epithelial origin of anaplastic carcinoma and that epithelial migration activity (EMA) is positive in those cases of anaplastic carcinoma. In many instances, the EMA and keratin studies were demonstrated in the same case, or even in the same cell. Alpha chymotrypsin was studied in 15 cases and indicated positivity in both epithelial and sarcomatous tumor cells. Desmin, considered to be a marker for muscle, was not present in Livolsi's studies. Indeed, there was no indication of desmin even in the cases of anaplastic carcinoma that were totally composed of spindle cells or that were completely sarcomatous. Rosai[20] reported that cytokeratin studies were superior to thyroglobulin in detecting the epithelial origin of tumor. In his ultrastructural markers, there were specific intracellular junctions visible on electron microscopy that had complex microvillus structures: filaments with intracellular laminae. He maintains that there are pitfalls in these criteria that were used in these studies, since reports varied from lab to lab, tumor to tumor, and technique to technique. In addition, the antibodies may vary, and the interpretation of the results may vary.

Intermediate Filaments and Other Markers

In 1988, Kawahara indicated that the study of intermediate filaments could prove to be a useful tool in the differential diagnosis of anaplastic carcinoma.[30] Rosai indicated that immunocytochemical reactions combined with electron microscopy could provide the kind of evidence that would prove the reliability of intermediate filaments for diagnosis.[20] Five subtypes of intermediate cytoplasmic filaments were defined both biochemically and immunologically: keratin is a marker for epithelial tissue, vimentin for mesenchymal tissue, desmin for muscle tissue, glial fibrillary acidic protein for glial tissue, and neural filaments for neuronal cells. The most useful epithelial marker using monoclonal antibodies is cytokeratin. This seems to delineate the epithelial origin of anaplastic carcinoma. Makinen utilized epithelial growth factor (EGF)-binding in two cases of anaplastic carcinoma and demonstrated a higher than normal degree of binding in malignant tissue as compared with normal tissue.[31] There also was a higher degree of binding than in the adjacent normal tissue. In other tumors, no such correlation of EGF binding and prognosis could be demonstrated.

Klemi[32] studied the DNA aneuploidy in 19 cases of anaplastic thyroid carcinoma. Of these cases, 15 were large cell and 4 spindle cell. Thirteen cases demonstrated DNA aneuploidy. He posited that coexisting cell lines with different DNA content may occur in anaplastic carcinoma, and that a change in DNA content is probably an early and common event in carcinogenesis. Aneuploidy was positive in anaplastic carcinoma in 15 of 19 cases. Ekman[12] studied 36 cases for DNA content using immunocytology and found that all patients had 82% to 100% aneuploid cells. It was believed that this was an index of higher grade malignancy. In 7 cases the DNA content did not change before or after therapy with chemotherapy and radiotherapy. His conclusion was that DNA analysis could not be helpful in providing better prognostic information beyond that which was obtained by histopathologic techniques, and there were no means to determine which patients with anaplastic thyroid carcinoma might survive longer in a palliative state.[12]

Aasland, in 1988, reported a recent finding that EGF induces proliferation and dedifferentiation in normal thyroid epithelial cells in vitro. He posited that epithelial growth factor may contribute to the development or the maintenance of the malignant phenotype in papillary carcinoma of the thyroid. Whether EGF has any role to play in anaplastic carcinoma remains to be seen.[33] Makinen, however, did study the receptors for EGF and thyrotropin in thyroid carcinoma[31]. He reported that in 10 patients with papillary and anaplastic carcinoma there was more EGF receptor found in the neoplasms than in adjacent normal tissue, and that indeed there was a very low content of EGF receptor found in medullary and follicular carcinoma. Therefore, the amount of EGF receptor was significantly higher; its distribution in papillary and anaplastic tissue was different from its distribution in follicular and medullary tissue. Moreover, the alteration in the EGF-receptor content was independent of the thyroid-stimulating hormone (TSH)-receptor content. It was found that there was a very low level of high-affinity TSH-receptor sites in anaplastic, medullary, or follicular cell carcinoma.

Pathophysiology

There have been many speculations concerning the relationship of previous radiation exposure, iodine deficiency, and the presence of well-differentiated thyroid carcinoma in the development of ATC.

In Aldinger's paper,[2] 960 cases of thyroid disease were studied in which 243 were treated with ^{131}I therapy. In the follow-up study of these 243 patients, a transformation to anaplastic thyroid carcinoma was demonstrated in only 10 patients. Spires has commented that any speculation with regard to the effects of previous irradiation of the thyroid gland, whether it be by external radiation or radioactive iodine, is difficult to evaluate because of the small number of patients that have been involved in these transformations.[11] There have been no adequate control groups for comparison, nor decent prospective studies made to answer these important questions. Therefore, all conclusions about the role of irradiation, whether external or radioactive iodine, must still be speculative. Kapp[34] in a study reported in the *Yale Journal of Biology and Medicine* cites an M.D. Anderson report from Houston of 352 cases treated with ^{131}I in which no transformation was demonstrated and another study of 359 cases treated with external radiation or ^{131}I cited by Tubiana,[35] again without providing evidence of transformation to anaplastic carcinoma. In the literature, there are interesting isolated case reports. Bridges[36] reports a case of anaplastic thyroid carcinoma that developed in an individual who had a heart valve replacement, had a multinodular goiter and became thyrotoxic after treatment with amiodarone. The thyrotoxicosis was treated with carbimazole and, subsequently, radioactive iodine. Apparently, 30 weeks after the induction of ^{131}I therapy, the patient was noted to have developed an anaplastic thyroid carcinoma. What the effect of low-dose exposure on the gland from ^{131}I therapy might be is an intriguing question. In particular, one would like to know the thyroid gland uptake of ^{131}I and the effect of this ionizing radiation after treatment with carbimazole. It has also been noted that an irritation phenomenon can occur with lower doses of radiation as opposed to higher doses. However, one such case does not prove or reinforce the concept that radiation has a role in the production of anaplastic thyroid carcinoma. Nevertheless, the literature is replete with reports of a possible relationship between anaplastic thyroid carcinoma and radiation.[11,17,37,38]

The role of iodine deficiency is complex and speculative; it has been discussed at greater length in the European literature. In some cases, a history of goiter has been demonstrated in 50% of patients who subsequently develop anaplastic carcinoma. Jereb found that 33 of 39 cases had a history of goiter,[4] and in another 22 of these cases there was a history of nontoxic goiter. He cites five patients with goiters in childhood who eventually developed anaplastic thyroid carcinoma in adult life. In a report from Taiwan, Chang cites 14 cases of longstanding goiter out of 24 cases of anaplastic thyroid carcinoma; and the median duration of these cases of goiter was 20 years.[15] He states that 3 out of 10 patients received radiation to the neck. Nel, in the *Mayo Clinic Proceedings* in 1985, reported that the incidence of anaplastic thyroid carcinoma was 15% to 50% in the European literature.[13] One is compelled to state that some of the diagnoses were not accurate with reference to the anaplastic type, but represented an increasing incidence of papillary carcinoma in the European literature, which then underwent transformation and dedifferentiation into anaplastic forms. Hofstadter, in 1980, discussed endemic goiter in Switzerland and the effect of iodine prophylaxis upon the development of goiter and carcinoma.[39] He found a remarkable difference between endemic and nonendemic goiters. There was a higher incidence of papillary carcinoma in the endemic areas, and iodine prophylaxis improved the survival rate in these thyroid carcinomas. With iodine prophylaxis, there was a decrease in the percentage of undifferentiated carcinoma, and there was an absolute decrease in total carcinoma cases from 1974 to 1980. Kapp also alludes to the observation that in areas of iodine deficiency, anaplastic carcinoma incidence rises.[34] Moreover, he reports that most often anaplastic carcinoma developed in patients without any effect from ^{131}I or external radiation.

The concept that radiation is contributory to the development of anaplastic carcinoma is based on the speculation that more than one cell type exists in well-differentiated thyroid carcinomas. These cells vary in their susceptibility to the effect of radiation. This is a selection process, with cells less responsive to radiation cloning during therapy, thus creating a new cell line that becomes dedifferentiated. It is also believed that perhaps viruses, environmental pollutants, and TSH might all be factors in dedifferentiation. Carcangiu reports that in Florence, 30% of anaplastic carcinomas were found in patients with goiter, as opposed to a 3.2% incidence of ATC and goiter in

Minnesota.[14] This was attributed to the fact that in Minnesota there was iodine prophylaxis as opposed to the cases in Florence, and that the decrease in frequency was secondary to the use of iodine prophylaxis. In those patients, Carcangiu reported no previous radiation exposure in childhood or adolescence.[14] All were euthyroid at the time of diagnosis. However, goiters or nodules were present in a substantial number of the cases, and some had indeed had surgery for adenoma and papillary carcinoma.

A more frequently observed phenomenon is the existence of a well-differentiated thyroid carcinoma that probably undergoes transformation or conversion into the anaplastic form. Livolsi discusses the evidence of 4 cases out of 29 with preexisting papillary carcinoma at the edge of anaplastic thyroid tumors.[7] This suggests that ATC may have its origin in an abnormal thyroid that may very well have been the locus for adenomatous goiter, preexisting adenoma, or well differentiated carcinoma. It has been said that goiter is present in some form in 80% of these cases, and that a low grade or benign process is transformed into a highly malignant process. Again, our ability to answer whether or not external radiation enhances the potential for transformation still eludes us, but the question is nevertheless a fruitful one for further investigation. In 1972, Nishayama discussed 68 cases of anaplastic carcinoma but immediately excluded 15 cases, 14 of which were small cell and one of which was fibrosarcoma.[8] Of the 53 cases of anaplastic thyroid carcinoma, 42 had well-differentiated carcinoma either coexisting with or preceding the anaplastic transformation. These 42 cases originated with papillary, follicular, Hürthle cell, clear cell, and medullary carcinomas. Silverberg reported that 6 out of 23 cases had previous papillary or follicular carcinoma that then transformed into anaplastic carcinoma.[17] He cites the fact that 5 of these 6 cases had had previous irradiation to the neck.

Harada in 1977 reported that 9 of 27 cases had coexistent well-differentiated carcinoma with anaplastic thyroid carcinoma and that 4 had apparently an association of well-differentiated carcinoma with squamous cell carcinoma.[38a] He posited that the malignant transformation of the well-differentiated carcinoma was part of the natural history of thyroid carcinoma, and that it was possible for a well-differentiated carcinoma to be transformed by dedifferentiation into either anaplastic or squamous cell carcinoma. At that time, Harada again raised the question of the possible role of external radiation or ^{131}I therapy in the dedifferentiation process and posed the problem of the existence of a more likely phenomenon; namely, natural transformation. Spires, in a report of 14 cases, indicated that 8 had had previous thyroid disease: 3 with papillary carcinoma, 3 with goiter, 2 with thyroid nodule, and 1 with adenoma.[11] He too alluded to the fact that 6 of these 14 cases had some form of radiation exposure prior to the onset of the ATC: 4 had been exposed to radioactive iodine and 2 to external radiation. Kapp found that an astounding 75% of patients with ATC had previously had goiter.[34]

Livolsi discusses the experimental work of Ueda and Furth,[40] in which papillary carcinoma after successive passages and tissue culture underwent sarcomatous transformation into a dedifferentiated anaplastic carcinoma. The distinction of anaplastic thyroid carcinoma from highly malignant sarcoma must be made by electron microscopy. Hirabayashi indicated that thyroiditis was very uncommon in localized follicular carcinoma, and did not occur in invasive follicular or medullary carcinoma, and was extremely uncommon in anaplastic thyroid carcinoma. This inflammatory reaction was most commonly seen in papillary carcinoma.[41] Aldinger found foci of well-differentiated thyroid carcinoma in 66 of 84 cases, and the metastases showed both differentiated and undifferentiated cells.[2] In some cases, the primary tumor showed no dedifferentiation, but the metastases showed undifferentiated cells. Aldinger refers to the confusion between squamous cell carcinoma on one hand and thyroid sarcoma on the other, and states that it is vital to evaluate these other entities with reference to etiology and survival data.[2] He too mentions the transformation in tissue culture of well-differentiated carcinoma into dedifferentiated cells, and mentions that these cells can coexist with differentiated carcinoma.

Mention is also made of the role of TSH stimulation and external and ^{131}I radiation. It has been claimed in the literature that ATC does develop in TSH-dependent, well-differentiated tumors after serial transfers. This has occurred in mice 3 to 7 years after a continuous TSH stimulation; in these animals the TSH-dependent tumors eventually become autonomous and undifferentiated. In Thomas' paper, 65 patients out of 84 had goiter.[16] He also mentions that some patients with small cell and clear cell carcinoma had goiter, and that this goiter was an underlying factor before the onset of ATC. In the 65 patients with goiter, 28 had had it for more than a year. Schneider[42] reports that spindle cell and giant cell tumors arise from previously differentiated tumor through anaplastic transformation and cites the study at M.D. Anderson Hospital (Houston, Texas) where, after thorough sectioning of the pathologic material, 7.5% revealed foci of differentiated lesions.[42] This was true at Memorial Hospital (New York) in 5.5% and at Capetown University in 12.2% of the cases. Getaz speculates about patients who had had Hodgkin's disease and received irradiation, subsequently developing anaplastic thyroid carcinoma. He cites the well-observed fact that thyroid radiation in infancy can lead to thyroid carcinoma, that at Hiroshima and Nagasaki, an increased incidence of thyroid carcinoma was present because of external radiation from the atomic bombs, and that patients given radiation to the face in adolescence develop a higher incidence of thyroid carcinoma.[43] Most often these carcinomas are papillary, follicular, or mixed. In Getaz's report in 1979, two patients developed anaplastic thyroid carcinoma following external radiation. No threshold dose is known for the induction and it is known that children have a greater propensity for development of nodules in the thyroid. The question of TSH suppression in patients given irradiation for other causes is raised: can hypothyroidism that results in an elevated TSH for prolonged periods of time, contribute over a period of years to the production of carcinoma and to the process of dedifferentiation (although this is highly speculative), and to the role this process plays in the production of anaplastic transformation? Throughout the literature there is reference made to Crile's seminal 1959 paper[44] in which he reported the transformation of a low grade papillary carcinoma into an anaplastic carcinoma after therapy with radioiodine. He reported a patient with a low grade papillary carcinoma, who had been given some small doses of radiation 28 years previously, and who was then subsequently treated with ^{131}I. There was no change in the tumor nor any regional metastases to the cervical nodes for years. Then suddenly there was a change from differentiated papillary carcinoma to undifferentiated autonomous carcinoma. At that time Crile posited the possibility of an increased output of TSH induced by ^{131}I therapy, which may have contributed to the initiation of the transformation process or to the possibility of growth of autonomous dormant carcinoma cells. He advocated, at that time, suppression therapy with thyroid hormone for papillary carcinoma, in the hope that this would prevent TSH stimulation; he also suggested an operation on papillary carcinoma that would remove most of the tissue that might provide the cells with materials for transformation and dedifferentiation of the tissue. Spires[11] also cites Ueda and Furth's experiments[40] of transformation of thyroid epithelial tissue in mice, into spindle and giant cell carcinomas over a 7-year period, considering these to be TSH-induced tumors. He also cites Fisher[22] who reported the conversion of giant cells from mixed giant and spindle ATC to a specific spindle cell form. He hypothesizes the existence of a prototypic cell element common to all thyroid tumors. This is similar to the idea that there are prototypic cell elements in the bone marrow that produce all forms of malignant cellular hematologic disease. Rosai posited that all thyroid carcinoma has the potential for dedifferentiation into highly aggressive neoplasms.[20] In Carcangiu's series,[14] 30% of the anaplastic carcinomas developed from, or at least they coexisted with well-differentiated carcinoma; this relationship could also be seen in metastatic foci. Spires maintained that 10 of 14 cases of anaplastic carcinoma were found to have well-differentiated thyroid carcinoma.[11] Rieger,[45] in Austria, studied thyroid carcinoma over a

17-year period, analyzing 1848 patients with thyroidectomy. Fourteen patients had coexisting thyroid malignancy, of which 5 were papillary, 4 follicular, 3 ATC, and 2 medullary. Ten cases were found in cold nodules, two in unidentifiable areas and two in hot areas. He found no thyroid carcinoma in cases of Graves' disease; indeed there were none out of 64 cases. In multinodular toxic goiter, 7 of 676 had carcinoma; in patients with uninodular toxic goiter, there was a very low rate, 3 of 1108 (0.279%). He concluded that coexisting malignancy and hypothyroidism was rare in endemic iodine deficient goiter areas. Of 126 cases of ATC, Wallin demonstrated 17 cases with well-differentiated tumor foci.[46] By using DNA analysis he attempted to demonstrate the autonomous and independent nature of ATC and that there was no real patterning for the coexistence of dedifferentiation and well-differentiated thyroid carcinoma. He states that in the majority of cases of ATC, the malignant cells arose *de novo* and were not a transformation of well-differentiated cells. Williams[47] states that since these carcinomas of an anaplastic nature (spindle and giant cell) arise from an epithelial origin, evidence implicating follicles has been demonstrated in small areas of differentiated carcinoma in a proportion of anaplastic carcinoma cases. He cites the fact that the incidence of anaplastic carcinoma can vary from 5% to 25% and reiterates the thesis of an origin from preexisting thyroid disease with a rapid transformation, as opposed to the papillary and follicular carcinomas that show slow growth. It is his thesis that ATC arises more from follicular than from papillary carcinoma. He mentions the increased incidence of ATC in Switzerland as compared with the United States.[47] He also cites the relatively inconsequential nature of radiation: a group study of more than 21,000 patients revealed only five cases that might have had transformation based upon therapy with ^{131}I. Treatment with ^{131}I was followed from 4 to 22 years.

Only a very small proportion of papillary or differentiated carcinoma goes on to become undifferentiated carcinoma and, therefore, the treatment of differentiated carcinoma should not be influenced by potential transformation since this is a rare phenomenon. Moreover, there is no known rationale for considering genetic factors to play a role in the incidence of anaplastic thyroid carcinoma or its propensity to dedifferentiate from well-differentiated carcinoma. Autoimmune thyroiditis and hyperthyroidism are not factors of any consequence in the understanding of this phenomenon. There is still some thought given to the role of TSH in neoplastic transformation. There seems to be experimental evidence connecting malignant changes, the influence of low iodine diet, and possibly partial thyroidectomy, all of which can lead to increased TSH levels and TSH stimulation. The data, are nevertheless inconclusive with regard to iodine deficiency and the incidence of thyroid carcinoma. Williams is quoted as saying that relating the development of ATC to continued stimulation by TSH has an attractiveness about it without the solidity of supporting evidence.[47] Thus our understanding of the etiology of anaplastic thyroid carcinoma and its interrelationship with the well-differentiated forms of thyroid carcinoma is not yet fully understood.

Diagnosis

The diagnosis of anaplastic carcinoma is made initially by adequate examination of the neck, disclosing a large, rock-like, indurated mass fixed to tissue, primarily the soft tissues of the neck. There may be cervical node involvement in an appreciably significant number of cases. Inspection and palpation of the neck are the first modalities to be used. In the past, soft tissue x-rays of the neck were performed, together with chest x-rays and skeletal surveys, all of which were utilized to pinpoint distant metastases secondary to the primary carcinoma in the neck. The mass has been described as multinodular, with adjacent cervical nodes palpable. Routine diagnostic techniques of uptake and thyroid scan, or even sonography, are not of any great diagnostic importance as the space-occupying lesion is readily apparent to the examiner.[48,49] Aspiration biopsy with a fine needle and cytologic evaluation of the material is the best possible diagnostic technique and usually has a high yield,[4,48,49] primarily because of the overwhelmingly neoplastic nature of the tumor. It is rare for this tumor to only have local foci (which may be missed on an aspiration needle biopsy). Despite the fact that areas of well-differentiated carcinoma may be found coexisting with anaplastic tissue, the cytology is quite accurate in diagnosing this condition. Ekman found that fine needle aspiration biopsy was positive in 32 of 36 cases.[12] At times, multiple aspirations are necessary because of the presence of inflammatory cells and necrotic tissue, edema, and hemorrhage. Therefore, one particular instance of aspiration may yield non-neoplastic tissue. Indeed, in the differential diagnosis of this condition, one must consider the possibility of hemorrhage into a benign tumor producing massive and acute enlargement of the tumor mass, or the presence of other aggressive malignant tumors of the thyroid. Walfish[49] has proposed that a combined sonographic study of the thyroid mass together with fine needle aspiration cytology be performed in these cases and Casterline has seconded this approach to the delineation of the anaplastic nature of the thyroid cancer.[50] Vickery in 1981 proposed that large needle biopsy should be utilized in the study of the thyroid, and felt this was the most successful approach, especially in single nodules.[51] He cites the experience at Massachusetts General Hospital from 1952 to 1980, when the Vim-Silverman technique was employed; during this period 123 malignancies were so studied, of which 73 were papillary; 13, follicular; 6, medullary; and 19, undifferentiated. The tissue obtained was more than adequate in over 90% of the nodules. It is his contention that the Vim-Silverman approach is very helpful in confirming the clinical suspicion of anaplastic carcinoma. In three cases, a fibrotic central core was aspirated, leading to a benign diagnosis. A re-biopsy was performed and confirmed the clinical impression favoring a malignancy. Vickery goes on to compare the histologic and cytologic needle biopsy techniques; he obviously favors the obtaining of a solid plug or core of tissue by large needle biopsy[51]. He reiterates the high success rate for obtaining excellent tissue for study. He states that although the fine needle biopsy has a similar rate of false negatives, it also has an increasing rate of false positives. Unfortunately, malignant cells from the thyroid differ from the cells of other malignancies found in the lung, uterus, and pancreas. They are endocrine neoplasms and may be composed of cells that are indistinguishable from normal cells. The interpretation of cytologic material on biopsy specimens may prove more difficult than a histologic preparation from a solid core specimen. Willems,[52] in a review of fine needle aspiration cytology, indicates that adequate material can most often be obtained with a cellular pattern that is variable. He describes clusters of oval or spindle-shaped cells; pleomorphic nuclei are a common finding. There are also mitotic figures and multinucleated giant cells. He mentions a variant which has been discussed, a malignant osteoclastomalike giant cell tumor also associated with high mortality.[52] He states, in contrast to Vickery, that the false-negative rate in cytology is about 10% of cases, but that there are very rare false-positive cytologic reports based upon the experience of well-trained cytologists. It is also important to note that in a number of thyroid carcinomata, probably up to 10% of cases, there is no way of specifying the specific cell type even in anaplastic carcinoma, because the cellular features are not distinctive, and there is a fair amount of edema and fibrosis. Of greater interest, of course, is the well-documented finding that at autopsy there is a group of nonpalpable carcinomas that are not even detected by scan in 8% to 28% of thyroid specimens at the postmortem table. An interesting clinical note is reported by Wang[53] on needle biopsy pathology of solitary cold nodules in an ongoing series from 1960 through 1979. Of 1874 cold nodules, 53 were malignant; of these 53, there were 41 that were papillary; 3, follicular; 2, medullary; 4, metastatic carcinoma; and 3, undifferentiated or anaplastic. The surprising observation here is that only 3 of 53 malignant lesions were anaplastic in nature.[53]

There have been scanning techniques employing gallium 67 to attempt imaging of thyroid carcinoma. Higashi[54] reports on 136 cases of suspected tumor in which this technique was applied. The purpose of the attempt was

(1) to define suspected anaplastic carcinoma or malignant lymphoma of the thyroid in order to detect distant metastases in either of these carcinomas; (2) to help in the evaluation of therapy; (3) to detect suspected metastases to the thyroid from other malignancies, namely a secondary involvement of the thyroid gland; and (4) to differentiate lymphoma from chronic thyroiditis. However, this kind of scanning has not proved to be successful.

Computed tomography (CT) scanning and magnetic resonance imaging (MRI) scanning of the thyroid have been utilized to define the nature of the mass and its contiguity and involvement with soft tissues of the neck, primarily to determine the efficacy of palliative surgery. Palliation that prevents respiratory obstruction is of value. Takashima[55] discusses CT scanning in 19 patients who had positive palpatory findings—most likely carcinoma of a fixed nature. Fifty-eight percent of these presented with a large mass of low attenuation with dense calcification, and 74% revealed necrosis within the mass. Adjacent structures were infiltrated. The carotid artery was involved in 8 of 10 cases, the esophagus in 4 of 5, the mediastinum in 5 of 5, with regional cervical nodes in 14 out of 16 cases. Seven had the aforementioned necrotic material, but only in nodes. In only one patient was the CT scan deemed to be superior to palpation because of the presence of metastatic nodes. The CT scan altered surgical plans in five of these patients because of the greater definition it provided of the intrathoracic extension of the tumor. Thus the CT scan or the MRI can increase diagnostic accuracy and make it more likely to choose the correct site for aspiration needle biopsy or Vim-Silverman biopsy. Again, any plan for surgery will be modified by CT-scan findings, and any other therapeutic modality will be enhanced by the anatomic detail provided by the imaging techniques.

Immunohistochemical techniques have been applied to the cytologic material obtained in aspiration biopsy material, and attempts also have been made to determine the CEA content of body fluids. There has been a more refined diagnosis of the small-cell carcinoma or large-cell anaplastic carcinoma by means of these techniques.

Therapy

Surgery

Surgery has been employed in the treatment of thyroid carcinoma as the first line of attack. It has been utilized in the treatment and cure of papillary, follicular, mixed papillary-follicular, and medullary carcinoma. However, the surgical therapy directed toward anaplastic carcinoma has proved to be most disappointing, dismal and frustrating. The surgery can be considered only of palliative importance directed to the relief of symptoms related to the airway and to the amelioration of dyspnea and respiratory embarrassment. There is a controversy as to the efficacy of total versus subtotal thyroidectomy, and whether or not there is any value to a total thyroidectomy because of the higher complication rate.

Therefore, the question that immediately arises is whether surgery is appropriate as a therapy for anaplastic thyroid carcinoma. The incidence of anaplastic carcinoma is fairly low in the solitary nodule, and the experience at Massachusetts General Hospital in Boston confirms this. In a series of 1249 nodules, 241 proved to be malignant; of these 241, twenty-three were anaplastic.[56]. If the discussion about surgical therapy indicates the existence of a major principle in the attack upon this tumor, it is the belief that—from the very inception of disease—this is a disseminated tumor and not a localized one. Nishayama[8] has gone so far as to suggest that a total thyroidectomy in thyroid carcinomas due to other etiologies might possibly prove to be helpful in the prevention of the phenomenon of transformation or dedifferentiation into anaplastic cancer. We have already discussed the relatively small incidence of anaplastic carcinoma due to dedifferentiation from a well-differentiated papillary or follicular carcinoma; hence, this may prove to be a very radical approach in terms of cost-benefit to patients with thyroid carcinoma. In essence, surgical principles are an attempt to limit the extent of disease and debulk the tumor in order to provide some symptomatic relief. It should be considered a case of wish-fulfillment to talk about complete extirpation of the tumor by surgical means.[16] However, if one can spare the parathyroids and limit recurrent laryngeal damage, then a more extensive procedure can be undertaken. Surgery, of course, has been used as the first step in a multi-modality approach to the treatment of anaplastic carcinoma; that is, after debulking has occurred, then external radiation can be employed, together with a multitude of chemotherapeutic agents. The role of chemotherapy in the treatment of anaplastic thyroid carcinoma is discussed later in this chapter. Sarda in 1989[57] opted for near total thyroidectomy as a preventive measure in the surgery of thyroid carcinoma. He again restates the hypothesis of the role of TSH in initiating thyroid carcinoma in endemic areas, and states that this occurs in younger patients with a fast growth and is more likely to dedifferentiate into anaplastic thyroid carcinoma. Again, he cites Crile's work[44] on the evidence that continuous TSH stimulation leads to the transformation of a differentiated, endocrine-dependent carcinoma into a rapid, autonomous, vigorous, and primitive tumor. B. Werner,[58] in contradistinction to Sarda[57] and Nishayama,[8] believes that total thyroidectomy is not required, since by the time of autopsy 28% of thyroid carcinomas have previously shown metastatic seeding; in addition, so many of the thyroid carcinomas detected at autopsy have proved not to be clinically meaningful.

Radiation Therapy

X-ray radiation has been employed for the treatment of the primary mass, especially if it is localized, and a technique known as hyperfractionation has been used in which the dose has been divided over a short period of time, in combination with the use of chemotherapy. Kim and Leeper use hyperfractionation radiotherapy with Adriamycin as a chemotherapeutic adjunct.[59] In the Mayo Clinic report, 55 of 82 patients received external radiation of 2000 to 5000 rads and 14 to 18 received more than 5000 rads.[13] Aldinger employed 6000 rads together with actinomycin-D in 84 patients and stated that 6 of the 84 had a 5-year survival.[2] He again describes the presence of both differentiated and undifferentiated thyroid carcinoma in metastatic disease, stating that 18 cases of his 84 dedifferentiated into anaplastic thyroid carcinoma. Thirteen of these were papillary, mixed, or follicular, and five were Hürthle cells.

Chemotherapy

In any discussion of therapy for anaplastic thyroid carcinoma, there can be no hard and fast compartmentalization of the therapeutic modalities, described in this section. The uses of surgery, radiation therapy, and/or chemotherapy are intermixed and combined because of the failure by any individual therapeutic modality to achieve a decent result, or even palliation. Many chemotherapeutic agents have been employed: bleomycin, doxorubicin, vincristine, actinomycin-D, cyclophosphamide, and 5-FU. Some authors have stated that combined modalities are promising. Sometimes preoperative radiation was first employed, followed by surgery. Nevertheless, if one reviews the survival data, a dismal outlook is seen with all of the protocols. One judges the efficacy of these protocols by a time factor of months, not years, and the relief of local symptoms caused by airway obstruction. In the hands of some investigators, radiation has been used postoperatively. In others, there has been an attempt to radiate preoperatively and then employ chemotherapy without the use of surgery. In other groups, radiation and chemotherapy have been used and surgery employed after debulking by the first two modalities.[56] Radiotherapy has also been used by itself, followed by surgery, and then followed-up postoperatively with chemotherapy. There has been a group which decided against employing any therapy, whether it be radiotherapy, chemotherapy, or surgery. Survival is always measured in months, with a maximum of twelve months. A case in which there was survival for several years has brought into question, as mentioned previously, whether the original diagnosis of anaplastic carcinoma was correct; that is, was it true spindle or giant cell? Spanos reports a 24-year-old man (in a case report), with inoperable giant cell, in whom preoperative bleomycin, Adriamycin, and cisplatin were employed, followed by surgery[60] and then postoperative radiation. The patient apparently survived two and a half years, developed pulmonary metastases, and was once again given Adriamycin and cisplatin for the metastatic disease. What one gleans from the literature on the use of combined modalities is that on occasion death, which still will occur in a period of months, is not attributable to local invasion and growth, but rather to the effect of distant metastases on the body chemistry. In Werner's group of 19 patients with combined radiotherapy and chemotherapy, no patient required a tracheostomy.[58] The most pronounced side effect, of course, was mucositis, which developed at the end of radiation. Attempts have been made to employ Bacillus Calmette-Guérin vaccine (BCG) as a form of immunotherapy together with the aforementioned surgery, radiation, and chemotherapeutic techniques. Neither sufficient case material nor sufficient groups have been explored with reference to this possible adjuvant therapeutic approach.

In a paper by Tallroth in 1987, he referred to a multimodality approach for anaplastic thyroid carcinoma involving bleomycin, cyclophosphamide, 5-FU, with occasional use of Adriamycin.[61] Radiotherapy was given in hyperfractionated doses. Of a group of 34 cases so treated, 4 apparently survived for more than two years.

In summary, this is a most difficult, frustrating, and disappointing carcinoma to contend with. The lack of progress in terms of survival, remission, and palliation (or whatever category of cancer statistics we wish to utilize) leaves us with unanswered questions about our approach to controlling this malignant and fulminating tumor.

Survival Data

The prognosis in ATC is dismal. Livolsi reported that 21of 23 cases died within one year, and 15 of the 21 had additional metastases to the lung, lymph nodes, and liver. Seven had tracheal invasion, and 4 of the 15 cases died of growth into the neck and trachea.[7] Indeed, the term "5-year survival" is still inappropriate in the study of anaplastic thyroid carcinoma; should anyone survive five years, one would question the original diagnosis. Aldinger reported somewhat optimistically that a small focus of spindle and giant cells at the time of diagnosis might offer a better chance of some prolonged survival.[2] Admittedly, if the tumor is bulky and aggressive, it is uniformly fatal. In his series which I previously cited,[2] of 1174 cases of which 84 were anaplastic thyroid carcinoma, 6 apparently survived 5 years, but mean survival was 2.8 months from the time of diagnosis, and at best 6.5 months from the time of symptom development. The overall duration of life from the time of diagnosis was 6 months, and from the time of symptoms, 11 to 12 months. Nishayama cited 49 deaths within one year of a total of 53 cases.[8] Patients died of respiratory obstruction, both to the trachea and the bronchial tree, and suffered from widespread metastases to the lungs and pneumonia. In Silverberg's group of 23 cases,[17] mean survival was 3.2 months. One patient apparently survived more than 30 months and three for about a year. Ibanez categorically stated that ATC produced fatality in one year or less in all his cases.[62] In a study at the Mayo Clinic of 160 patients, the average duration of survival was 6 months, with one patient cited as having survived for more than 2 years.[16] However, this may have been a small cell carcinoma. Whether there are any attributes of these tumors that can affect survival is very questionable, but at one time it was felt that perhaps a difference in the origin of the tumor, its biologic characteristics, its natural history, or its response to therapy might affect survival. This has proved to be most disappointing. In Jereb's experience, 78 of 79 patients died: an average survival of $2\frac{1}{2}$ months.[4] He too believed that survivors usually do not have anaplastic thyroid carcinoma. Elman's group of 36 demonstrated 31 fatalities within 22 months.[12] Eighteen died of distant metastases and 13 of local extension. Four patients were alive and apparently disease-free $2\frac{1}{2}$ to 14 years after diagnosis. Spires' group of 14 showed a median survival time of 4 months with 3 surviving more than a year.[11] In Carcangiu's 57 cases,[14] 12 died immediately postoperatively and 35 within 6 months; 10 died within 2 years. Of the 57, there were 44 with massive local growth into vital structures, 7 with distant metastases, and 6 with combined local and distant metastases. In all, the mean survival from the time of diagnosis was 4 months. Casterline states it most succinctly: any patient surviving more than two years with anaplastic thyroid carcinoma merits further close investigation and pathologic analysis.[50]

Summary

One is left with a feeling of emptiness concerning the therapeutic assault on this carcinoma. Although much is known about the origin and pathogenesis of the tumor and the cell type or types, and although there has been much speculation as to its formation; one is left with a nagging feeling that we have only touched on some small facets of this problem. We have to know more about the nature of the prototypic cell type that produces these carcinomas. We have to delineate the process of dedifferentiation—the basic cell reactions (even if the enzymatic changes are due to a genetic predisposition). We do not understand the biologic and biochemical processes that fuel the anaplastic process; indeed, the primitiveness of this tumor makes it most difficult to investigate. Even with sophisticated electron microscopic techniques and cytochemical and immunohistochemical techniques, we have a subgroup within this particular group that defies any classification. This subgroup is so primitive in its dedifferentiation that no markers are available. This presents a massive difficulty in any investigate assault on this tumor. The future must lie within the realm of molecular biology and the unravelling of cell dynamics and intracellular biochemical processes of these primitive cell types. One should look at anaplastic thyroid carcinoma as one variant of the extremely complex maze and puzzle that is posed by cancer genesis. The question to answer, of course, is: are all the carcinomas of the thyroid interrelated, or is that a fiction of pathology? If they are related, then where is the origin for the change from benignity to malignancy, and then from well differentiated cells to dedifferentiated cells? Where is the intracellular key to the genesis of anaplastic cancer?

References

1. Livolsi VA, Merino MJ. Histopathologic differential diagnosis of the thyroid. Path Ann 1981;16:357–406.
2. Aldinger KA, Samaan NA, Ibanez M, Hill CS Jr. Anaplastic carcinoma of the thyroid: a review of 84 cases of spindle and giant cell carcinoma of the thyroid. Cancer 1978;41:2267–2275.
3. Shields JA, Farringer JL Jr. Thyroid cancer: twenty three years' experience at Baptist and St. Thomas hospitals. Am J Surg 1977;133:211–215.
4. Jereb B, Stjernswärd J, Löwhagen T. Anaplastic giant cell carcinoma of the thyroid. Cancer 1975; 35:1293–1295.
5. Woolner LB. Thyroid carcinoma: pathologic classification with data on prognosis. Sem Nucl Med 1971; 1:481–502.
6. Schneider V, Frable WJ. Spindle and giant cell carcinoma of the thyroid: cytologic diagnosis by fine needle aspiration. Acta Cytol 1980;24:184–189.
7. Livolsi VA, Brooks JJ, Arendash-Durand B. Anaplastic thyroid tumors, immunohistology. American J Clin Path 1987;87:434–442.
8. Nishayama RH, Dunn EL, Thompson NW. Anaplastic spindle-cell and giant-cell tumors of the thyroid gland. Cancer 1972;30:113–127.
9. Shvero J, Gal R, Avidor I, Hadar T, Kessler E. Anaplastic thyroid carcinoma. A clinical, histologic, and immunohistochemical study. Cancer 1988;62:319–325.
10. Hrafnkelsson J, Jonassen JG, Sigurdsson G, Sigvaldason H, Tulinius H. Thyroid cancer in Iceland 1955–1984. Acta-Endocrinol 1988;118:566–572.
11. Spires JR, Schwartz MR, Miller RH. Anaplastic thyroid carcinoma. Association with differentiated thyroid cancer. Arch Otolaryngol Head Neck Surg 1988;114:40–44.
12. Ekman ET, Wallin G, Backdahl M, Löwhagen T, Auer G. Nuclear DNA content in anaplastic giant-cell thyroid carcinoma. AM J Clin-Oncol 1989;12:442–446.
13. Nel CJ, van Heerden JA, Goellner JR, Gharib H, McConahey WM, Taylor WF, Grant CS. Anaplastic carcinoma of the thyroid: a clinico-pathologic study of 82 cases. Mayo Clin Proc 1985;60:51–58.
14. Carcangiu ML, Steeper T, Zampi G, Rosai J. Anaplastic thyroid carcinoma-a study of 70 cases. Am J Clin Path 1985;83:135–158.
15. Chang TC, Liaw KY, Kuo SH, Chang CC, Chen FW. Anaplastic thyroid carcinoma: review of 24 cases with

emphasis on cytodiagnosis and leucocytosis. Taiwan I Hsueh Hui Tsa Chih 1989;88:551–556.

16. Thomas CG Jr, Buckwalter JA. Poorly differentiated neoplasms of the thyroid gland. Ann Surg 1973; 177:632–642.
17. Silverberg SG, Hutter RV, Foote FW Jr. Fatal carcinoma of the thyroid: histology, mestastases, and causes of death. Cancer 1970;25:792–802.
18. Simpson WJ, McKinney SE. Canadian survey of thyroid cancer. Can Med Assoc J 1985;132:925–931.
19. Werner S. Letter to the editor. J Clin Endo 1969; 29:860–862.
20. Rosai J, Saxen EA, Woolner L. Undifferentiated and poorly differentiated carcinoma. Sem In Diagn Path 1985;2:123–136.
21. Gaal JM, Horvath E, Kovacs K. Ultra structure of two cases of anaplastic giant-cell tumor of the human thyroid gland. Cancer 1975;35:1273–1279.
22. Fisher ER, Gregorio R, Shoemaker R, Horvat B, Hubay C. The derivation of so-called "giant-cell" and "spindle-cell" undifferentiated thyroidal neoplasms. Am J Clin Path 1974;61:680–689.
23. Jao W, Gould VE. Ultrastructure of anaplastic (spindle and giant cell) carcinoma of the thyroid. Cancer 1975;35:1280–1292.
24. Taylor S. Clinical features of thyroid tumors. Clin Endo Metab 1979;8:209–221.
25. Rayfield EJ, Nishiyama RH, Sisson JC. Small-cell tumors of the thyroid. A clinicopathological study. Cancer 1971;28:1023–1030.
26. Vizel-Schwartz M. Osteoclastome-like giant-cell thyroid carcinoma controlled by extensive radiation and adriamycin, in a patient with meningioma and multiple myeloma treated by radiation and cytoxan. J Surg Oncol 1981;17:57–61.
27. Nicolaides AR, Rhys EP, Parker C. Adenosquamous carcinoma of the thyroid gland. J Laryngol Otol 1989;103:978– 979.
28. Böcker W, Dralle H, Husselmann H, Bay V, Brasso WM. Immunohistochemical analysis of thyroglobulin synthesis in thyroid carcinomas. Virchows-Arch (Path Anat) 1980;385:187– 200.
29. Beitrami CA, Criante P, Diloreto C. Immunocytochemistry of anaplastic carcinoma of thyroid gland. Appl Path 1989;7:122–133.
30. Kawahara E, Nakanishi I, Terahata S, Ikegaki S. Leiomyosarcoma of the thyroid gland. A case report with a comparative study of 5 cases of anaplastic carcinoma. Cancer 1988;62:2558–2563.
31. Makinen T, Pekonen F, Franssila K, Lamberg BA. Receptors for epithelial growth factor and thyrotropin in thyroid carcinoma. Acta Endocrinol 1988;117:45–50.
32. Klemi PJ, Joensuu H, Elerola E. DNA aneuploidy in anaplastic carcinoma of the thyroid gland. Am J Clin Path 1988;89:154–159.
33. Aasland R, Lillehaug JR, Male R, Josendal O, Varhaug JE, Kleppe K. Expression of oncogenes in thyroid tumors: coexpression of c-erbB2/neu and c-erb B. Brit J Cancer 1988;89:154–159.
34. Kapp DS, Livolsi VA, Sanders MM. Anaplastic carcinoma following well-differentiated thyroid cancer: etiological considerations. Yale J Biol Med 1982; 55:521–528.
35. Tubiana M, Lacour J, Monnier JP. External radiotherapy and radioiodine in the treatment of 359 thyroid cancers. Brit J Radiol 1975;48:894–907.
36. Bridges AB, Davies RR, Newton RW, McNeill GP. Anaplastic carcinoma of the thyroid in a patient receiving radio-iodine therapy for amiodarone-induced thyrotoxicosis. Scot Med J 1989;34:471–472.
37. Leeper RD, Shimaoka K. Treatment of metastatic thyroid cancer. Clin Endo Metab 1980;9:383–404.
38. Harada T, Ito K, Shimaoka K, Hosoda Y, Yakumara K. Fatal thyroid carcinoma. Anaplastic transformation of adenocarcinoma. Cancer 1977;39:2588–2596.

38a. Harada T, Shimaoka K, Yakumara K, Ito K. Squamous cell carcinoma of the thyroid gland—transition from adenocarcinoma. J Surg Oncol 1982;19(1):36–43.

39. Hofstadter F. Frequency and morphology of malignant tumors of the thyroid before and after the introduction of iodine-prophylaxis. Virchows Arch (Pathol Anat) 1980;385:263–270.
40. Ueda G, Furth J. Sarcomatoid transformation of transplanted thyroid carcinoma. Arch Path 1967;83:3–12.
41. Hirabayashi RN, Lindsay S. The relation of thyroid carcinoma and chronic thyroiditis. Surg Gynec Obstet 1965;121:243–252.
42. Schneider V, Frable WJ. Spindle and giant cell carcinoma of the thyroid: cytologic diagnosis by fine needle aspiration. Acta Cytol 1980;24:184–189.
43. Getaz EP, Shimaoka K, Rao U. Anaplastic carcinoma of the thyroid following external irradiation. Cancer 1979;43:2248–2253.
44. Crile G Jr, Wilson DH. Transformation of a low grade papillary carcinoma of the thyroid to an anaplastic carcinoma after treatment with radioiodine. Surg Gyn and Obstet 1959;108:357–360.
45. Rieger R, Pimpl W, Money S, Rettenbacher L, Galvan G. Hyperthyroidism and concurrent thyroid malignancies. Surgery 1989;106:6–10.
46. Wallin G, Backdahl M, Tallroth-Ekman E, Lundell G, Auer G, Löwhagen T. Co-existent anaplastic and well differentiated thyroid carcinoma: a nuclear DNA study. Eur J Surg Oncol 1989;15:43–48.
47. Williams ED. The aetiology of thyroid tumors. Clin Endo Metab 1979;8:193–207.
48. Walfish PG, Hazani E, Strawbridge HTG, Miskin M, Rosen IB. Combined ultrasound and needle aspiration cytology in the assessment and management of hypofunctioning thyroid nodule. Ann Int Med 1977; 87:270–274.
49. Walfish PG, Miskin M, Rosen IB, Strawbridge HTG. Application of special diagnostic techniques in the management of nodular goiter. Can Med Assn J 1976;115:35–40.
50. Casterline PF, Jacques DA, Blom H, Wartofsky L. Anaplastic giant and spindle cell carcinoma of the

thyroid: a different therapeutic approach. Cancer 1980; 45:1689–1692.

51. Vickery AL Jr. Needle biopsy pathology. Clin Endo Metab 1981;10:275–292.
52. Willems JS, Löwhagen T. Fine-needle aspiration cytology in thyroid disease. Clin Endo Metab 1981;10:247- 266.
53. Wang C. Management of thyroid disease based on needle biopsy pathology. Clin Endo Metab 1981;10:293- 298.
54. Higashi T, Ito K, Nishikawa Y, Everhart FR Jr, Ozak O, Manabe Yi, Suzuki A, Yashiro T, Hasegawa M, Mimura T. Gallium 67 imaging in the evaluation of thyroid malignancy. Clin Nucl Med 1988;13:792–798.
55. Takashima S, Morimoto S, Ikezoe J, Takai S, Kobayashi T, Koyama H, Nishiyama K, Kozuka T. CT evaluation of anaplastic thyroid carcinoma. AJNR 1990; 11:361–367.
56. Brooks JR, Starnes HF, Brooks DC, Pelkey JN. Surgical therapy for thyroid carcinoma: a review of 1249 solitary thyroid nodules. Surgery 1988;104:940–946.
57. Sarda AK, Bal S, Kapur MM. Near total thyroidectomy for carcinoma of the thyroid. Br J Surg 1989;76:90–92.
58. Werner B, Abele J, Alveryd A, Bjorklund A, Franzen S, Grandbery PO, Landberg T, Lundell G, Löwhagen T, Sunblad R et al. Multimodal therapy in anaplastic giant cell thyroid carcinoma. World J Surg 1984;8:64–70.
59. Kim JH, Leeper RD. Treatment of anaplastic giant and spindle cell carcinoma of the thyroid gland with combination adriamycin and radiation therapy. A new approach. Cancer 1983;52:954–957.
60. Spanos GA, Wolk D, Desner MR, Khan A, Platt N, Khafif R, Cortes EP. Preoperative chemotherapy for giant cell carcinoma of the thyroid. Cancer 1982;50:2252–2256.
61. Tallroth E, Wallin G, Lundell G, Löwhagen T, Einhorn J. Multimodality treatment in anaplastic giant cell thyroid carcinoma. Cancer 1987;60:1428–1431.
62. Ibanez ML, Russell WO, Albores-Saavedra J, Lampertico P, Whlte EC, Clark RL. Thyroid carcinoma—biologic behavior and mortality. Postmortem findings in 42 cases, including 27 in which the disease was fatal. Cancer 1966;19:1039–1052.

10

Lymphoma of the Thyroid Gland

DAVID K. SIROTA

Introduction

At one time, primary (non-Hodgkin's) lymphoma of the thyroid gland was considered to be a rare thyroid malignancy. However, in recent years it has been estimated that it may account for 5% to 10% of thyroid cancers. Among patients with a solitary discrete nodule of the thyroid gland, the incidence of primary lymphoma is 1 in 1000. In patients with diffuse goiters, the incidence of primary lymphoma is 1 in 100. Primary lymphomas of the thyroid gland are said to constitute only 1.3% to 6.5% of all extranodal lymphomas. The reported mean age at the time of diagnosis is approximately 60 to 65 years with a range of 10 years to 90 years. The female-to-male ratio ranges from 3:1 to 18:1 but in the subgroup aged 60 years or less the ratio narrows toward 1:1. Approximately 40% of patients are under the age of 60 years at the time of diagnosis.[1–18]

Clinical Features

A discrete thyroid mass or diffuse thyromegaly is present in all cases of primary lymphoma of the thyroid gland. Rapid enlargement of the mass is very common and is an hallmark of the disease. In approximately 75% of cases, the mass has been present for 3 months or less—typically 3 to 6 weeks. Fever, sweats or weight loss at the time of presentation are uncommon. Symptoms of local compression, such as stridor and dysphagia, are common and are associated with a marked adverse effect on survival. Local pain may occur in 5 to 33% of patients.[8,10,12,15,17–19] Hoarseness occurs in approximately 50% of patients. Of these, approximately 60% have demonstrated vocal cord paralysis.[10,12] The reason for hoarseness in patients without vocal cord paralysis is unclear, but it has been suggested that local extension of the lymphoma into the subglottic larynx along with occlusion of the lymphatic outflow of the subglottic trachea, edema of the vocal cords, and limitation of cricothyroid motion may combine to cause hoarseness in this group of patients.[20–22]

On physical examination, a firm to stoney-hard anterior neck mass, usually larger than 6 cm in diameter, is present. Most masses are solitary and unilateral but up to 25% are diffuse. The mass is fixed to surrounding structures in approximately 50% of cases and is tender in 10% to 30% of cases. Palpable local lymphadenopathy at the time of presentation is rare, occurring in only 10% to 20% of cases. Hepatomegaly and splenomegaly at the time of presentation is also rare.[10–12] A clinical picture of hypothyroidism may be present in patients with primary lymphoma of the thyroid gland;[12,15] hyperthyroidism associated with thyroid lymphoma is rare.[11,23]

Many laboratory features of primary lymphoma of the thyroid are nonspecific. Nuclear scanning usually shows the mass to be cold or cool with patchy uptake.[10,15] On ultrasonography (US) primary lymphomas of the thyroid gland are seen as extremely hypoechoic (pseudocystic) areas intermingled with echogenic structures. It is always necessary to perform sonograms at a high-gain setting to demonstrate internal echoes in the mass. Adjacent, nontumorous areas of lymphocytic thyroiditis also have an heterogeneous, hypoechoic appearance on US, but their echogenicity is higher than that of the tumor, thus allowing a clear delineation between the lymphoma and the adjacent thyroid tissue. When the lymphoma involves the entire thyroid gland the US findings appear to be of little value since there is no adjacent normal tissue for comparison of echogenicity. Because the echogenicity observed in lymphocytic thyroiditis is closely related to the degeneration of the thyroid follicles, cases of advanced lymphocytic thyroiditis with severe follicular degeneration or no follicles will have echogenicity similar to that seen in lymphoma of the thyroid gland, making it impossible to distinguish lymphoma from lymphocytic thyroiditis. In general, the US findings in thyroid lymphoma are not specific enough to be diagnostic on their own.[24,25]

On plain computerized tomographic (CT) scanning, lymphomas of the thyroid show either low attenuation or intermediate attenuation areas. The tumors become more clearly recognizable as low attenuation zones on contrast-enhanced CT scans. When the lymphoma involves the entire gland, reduced attenuation is present diffusely but no discrete tumor can be demonstrated. Lymphocytic thyroiditis also shows low attenuation on CT scans when compared to normal thyroid tissue. Since lymphocytic thyroiditis is usually present adjacent to lymphomas of the thyroid, precise definition and diagnosis of lymphoma of the thyroid by CT scanning is not possible without additional supportive clinical and histologic data. The CT findings are not specific enough to differentiate lymphoma from other malignant lesions of the thyroid. CT is useful in delineating local compression and infiltration by the lymphoma and is helpful in staging.[26] In a study comparing computer tomography and ultrasonography as techniques for assessing primary lymphoma of the thyroid in 16 patients, CT was found to be the more important modality for diagnosis and staging while US was felt to be more useful for local follow-up. In that series there was one lymphoma that was not detected by either technique.

Though there are several reports on magnetic resonance (MR) imaging in benign and maligant diseases of the thyroid in the literature, there is only one case report of MR findings in primary lymphoma of the thyroid. In this report the T-1–weighted images had similar intensity to that of lymphocytic thyroiditis, that is, an enlarged thyroid gland with overall increased intensity, often accompanied by linear bands of decreased signal on long Repetition Time/Echo Time (TR/TE) images. However, on T-2–weighted images, the thyroid lymphoma was seen as an homogeneous area of high intensity as compared to lymphocytic thyroiditis. Unfortunately, as with CT scanning and ultrasonography, the MR findings in the one case studied were similar to those seen in other thyroid cancers and thyroid adenomas. Although MR is useful in defining the full extent of the mass and extrathyroidal nodal involvement without the use of contrast, at the present time it has no value as a modality to help distinguish primary lymphoma of the thyroid gland from other thyroid malignancies.[27]

Gallium 67 imaging, which has been shown to be negative in cases of papillary and follicular carcinoma and positive in 40% of patients with chronic thyroiditis, is positive in 85% of anaplastic carcinoma of the thyroid and in 100% of patients with primary lymphoma of the thyroid. Though these findings are nonspecific, a positive Gallium 67 scan performed in the clinical setting of a rapidly growing thyroid mass is highly suggestive of either primary lymphoma or anaplastic carcinoma.[28]

In most patients with primary lymphoma of the thyroid, thyroid function studies are in the euthyroid range. However, as previously mentioned, hypothyroidism has been reported. Although there is one study that reported that 50% of patients with lymphoma of the thyroid have hypothyroid laboratory parameters,[17] most reports suggest a lower incidence.[12,15,29] Between 25% and 100% of patients with primary lymphoma of the thyroid have serologic evidence of autoimmune thyroiditis.[3,5,8,29,30,31]

Although fine needle aspiration of thyroid

masses has become popularized in recent years, its usefulness in the diagnosis of primary lymphoma is open to question. In 1979 we speculated that blind needle aspiration or core biopsy could easily miss an area of lymphoma of the thyroid while obtaining benign lymphocytic cells because of the high incidence of areas of lymphocytic thyroiditis one finds adjacent to primary lymphomas. Alternatively, lymphomas could be misdiagnosed as lymphocytic thyroiditis or small cell anaplastic carcinoma.[10] Although several authors have reported a high percentage of correct diagnoses of primary lymphoma of the thyroid based on needle biopsy[3,15] and/or aspiration findings,[32] there are several studies that confirm that needle biopsy and aspiration can easily miss the correct diagnosis.[12,17,33-35] A report reviewing the fine needle aspiration cytology in 5 patients with proven primary lymphoma of the thyroid observed that in only one of the 5 cases was the correct diagnosis made. In 3 of the 5 cases a diagnosis of anaplastic carcinoma of the small cell type was made. The final case in this series was misdiagnosed as thyroiditis twice before being correctly diagnosed as primary lymphoma the third time around.[34] Another study has pointed out that, although fine needle aspiration seems to reliably differentiate between primary thyroid carcinoma, anaplastic carcinoma, and malignant lymphoma, difficulties can arise when attempting to differentiate between malignant lymphoma and lymphocytic thyroiditis.[33]

The cytologic features of malignant lymphoma of the thyroid include large numbers of malignant cells distributed as isolated cells with monotonous features, malignant cells slightly larger than normal lymphocytes, and the possible presence of cleaved cells or large nucleoli.[34] These findings are vague enough to account for the difficulties encountered in distinguishing malignant lymphoma from lymphocytic thyroiditis. Though immunocytochemical analysis may improve the chances of correctly identifying thyroid lymphomas on aspiration cytology specimens, errors in making the diagnosis by this technique still occur.[32] Therefore, it is our recommendation that one should be guided more by the clinical picture and open biopsy than by needle aspiration in making this difficult diagnosis.

Table 10.1. Differential diagnosis of primary lymphoma of the thyroid gland

Benign goiters and tumors
Papillary, follicular, or medullary carcinoma
The fibrous variant of lymphocytic thyroiditis
Reidel's struma
Pseudolymphoma of the thyroid
Small cell anaplastic carcinoma
Plasmacytoma
Carcinoma metastatic to the thyroid from non-thyroidal primaries

Differential Diagnosis

Table 10.1 lists the differential diagnosis of primary lymphoma of the thyroid gland. Benign goiters and tumors are usually slow-growing and nonaggressive, rarely causing compression symptoms. Papillary, follicular, and medullary carcinomas are characterized by an indolent growth pattern. Their doubling times may be years, while that of primary Iymphoma is weeks to months. Pathologically, there is no similarity.

The fibrous variant of lymphocytic thyroiditis closely mimics the clinical picture of primary lymphoma of the thyroid. The age and sex incidence are similar. Both are characterized by a rapidly enlarging stoney-hard goiter. In both cases the patients may be hypothyroid. On examination of the gross pathology, however, the fibrous variant of lymphocytic thyroiditis has a clearly demarcated capsule that is not adherent to surrounding structures. Microscopically, lesions contain areas of typical lymphocytic thyroiditis, but the fibrous variant of lymphocytic thyroiditis is characterized by replacement of thyroid parenchyma by broad dense bands of fibrous connective tissue, often hyalinized, separating zones of degenerating thyroid tissue.[36]

Reidel's struma also has a sex and age incidence similar to primary lymphoma of the thyroid and is associated with approximately the same incidence of hypothyroidism. It also presents as a rapidly enlarging stony-hard thyroid mass that is invasive and adherent to adjacent cervical structures. It frequently causes respiratory compromise secondary to tracheal compression. However, microscopically, thick fibrous tissue extends beyond the thyroid capsule. There are no changes suggestive of lymphocytic thyroiditis and no malignant cells are present. A characteristic vasculitis involving only veins is always present. Clinically, along with small-cell carcinoma and metastatic carcinoma to the thyroid, Reidel's struma most closely resembles primary lymphoma of the thyroid. Surgical resection of the lesion usually leads to complete recovery.[37]

Pseudolymphoma of the thyroid can be distinguished histologically from true lymphoma by good demarcation, the presence of mature lymphocytes with prominent follicle formation and germinal centers, and mature plasma cells. Immunohistochemically, pseudolymphoma shows a distribution of T cells and B cells similar to that seen in reactive lymph nodes.[38]

Small-cell anaplastic carcinoma of the thyroid is being diagnosed less in recent years than it has been in the past, while primary lymphoma of the thyroid is being diagnosed with greater frequency.[5,11,15,19,39-41] It appears that this trend is not a result of changing patterns of occurrence of the two entities, but rather the result of more accurate histochemical techniques that have allowed more accurate differentiation between them. In one study, one third of cases originally diagnosed as small-cell thyroid carcinoma were reclassified as primary lymphomas when restudied with appropriate techniques.[42] The therapeutic implications of this are obvious, as will be seen in the section on treatment and survival.

Plasmacytoma of the thyroid is much rarer than primary lymphoma. It may also occur in the setting of pre-existing lymphocytic thyroiditis. This entity will be discussed separately in greater detail later in this chapter.

Carcinoma that metastasizes to the thyroid frequently presents with the same clinical picture as primary lymphoma. It is usually seen in patients who are known to have previously existing nonthyroidal malignancies, but may be the presenting symptom. This entity will be discussed in greater detail in Chapter 11.

Pathology

Gross Pathology

In one large study of 245 cases of primary lymphoma of the thyroid gland, the size of the tumor at surgery or autopsy ranged from 1 cm to 14 cm in greatest diameter, with a mean of 6.9 cm. The tumors are usually gray-tan or gray-white in color, fleshy and homogeneous in character, and rubbery to firm or stony-hard. The tumors are frequently adherent to adjacent structures and are rarely necrotic grossly. The overall appearance of the tissue is suggestive of lymphoid tissue. When uninvolved thyroid tissue is present, it has the appearance of a compressed rim along the periphery of the expanding mass.[11]

Histopathology

Microscopically, by the Rappaport classification, most lymphomas of the thyroid are of the diffuse histiocytic type, although some follicular lymphomas have been reported.[8,18,43,44] When classified by the "Working Formulation,"[45] 14% of lymphomas are classified as low-grade, 71% as intermediate-grade and 10% as high-grade. Further breakdown by the working formulation shows that among the patients with low-grade lymphomas, 54% are of the small lymphocytic type, 19% are of the follicular, predominantly small cleaved cell type, and 27% are of the follicular, mixed small cleaved cell and large cell type. Among the intermediategrade lymphomas, 7% are of the follicular, predominantly large cell type, 14% are intermediate lymphocytic lymphomas, 11% are of the diffuse small cleaved cell type, 5% are of the diffuse, mixed small and large cell type and 63% are of the diffuse large cell type. Among the high-grade lymphomas, all are immunoblastic. Five percent of the thyroid lymphomas are undefined by the "Working Formulation."[30]

By the Kiel classification,[46,47] 65% of patients have low-grade thyroid lymphomas and 35% have high-grade lymphomas. Among the low-grade lymphomas, 14% are of the lymphoplasmacytic/lymphoplasmocytoid type, 16% are of the intermediate lymphocytic type,

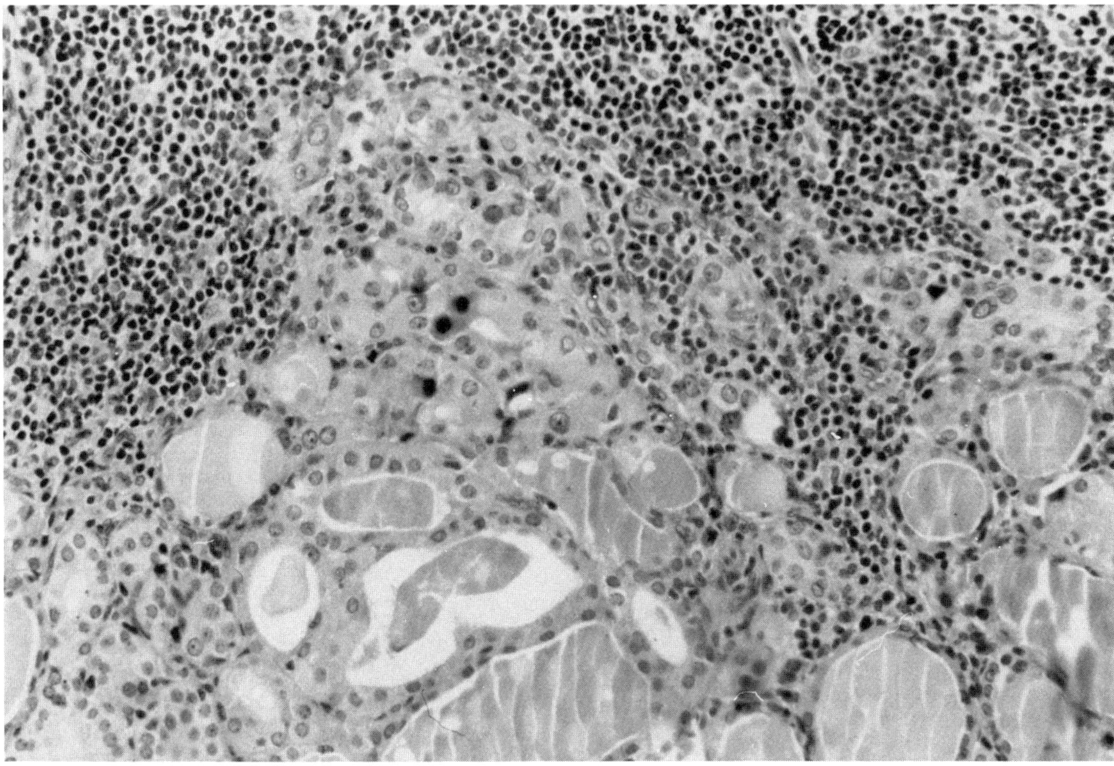

Figure 10.1. Primary lymphoma of the thyroid gland adjacent to areas of lyrnphocytic thyroiditis containing granular, oxyphylic changes in the cytoplasm of the follicular epithelium (Askanazy cells). (original magnification ×200)

17% are of the centrocytic type, 10% are of the follicular type, 40% are of the diffuse type and 8% show combined follicular and diffuse characteristics. Among the high-grade lymphomas of the thyroid, 58% are centroblastic, 29% are immunoblastic, and 13% are undetermined.[30] As will be shown later, survival rates depend strongly on the histologic characteristics of the tumor.

Histologically, complete or partial nodular proliferation is present in 10% to 17% of patients with primary lymphoma of the thyroid whereas germinal center cell tumors account for 50% to 72% of cases. Less frequently, intermediate lymphocytic lymphoma is seen in the thyroid. Monomorphous infiltrates, which show effacement of the thyroid architecture with isolation and destruction of the follicles, is also an important histologic feature of malignant lymphoma of the thyroid. "Packing" of thyroid follicles and infiltration of whole blood vessel walls by tumor cells is also a common characteristic seen in primary lymphoma of the thyroid.[11,17,18,30,48–50] This is an unfavorable prognostic indicator, as are extrathyroidal extension and tumor necrosis.

A most striking histologic finding in primary lymphoma of the thyroid is the presence in most of the cases studied of chronic lymphocytic thyroiditis adjacent to the lymphoma (see Figs. 10.1 and 10.2). Lymphocytic infiltration is usually present ordinarily forming lymphoid follicles with germinal centers showing varying degrees of fibrosis and oxyphillic changes or squamous metaplasia in epithelial cells of thyroid follicles. In some cases, marked secondary follicles, probably residual of chronic lymphocytic thyroiditis, are observed in the diffuse proliferation of small lymphoid cells, giving the impression that these cases might be reactive.

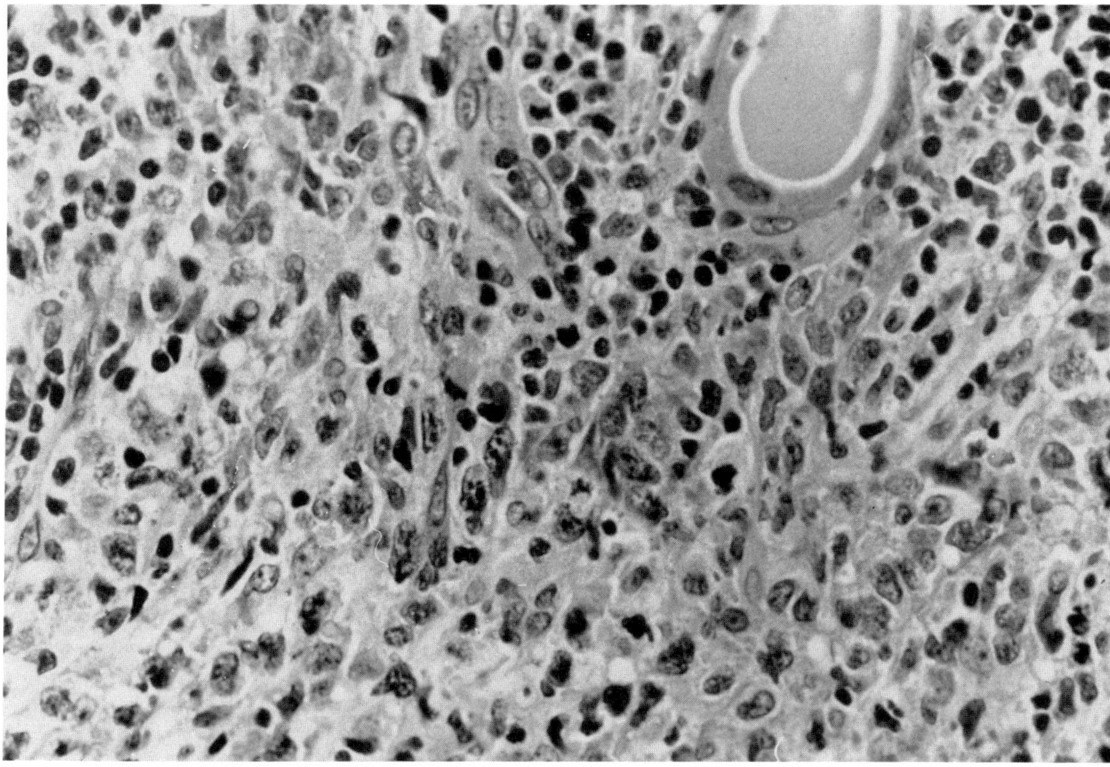

Figure 10.2. Primary lymphoma of the thyroid gland adjacent to areas of lymphocytic thyroiditis containing granular, oxyphylic changes in the cytoplasm of the follicular epithelium (Askanazy cells). (original magnification ×400)

Of interest is the finding that most patients who are serologically negative for antithyroid antibodies have histologic evidence of chronic lymphocytic thyroiditis.*

Immunocytology and Immunohistology

Cell suspension and tissue immunohistochemical studies show a restricted expression of immunoglobulin light chain by the neoplastic cells in most patients. The majority exhibit kappa and a smaller percentage exhibit lambda. Approximately 20% of patients show no light chain expression. Surface staining on cell suspension and in tissue section is usually present in the neoplastic cells. Thyroid lymphomas are frequently infiltrated by large numbers of E rosettes. On tissue sections Leu-1^+, Leu-4^+ small lymphocytes are generally abundant in tumors, with a preponderance of Leu-$3a + 3b^+$ cells (helper/inducer cells) to Leu-$2a^+$ (suppressor/cytotoxic cells.) In cases of follicular lymphoma of the thyroid, Leu-1^+, Leu-4^+ cells are mainly distributed around the neoplastic follicles and strengthen the follicular arrangement of tumor cells. In cases of diffuse lymphoma of the thyroid, vague nodular structures that could be overlooked by routine histologic techniques are clearly shown by staining with Leu-1 and Leu-4. In general, neoplastic follicles contain much larger numbers of Leu-$3a + 3b^+$ cells than Leu-$2a^+$ cells. The thyroid follicular epithelium consistently stains positive for HLA-DR.[29,48–50,52,53].

Most authors agree that there is close homology between the lymphoplasmacytic infiltrates seen in lymphocytic thyroiditis and normal

*References 10, 11, 15, 17, 19, 29, 30, 31, 44, 48–51

mucosa-associated lymphoid tissue and that, like lymphomas that originate at mucosal sites, primary lymphomas of the thyroid are derived from the parafollicular ("centrocyte-like") B cells. High-grade thyroid lymphomas appear to be derived from low-grade tumors. There are close histologic, immunohistologic and clinical similarities between low- and high-grade non-Hodgkin's lymphomas of the thyroid and those originating at mucosal sites.[29,48]

Pathophysiology

The etiology of primary lymphoma of the thyroid has been a topic of considerable interest in the literature. Primary lymphoma has been reported in patients who had undergone radiotherapy to the head or neck during childhood or adolescence.[54] There is at least one case report of lymphoma presenting many years after treatment with I 131 for hyperthyroidism.[17] Rare cases of primary lymphoma of the thyroid have been reported in association with follicular carcinomas of the thyroid and plasmacytoma of the thyroid.[55] However the major focus of the etiology of primary lymphoma of the thyroid gland has clearly been the finding of concomitant lymphocytic thyroiditis accompanying the majority of thyroid lymphomas.* It has been estimated by some that primary lymphoma of the thyroid gland occurs in 1.4% of patients with lymphocytic thyroiditis.[10]

In 1985, a group from Sweden reported that the risk of developing primary lymphoma of the thyroid in patients with lymphocytic thyroiditis is 67 times greater than expected statistically.[56] In the same year a group from Japan also reported a significantly higher incidence of primary lymphoma of the thyroid among patients with lymphocytic thyroiditis compared to the incidence of lymphoma among a control group with Basedow's disease. There were 8 cases of primary lymphoma of the thyroid in the lymphocytic thyroiditis group versus none in the control group. All of the lymphomas were of the B cell type. The average interval between the diagnosis of lymphocytic thyroiditis and the development of lymphoma was 9.2 years.

Most primary lymphomas of the thyroid are of B cell derivation and of follicular center origin. It is believed that the chronic antigenic stimulation of the lymphocytes in lymphocytic thyroiditis makes these lymphocytes more susceptible to neoplastic change.[51,56] Several studies suggest that primary lymphomas of the thyroid gland are derived from mucosa-associated lymphoid tissue, specifically from the parafollicular ("centrocyte-like") B cells. Further proof of the B cell derivation of most thyroid lymphomas is the expression of restricted immunoglobulin light chains in most lymphomas studied.[29,30,48,50–53,56]

A 1986 report from Kobe, Japan has shown that, when using an immunoperoxidase staining method on thyroid tissue sections from patients with Hashimoto's thyroiditis, polyclonal intracytoplasmic immunoglobulins were usually present; whereas the thyroid tissue sections of patients with primary lymphoma of the thyroid showed monoclonal intracytoplasmic immunoglobulins. This group has also shown that in some of the patients with malignant lymphoma with demonstrable intracytoplasmic monoclonal immunoglobulins, monoclonal gammopathy was demonstrable by serum protein electrophoresis. They recommend that patients with Hashimoto's thyroiditis be screened with fine needle aspiration biopsy and with serum protein electrophoresis.[52]

Also of interest is a 1989 study from Japan in which karyotypes from 7 patients with thyroid lymphoma were studied before treatment. They identified two distinct groups of patients with thyroid lymphoma. In a group of 4 patients who had solely numerical abnormalities in their chromosomal analysis, there was a long interval from the time of onset of goiter to the time of surgery for thyroid lymphoma. This group of patients had abnormal thyroid function studies and tested positive for antithyroidal autoantibodies. Two of these patients showed trisomy 22 and two patients showed loss of a sex chromosome. The second group of patients with solely structural chromosome abnormalities had lymphoma that followed a more rapid course from onset of goiter to

*References 10, 11, 15, 17, 19, 29, 30, 31, 44, 48–51

time of surgery. These patients had normal thyroid function studies and negative antithyroidal autoantibodies. Two of the three patients in this group showed a 14q+ abnormality. What role these genetic changes play etiologically is still unclear, but the authors theorize that the chronic stimulation of the lymphocytes in chronic lymphocytic thyroiditis by thyroid autoantigen may lead to a population of B lymphocytes that are more susceptible to mitotic errors, resulting in the development of an aneuploid clone or other genetic abnormality. The 14q+ marker chromosome described in two of the patients in this study is characteristic of nodal B cell lymphomas and occurs in about 65% of such patients.[57]

A recent report by Matsubayashi et al. suggests the possibility that continuous or recurrent Epstein-Barr virus infection may influence B cell proliferation in the thyroid gland and could be a causative or potentiating factor in the development of malignant lymphoma of the thyroid.[58]

Therapy

The treatment of primary lymphoma of the thyroid gland is a controversial area; the choice of an appropriate treatment is dependent on many criteria. As with non- thyroidal lymphomas, surgery, radiation therapy, and chemotherapy, separately or in combination, have been used with varying degrees of success. Much of the confusion in the literature results from authors with particular fields of interest and expertise endorsing their own formula for treatment. Clearly, there are several features of tumor biology and behavior that impact on the selection of a therapeutic regimen and upon the outcome of treatment. These include staging of the tumor, cell type, and tumor bulk. To best assess the value of the available modalities of therapy, each will be discussed separately.

Surgery

Most authors agree that surgery alone is not an effective approach in the management of primary lymphomas of the thyroid. Standard practice has been to do nothing surgical beyond a biopsy in stage III and IV disease. Some authors also believe that surgery has no significant place in the management of stage I and II disease.[15,17] However, several recent studies suggest that aggressive surgery in stage I and II disease may have a favorable effect on survival.

Rosen et al. reported that the effectiveness of surgery in patients with primary lymphoma of the thyroid gland depends on the amount of tumor left behind following surgery. If less than 2.5 cm of residual disease is left postoperatively, 80% of patients have lifelong disease control as compared to 40% lifelong disease control if more than 2.5 cm of tumor is left postoperatively. Distant metastases occur in 7% of patients who have less than 2.5 cm of tumor tissue left; they occur in 23% of patients who have more than 2.5 cm of residual tumor tissue.[59]

Tupchong et al. reported that patients who had total macroscopic removal of tumor had the highest rate of local control and long-term survival. Though no statistically significant difference was seen between lobectomy, subtotal, and total thyroidectomy, 7 of the 9 long-term survivors (58 to 129 months) in their series of 46 cases had had total thyroidectomy. Patients who underwent definitive surgery with resection of tumor had a statistically significant greater survival than those who only underwent biopsy. In this series 60% of patients with total macroscopic removal of tumor had a 60% ten-year survival as compared to a 17% ten-year survival among patients who had post-surgical residual tumor.[18]

Several authors believe that there is an inverse relationship between tumor bulk and local control of thyroid lymphoma and that the reduction of tumor bulk may be a more significant factor in disease control than either histology or staging.[18,44,59]

Radiotherapy

Radiotherapy has assumed a more important role in the treatment of primary lymphoma of the thyroid gland in recent years. Although 5-year survival rates of 50% or less in patients treated with radiation therapy were the norm in the past, several authors have more recently reported considerably better results in stage IE and IIE disease. In the 1986 series of Vigliotti et al. from the University of Texas M.D. Anderson Hospital, the overall survival among 38 patients treated with definitive radiotherapy alone (15 patients), combination chemotherapy and radiotherapy (14 patients), chemotherapy alone (6 patients), and surgery alone (3 patients) was 72% with a 5-year disease-free survival of 64%. The patients with stage IE disease treated with radiation therapy alone had a 100% 5-year survival and an 83% disease-free survival. In patients with stage IIE disease treated with radiotherapy alone, the respective rates were 88% overall survival and 75% disease-free survival. In this group the survival rate was better if the mediastinum was not involved. Seven patients with stage IE and 10 patients with stage IIE disease underwent combination radiation and chemotherapy. Both the overall and disease-free 5-year survival rates were 77% in this group of patients. These authors concluded that radiation therapy alone is excellent treatment for lymphoma limited to the thyroid, with or without cervical adenopathy. If mediastinal extension was present, radiation therapy alone was not satisfactory and the addition of chemotherapy was indicated.[60]

Evaluation of 38 patients with primary lymphoma of the thyroid treated with radiation therapy at the Mayo Clinic between 1965 and 1979 showed an overall 5-year survival of 57% and 10-year survival of 50%. Disease-free survival was 59% at 5 years and 10 years. Among stage I patients, 5-year survival following radiation therapy was 83% if the lymphoma did not extend beyond the capsule but dropped to 59% if extension beyond the capsule was present. There was no correlation between overall disease-free survival and whether the course of treatment was continuous or split. No significant side effects of treatment occurred in this group. In this series, as in others previously cited, improved disease-free survival was noted among those patients undergoing gross total surgical resection prior to radiation therapy rather than only biopsy. Five-year survival among patients with no residual disease after surgery who subsequently received radiotherapy was 75% as compared with 49% 5-year survival among patients who did have residual disease after surgery.[44]

A 1987 study by Connors et al. from the Cancer Control Agency of British Columbia reported a complete initial response to a regimen consisting of a combination of brief chemotherapy with cyclophosphamide, doxorubicin, vincristine and prednisone (CHOP) followed by involved field radiation therapy in 11 of 11 (ie 100%) patients with primary lymphoma of the thyroid gland. In this group of patients, only 2 were noted to relapse over a median follow-up period of 30 months.[61] Ikeda reported that the 5-year survival rate among patients with primary lymphomas of the thyroid with a diameter of less than 11 cm who received radiotherapy is 83% while the survival among patients with lesions greater than 12 cm is only 61%.[62] All authors agree that careful staging of primary lymphomas of the thyroid improve the chances for survival with radiation therapy by identifying those patients who will require more extensive treatment and those who may benefit from adjunct chemotherapy.[18,44]

From the technical point of view the dose of radiation delivered to the tumor seems to be critical. For treatment of gross tumor there appears to be a threshold effect at 40 Gy. Patients receiving between 20 and 39 Gy may respond to radiation therapy if there is minimal residual disease postsurgery, or if radiotherapy is augmented by chemotherapy. Above 40 Gy, local control of thyroid lymphoma can be attained in 86% of patients.[18,44,62] One report suggests that there is no increase in survival of patients with lymphoma of the thyroid who receive doses which exceed 40 Gy; however, this study does not correlate the dosage with the degree of local control achieved.[44]

Treatment is usually delivered in 20 doses over a 4 to 5 week period. Methods of delivery range from irradiating the thyroid gland, the neck bilaterally and the mediastinum, to irradiating all of the preceeding with the inclusion of the axillae, to irradiating the neck only. Tupchong et al, who advocate the last approach, believe that patients with retrosternal or mediastinal disease have decreased survival that is not affected by radiation. However, in the study by Blair et al., those patients receiving radiation to the neck and mediastinum had a 5-year survival of 63% compared to a 40% 5-year survival among patients who underwent neck irradiation only.[18,44,62]

Chemotherapy

As has been stated above. until recently the role of chemotherapy used by itself in the treatment of primary lymphoma of the thyroid has been of limited value. In the study of Vigliotti et al. only 5 patients, all with stage II disease were treated with combined chemotherapy alone (CHOP with or without bleomycin.) Five-year survival was 60% and 5-year disease-free survival was 40%. In most other reports, chemotherapy has been used as an adjunct or salvage therapy. Salvage chemotherapy for primary lymphomas of the thyroid seems to have little, if any, impact on survival. As noted above, chemotherapy as adjunctive therapy, particularly prior to radiation therapy, appears to have a positive effect on survival. Regimens which include CHOP with or without bleomycin appear to have the greatest prospects.[18,60,61]

A recent report by Leedman et al. from the Royal Melbourne Hospital suggests that combination chemotherapy as a single modality therapy for stage IE and IIE thyroid lymphoma may hold promise for the future. They treated three women with primary lymphoma of the thyroid, two with the CHOP program (one for 8 cycles, 21 days apart and one for 6 cycles, 21 days apart) and one with a regimen consisting of methotrexate, adriamycin, cyclophosphamide, vincristine, prednisone, and bleomycin over a 12-week period. This last patient had previously undergone a hemithyroidectomy for removal of the tumor. The two CHOP-treated patients were alive and relapse-free at 26 and 28 months. The third patient was alive and relapse-free at 38 months. All three patients tolerated the therapy without difficulty. Since most thyroid lymphomas that recur do so within the first 12 months following initial treatment, the authors believed that the prognosis for this small group of patients was good. Pathologically, all three patients had tumors classified as diffuse large cell lymphomas and all showed evidence of lymphocytic thyroiditis. Of interest is the fact that all three patients had hoarseness secondary to vocal cord paralysis as one of their presenting findings, and that in at least one patient the hoarseness persisted through the follow-up period.[63]

We have not addressed the question of stage III and IV lymphomas of the thyroid in any detail. As previously mentioned, salvage chemotherapy has been the treatment of choice in these situations; however, the 5-year survival, no matter what regimen has been used, is less than 5%.[15]

Recommendations for Treatment of Primary Lymphoma of the Thyroid

Based on the data available at the present time, the following approach to the treatment of stage IE and IIE primary lymphoma of the thyroid gland is recommended after a full staging work-up that should include complete blood count and chemistries, chest x-rays, lymphoangiogram and/or abdominal and pelvic CT scan, Gallium scan and bone marrow biopsy:

1. Surgical removal of as much tumor tissue and involved lymph nodes as possible. Most studies strongly suggest that maximum debulking of the tumor improves survival rates.
2. Radiation therapy of the entire tumor bed area of the neck and lymph nodes with or without radiation of the mediastinum. A minimum dose of 40 Gy should be given in 20 treatments over a 4- to 5-week period. Massive tumors may require additional "booster" treatments to residual masses. Based on the most recent information available, it seems advisable that the radiotherapy be preceded by three courses of combination chemotherapy at three-week intervals, with a 3 to 4 week rest period after the third course, before beginning radiation therapy. At the present time, the most effective chemotherapeutic regimen appears to be CHOP with or without

Table 10.2. Adverse prognostic factors for survival in patients with primary lymphomas of the thyroid gland

Clinical
Age greater than 60 years
Mass present 6 months or less
Tumor size greater than 10 cm
Hoarseness
Dyspnea
Dysphagia
Stridor
Mediastinal enlargement/superior mediastinal mass
Tracheal deviation

Pathologic
Tumor fixation
Extracapsular extension
Vascular invasion
Tumor necrosis
High-grade histology (Kiel classification)

bleomycin. This approach should result in 85% to 100% 5-year survival and hopefully cure.

3. As for combination chemotherapy alone, earlier data suggest that it should only be used for salvage therapy. The promising recent report from Australia was based on an experience with only three patients. Treatment of many more patients over much longer follow-up periods will be necessary before this modality of therapy can be properly evaluated.

Factors Influencing Survival

Adverse prognostic factors for survival in patients with primary lymphomas of the thyroid are listed in Table 10.2. Although some authors feel that age is not a factor, most agree that patients above the age of 60 have a poorer chance of survival. Signs and symptoms of extrathyroidal extension including hoarseness, stridor, dyspnea, and dysphagia are also negative prognostic factors. Most authors agree that tumor bulk is important in determining outcome. They consider a size of 10 or 11 cm to be a cut-off point. Tumors larger than this have a poorer prognosis. Other negative prognostic factors include perithyroidal invasion, vascular invasion, tumor necrosis, tracheal deviation, mediastinal enlargement, and superior mediastinal mass. Presence of the thyroid mass for less than six months is associated with shortened survival.[18,19,30,44]

Factors that do not affect survival include sex, thyroid functional status, and presence or absence of lymphocytic thyroiditis. In the Mayo Clinic report, the presence of local pain was associated with improved prognosis.[44] As previously stated, tumors under 10 cm that have been present less than 6 months in an individual under 60 years of age also carry a better prognosis. Although some authors contend that histologic features do not impact on prognosis, most do find a correlation. Aozosa et al. reported 5-year survival rates as follows: immunoblastic lymphoma, 13%; Intermediate grade, 79%; and low grade, 92%.[30]

Plasmacytoma of the Thyroid Gland

Introduction

The first case of localized plasmacytoma of the thyroid gland was reported by Voeght in 1938.[64] Since then, approximately 60 cases have been reported in the English-language literature. Two studies which between them reported 14,870 thyroid tumors examined at surgery, identified only three primary plasmacytomas of the thyroid gland.[65,66]

Although primary thyroid plasmacytomas, like primary lymphomas, appear to develop in a setting of antecendent lymphocytic thyroiditis,[67–70] the clinical features and biologic behavior of the two entities are quite different. The age range at the time of diagnosis is 37 to 82 years, with a median of 48 to 57 years.[67,68] The male-to-female ratio has been reported as low as 1:1, but most authors report a higher incidence in males[67–70]; one report states that the male-to-female ratio is 15:1.[67] Hypothyroidism in plasmacytoma of the thyroid is rare, it has been reported in only 5 cases.[67,68] In addition to their frequent association with lymphocytic thyroiditis, there have been rare reports of primary plasmacytomas of the thyroid occurring concurrently with follicular lymphoma of the thyroid gland[71] and with dermatomyositis and palmar fasciitis.[72]

Clinical Features

All patients present with an enlarging goiter of 1 month to 10 years duration (median = 3 months).[67] Many of the tumors reported are slow growing. The goiter may be nodular or diffuse, and is usually painless. Dysphagia and vocal cord paralysis may be present, as may localized lymphoadenopathy. Bone lesions are not present at the time of diagnosis.[67,68]

Laboratory Findings

Routine hematologic and chemical studies are usually normal in primary plasmacytoma of the thyroid gland. Thyroid function studies are occasionally in the hypothyroid range but most patients have euthyroid parameters. Hyperthyroidism has not been reported. The tissue that is involved is usually cold on I 131 nuclear scanning.[67,68] In the only CT description published to date, the tumor tissue was homogeneous with lobular contours, and with an attenuation coefficient of about 30 Hounsfield units (lower than usually seen in normal thyroid tissue). This finding, although nonspecific, is similar to CT findings reported in extramedullary plasmacytomas of pancreas and kidney.[73] Antithyroglobulin and antimicrosomal antibodies are usually positive.[67–70]

Bence-Jones proteinuria has rarely been reported in patients with primary plasmacytoma of the thyroid gland. However, immunoelectrophoresis shows the presence of M protein in 17% to 33% of cases and serum protein electrophoresis may show a monoclonal peak in up to 33% of cases as well.[67,69,71]

Pathology

Gross Pathology and Histology

The tumors of primary plasmacytoma of the thyroid may be solitary or multiple. The cut surfaces usually have a lobulated, pale fleshy appearance with no capsule present. Juxtathyroidal lymph node involvement may or may not be present.[67–70]

Histologically, the plasmacytomas show large foci of infiltration of the thyroid parenchyma by sheets of plasma cells that are mature appearing in some tumors but which may show nuclear pleomorphism and frequent mitotic figures in others. The tumor cells generally have eccentric nuclei with a central eosinophilic nucleolus and marginal condensed chromatin. There is a moderate amount of cytoplasm with a pale paranuclear zone. Russell bodies may or may not be present. The cells either surround, destroy, or completely replace the thyroid follicles, which consist of columnar epithelium and contain eosinophilic colloid material, macrophages and/or tumor cells. Most histologic specimens show typical changes of lymphocytic thyroiditis adjacent to the tumor tissue. Marked lymphocytic infiltration and secondary lymphoid follicles, occasionally surrounded by oxyphilic changes in the follicular epitheilium are mixed with the plasmacytic infiltration. Mild, diffuse aggregates of small lymphocytes and a few plasma cells may be seen in the nonnodular portion of the thyroid gland. Electron microscopy shows typical features of plasmacytoma.[67–70]

Recently, plasma cell granulomas of the thyroid that sometimes resemble plasmacytomas have been reported; there is speculation that some early published cases of plasmacytoma of the thyroid may actually have been plasma cell granulomas. With the advent of immunohistochemical techniques, these two tumorous forms of plasma cell proliferation can easily be differentiated, because plasmacytomas demonstrate monoclonal proliferation whereas polyclonal proliferation is seen in plasma cell granulomas.[69–71]

Immunocytology and Immunohistology

Immunoperoxidase staining shows monoclonal staining in all cases in which the technique has been used, providing justification for the diagnosis of primary plasmacytoma of the thyroid. In most cases, IgG-kappa has been present but cases showing IgA-kappa and cells staining for monoclonal lambda chains have also been reported. In those cases in which bone marrow and other lymphoid tissue elements have been studied in patients with primary plasmacytoma of the thyroid, monoclonal-staining plasma cells have not been present in the non-thyroidal tissues, again confirming that the thyroid tumors are primary extramedullary plasmacytomas.[67–74]

Treatment

Most cases reported in the literature have been treated with total thyroidectomy or hemithyroidectomy, radiation therapy, or both. Extramedullary plasmacytomas tend to be highly radiosensitive. Of the cases reported in the literature, 31 were treated with radiotherapy alone after the diagnosis was made, while 14 were treated with radiation therapy after surgical removal of the tumor. When radiation therapy is used either alone or after surgical treatment, a dose of 5000 to 6000 rads appears to minimize the rate of failure while causing minimal complications. Surgery alone or low-dose radiation therapy (under 4000 rads) are not considered to be adequate treatment and will result in higher rates of recurrence. At the present time, the optimal treatment of primary plasmacytoma of the thyroid gland is total thyroidectomy followed by 4000 to 6000 rads of radiation therapy. Chemotherapy has no place in the initial management of the disease but may be useful in the secondary management of the rare cases that develop distant metastases.[67–73]

Survival

Localized primary plasmacytoma of the thyroid gland, with or without juxtathyroidal nodal involvement, has an excellent prognosis. In general, extramedullary plasmacytomas have a more favorable prognosis than does solitary myeloma or multiple myeloma. Multiple myeloma develops more frequently from solitary myeloma than from extramedullary plasmacytoma. When treated aggressively with surgery and radiation therapy as outlined above, primary plasmacytomas rarely metastasize to distant sites. When distant metastases do occur, they tend to develop after long, disease-free intervals and are usually controllable with chemotherapy. Local recurrence does not appear to affect survival significantly and can usually be controlled by local treatment. Because the number of cases of primary plasmacytoma of the thyroid reported in the literature is too small, it is not possible to present specific survival data at present.[67–69]

Primary Hodgkin's Disease of the Thyroid Gland

Less than 5% of all cases of Hodgkin's disease are extranodal.[75,76] Primary Hodgkin's disease of the thyroid gland, if it occurs at all, is very rare. Less than 25 cases have been reported in the literature; there is considerable question as to whether some of these were indeed primary in the thyroid or whether they were metastatic from other sites.[5,8,11,18,77–80] Furthermore, among the cases that did appear to be primary in the thyroid, there is the belief that they have been misdiagnosed and were really pleomorphic histiocytic lymphomas of the thyroid.[11] In any case, Hodgkin's disease involving the thyroid should be considered part of a more generalized process, and should be managed accordingly.

References

1. Welch JW, Chesky VE, Hellwig CA. Malignant lymphoma of the thyroid. Surg Gynecol Obstet 1958; 106:70–76.
2. Roberts L, Primary reticulosarcoma of the thyroid gland. Postgrad Med J 1961; 37:481–484.
3. Crile G Jr. Lymphosarcoma and reticulum cell sarcoma of the thyroid. Surg Gynecol Obstet 1963;116:449–450.
4. Mikal S. Primary lymphoma of the thyroid gland. Surgery 1964;55:233–239.
5. Woolner LB, McConahey WM, Beahrs OH, Black BM. Primary malignant lymphoma of the thyroid: review of forty-six cases. Am J Surg 1966;111:502–523.
6. Slimkin PM, Sagerman RH, Lymphoma of the thyroid gland. Radiology 1969;92:312–316.
7. Smithers DW. Malignant lymphomas of the thyroid gland. Eng Monogr Neoplast Dis Var Sites 1970; 6:141–154.
8. Burke JS, Butler JJ, Fuller LM. Malignant lymphomas of the thyroid: a clinical pathologic study of 35 patients including ultrastructural observations. Cancer 1977; 39:1587–1602.
9. Devine RM, Edis AJ, Banks PM. Primary lymphoma of the thyroid: a review of the Mayo Clinic experience through 1978. World J Surg 1981;5:33–38.
10. Sirota DK, Segal RL. Primary lymphoma of the thyroid gland. JAMA 1979;242:1743–1746.

11. Compagno J, Oertel JE. Malignant lymphoma and other lymphoproliferative disorders of the thyroid gland. Am J Clin Pathol 1980;74:1–11.
12. Grimley RP, Oates GD. The natural history of malignant thyroid lymphomas. Br J Surg 1980;67:475–477.
13. Williams ED. Malignant lymphoma of the thyroid. Clin Endocrinol Metab 1981;10:379–389.
14. Miller JM, Kini SR, Rebuck J, Hamburger JI. Is lymphoma of the thyroid a disease which is increasing in frequency? In: Hamburger JI, Miller JM, eds. Controversies in Clinical Thyroidology. New York: Springer-Verlag;1981:267–297.
15. Hamburger JI, Miller JM, Kini SR. Lymphoma of the thyroid. Ann Intern Med 1983;99:685–693.
16. DeGroot LJ, Larsen PR, Refetoff S, Stanbury JB. The Thyroid and Its Diseases. 5th ed. New York: John Wiley; 1984.
17. Rasbach DA, Mondschein MS, Harris NL, Kaufman DS, Wang CA. Malignant lymphoma of the thyroid gland: a clinical and pathologic study of twenty cases. Surgery 1985;98:1166–1170.
18. Tupchong L, Hughes F, Harmer CL. Primary lymphoma of the thyroid: clinical features, prognostic factors, and results of treatment. Int J Radiat Oncol Biol Phys 1986;12:1813–1821.
19. Butler JS, Brady LW, Amendola BE. Lymphoma of the thyroid-report of five cases and review. Am J Clin Oncol 1990;13:64–69.
20. Graham CP. Hoarseness associated with lymphoma of the thyroid gland. South Med J 1982;75:1566–1567.
21. Watson C. Laryngeal oedema complicating thyroid lymphoma. J Laryngol Otol 1988;102:947–948.
22. Van Ruiswyk J, Cunningham C, Cerletty J. Obstructive manifestations of thyroid lymphoma. Arch Intern Med 1989;149:1575–1577.
23. Jennings AS, Saberi M. Thyroid lymphoma in a patient with hyperthyroidism. Am J Med 1984;76:551–552.
24. Parulekar SG, Katzman RA. Primary malignant lymphoma of the thyroid: sonographic appearance. JCU 1986;14:60–62.
25. Hamada S, Ikeda H, Masaki N, Kozuka T, Matsuzuka F. Comparison of CT and US assessment. Radiology 1989;171:439–443.
26. Takashima S, Ikezoe J, Morimoto S, et al. Primary thyroid lymphoma: Evaluation with CT. Radiology 1988;168:765–768.
27. Takashima S, Ikezoe J, Morimoto S, Harada K, Kozuka T, Matsuzuka F. MR imaging of primary thyroid lymphoma. J Comp Assist Tomogr 1989;13:517–518.
28. Higashi T, Ito K, Nishikawa Y, et al. Gallium-67 imaging in the evaluation of thyroid malignancy. Clin Nucl Med 1988;13:792–799.
29. Hyjek E, Isaacson PG. Primary B cell lymphoma of the thyroid and its relationship to Hashimoto's thyroiditis. Hum Pathol 1988;19:1315–1326.
30. Aozasa K, Inoue A, Tajima K, Miyauchi A, Matsuzuka F, Kuma K. Malignant lymphomas of the thyroid gland. Analysis of 79 patients with emphasis on histologic prognostic factors. Cancer 1986;58:100-104.
31. Shinomiya S, Sumitomo M, Kudo E, Sakaki A, Hizawa K. Malignant thyroid neoplasms and coexistent lymphocytic thyroiditis. Tokushima J Exp Med 1988;35:91–100.
32. Willems JS, Lowhagen T. The role of fine-needle aspiration cytology in the management of thyroid disease. Clin Endocrinol Metab 1981;10:267–273.
33. Tani E, Skoog L. Fine needle aspiration cytology and immunocytochemistry in the diagnosis of lymphoid lesions of the thyroid gland. Acta Cytol 1989;33:48–52.
34. Limanova Z, Neuwirtovar R, Smejkal V. Malignant lymphoma of the thyroid. Exp Clin Endocrinol 1987;90:113–119.
35. Matsuda M, Sone H, Koyama H, Ishiguro S. Fine-needle aspiration cytology of malignant lymphoma of the thyroid. Diagn Cytopathol 1987;3:244–249.
36. Harasch HR, Williams ED. Fibrous thyroiditis—An immunopathological study. Histopathology 1983;7:739–751.
37. Schwaegenle SM, Bauer TW, Esselstyn CB. Riedel's thyroiditis. Am J Clin Pathol 1988;90:715–722.
38. Mizukami Y, Ikuta N, Hashimoto T et al. Pseudolymphoma of the thyroid. Acta Pathol Jpn. 1988;38:1329–1336.
39. Rayfield EJ, Nishiyama RH, Sisson JC. Small cell tumors of the thyroid: a clinicopathologic study. Cancer 1971;28:1023–1030.
40. Heimann R, Vannineuse A, De Sloover C, Dor P. Malignant lymphoma and undifferentiated small cell carcinoma of the thyroid: a clinicopathological review in the light of the Kiel classification for malignant lymphoma. Histopathology 1978;2:201–213.
41. Tobler A, Maurer R, Hedinger CE. Undifferentiated thyroid tumors of diffuse small cell type: histological and immunohistochemical evidence for their lymphomatous nature. Virchows Arch [A] 1984;404:117–126.
42. Schmid KW, Kroll M, Hofstadter F, Ladurner D. Small cell carcinoma of the thyroid. A reclassification of cases originally diagnosed as small cell carcinomas of the thyroid. Pathol Res Pract 1986;181:540–543.
43. Souhami L, Simpson WJ, Carruthers JS. Malignant lymphoma of the thyroid gland. Int J Radiat Oncol Biol Phys 1980;6:1143–1147.
44. Blair TJ, Evans RG, Buskirk SJ, Banks PM, Earle JD. Radiotherapeutic management of primary thyroid lymphoma. Int J Radiat Oncol Biol Phys 1985;11:365–370.
45. National Cancer Institute sponsored study of classifications of non-Hodgkin's lymphoma. Summary and description of a working formulation for clinical usage. Cancer 1982;49:2112–2135.
46. Gerard-Marchant R, Hamlin I, Lennert K, Rilke F, Stansfeld AG, Van Unnik JAM. Classification of non-Hodgkin's lymphomas. Lancet 1974;2:405–408.
47. Lennert K, Stein H, Kaiserling E. Cytological and functional criteria for the classification of malignant lymphomata. Br J Cancer 1975;31 (suppl II): 29–42.
48. Anscombe AM, Wright DH. Primary malignant lymphoma of the thyroid—a tumor of mucosa-associated lymphoid tissue: review of seventy-six cases. Histopathology 1985;9:81–97.

49. Aozasa K, Inoue A, Yoshimuru H et al. Intermediate lymphocytic lymphoma of the thyroid. An Immunologic and immunohistologic study. Cancer 1986; 57:1762–1767.
50. Aozasa K, Ueda T, Katagiri S, Matsuzuka F, Kuma K, Yonezawa T. Immunologic and immunohistologic analysis of 27 cases with thyroid lymphomas. Cancer 1987;60:969–973
51. Kato I, Tajima K, Suchi T et al. Chronic thyroiditis as a risk factor of B-cell lymphoma in the thyroid gland. Jpn J Cancer Res 1985;76:1085–1090.
52. Matsubayashi S, Tamai H, Keisuke N, Kuma K, Nakagawa T. Monoclonal gammopathy in Hashimoto's thyroiditis and malignant lymphoma of the thyroid. J Clin Endocrinol Metab 1986;63:1136–1139.
53. Faure P, Chittal S, Woodman-Memeteau F et al. Diagnostic features of primary malignant lymphomas of the thyroid with monoclonal antibodies. Cancer 1988;61:1852–1861.
54. Bisbee AC, Thoeny RH. Malignant lymphoma of the thyroid gland following irradiation Cancer 1975; 35:1296–1299.
55. Aozasa K, Inoue A, Yoshimura H, Miyauchi A, Matsuzuka F, Kuma K, Plasmacytoma of the thyroid gland. Cancer 1986;58:105–110.
56. Holm LE, Blomgren H, Lowhagen T. Cancer risks in patients with chronic lymphocytic thyroiditis. N Engl J Med 1985;312:601–604.
57. Taniwaki M, Nishida K, Misawa S et al. Correlation of chromosome abnormalities with clinical characteristics in thyroid lymphoma. Cancer 1989;63:873–876.
58. Matsubayashi S, Tamai H, Morita T et al. Malignant lymphoma of the thyroid and Epstein-Barr virus. Endocrinol Japan 1989;36:343–348.
59. Rosen IB, Sutcliffe SB, Gospodarowicz MK, Chua T, Simpson JK. The role of surgery in the management of thyroid lymphoma. Surgery 1988;104:1095–1099.
60. Vigliotti A, Kong JS, Fuller LM, Velasquez WS. Thyroid lymphomas stages Ie and IIe: comparative results for radiotherapy only, combination chemotherapy only, and multimodality treatment. Int J Radiat Oncol Biol Phys 1986;12:1807–1812.
61. Connors JM, Klimo P, Fairey RN, Voss N. Brief chemotherapy and involved field radiation therapy for limited-stage, histologically aggressive lymphoma. Ann Intern Med 1987;107:25–30.
62. Ikeda H, Masaki N, Aozasa K. Results of the treatment of localized non-Hodgkin's lymphoma originated in the thyroid gland. Gan No Rinsho 1988;34:637–643.
63. Leedman PJ, Sheridan WP, Downey WF, Fox RM, Martin IR. Combination chemotherapy for stage IE and IIE thyroid lymphoma. Med J Aust 1990;152:40–43.
64. Voegt H. Extramedullae plasmocytome. Virchows Arch Pathol Anat 1938;302:497–508.
65. Hazard JB, Schildecker WW. Plasmacytoma of the thyroid. Am J Pathol 1949;25:819–820.
66. Macpherson TA, Dekker A, Kapadia SB. Thyroid-gland plasma cell neoplasm (plasmacytoma). Arch Pathol Lab Med 1981;105:570–572.
67. Aozas K, Inoue A, Yoshimura H, Miyauchi A, Matsuzuka F, Kuma K. Plasmacytoma of the thyroid gland. Cancer 1986;58:105–110.
68. Chen KTK, Bauer V, Bauer F. Localized thyroid plasmacytoma. J Surg Oncol 1986;32:220–222.
69. Beguin Y, Boniver J, Buri J et al. Plasmactyoma of the thyroid: A case report, a study with use of the immunoperoxydase technique and a review of the literature. Surgery 1987;101:496–500.
70. Yashiro T, Aiba M, Obara T, Fujimoto Y, Hirayama A. IgG-Kappa-producing primary plasmacytoma of the thyroid gland with preoperative serum M protein. Acta Pathol Jpn 1988;38:371–381.
71. Aozasa K, Inoue A, Katagiri S, Matsuzuka F, Katayama S, Yonezawa T. Plasmacytoma and follicular lymphoma in a case of Hashimoto's thyroiditis. Histopathology 1986;10:735–740.
72. Caron P, Lassoued S, Thibaut I, Fournie B, Fournie A. Thyroid plasmacytoma with dermatomyositis and palmar fasciitis. J Rheumatol 1989;16:997–999.
73. Salazar JE, Nelson JF, Winer-Muram HT. Extramedullary plasmacytoma of the thyroid. J Can Assoc Radiol 1987;38:135–137.
74. Baba T, Watanabe M, Hotchi M, Miyagawa A. An autopsy case of plasmacytoma of the thyroid gland. Gan No Rinsho 1987;33:392–398.
75. Freeman C, Berg JW, Cutler SJ. Occurrence and prognosis of extranodal lymphomas. Cancer 1972; 29:252–260.
76. Kim YH, Fayos JV, Schnitzer B. Extranodal head & neck lymphomas: results of radiation therapy. Int J Radiat Oncol Biol Phys 1978;4:789–794.
77. Roberts TW, Howard RG. Primary Hodgkin's disease of the thyroid: Report of a case and review of the literature. Ann Surg 1963;157:625–632.
78. Gibson JM, Prinn MG. Hodgkin's disease involving the thyroid gland. Br J Surg 1968;55:236–239.
79. Abel WG, Finnerty J. Primary Hodgkin's disease of thyroid. NY State J Med 1969; 314–315.
80. Ackerman LV, del Regato JA. Cancer; diagnosis, treatment and prognosis. 2nd ed. St. Louis: MO The C.V. Mosby Company; 1954.

11

Carcinoma Metastatic to the Thyroid Gland

David K. Sirota

Introduction

Carcinomas metastasizing from other organs to the thyroid gland were considered to be rare[1,2] until the 1950s[3–5] when several authors began reporting a significant incidence of this entity at autopsy as well as sporadic clinically apparent cases. As more attention has been paid to this phenomenon, more has been learned about it.[6–32] The incidence, clinical picture, differential diagnosis, and treatment and prognosis are discussed below.

Incidence

The majority of cases of carcinomas metastatic to the thyroid gland have been reported as incidental findings at autopsy, in which the incidence ranges from 0% to 26.4%,[8] and as surgical findings, in which they make up 3% to 10% of all malignant thyroid tumors identified at surgery.[6] As greater awareness of this entity has developed, and with the advent of needle aspiration and biopsy of the thyroid gland, more cases in recent years have been diagnosed in life. Although most clinically recognizable cases are part of a more generalized picture of distant metastatic disease, there have been several cases reported in which the thyroid metastasis has been the initial presenting finding and has led to the discovery of a previously unsuspected primary tumor elsewhere.[16,18,24,25]

The wide range in the reported incidence of metastatic cancer to the thyroid at autopsy has been attributed to differences in techniques used to examine the thyroid gland post mortem. There are several large autopsy series in which the incidence has been reported to be under 2%.[3,32–34] On the other hand several authors have done meticulous examinations of the thyroid glands of patients who died of carcinomatosis; Brierre and Dickinson[8] and Silverberg and Vidone[9] found the incidence of metastatic cancer to the thyroid gland to be 26.4% and 24.2%, respectively. The average incidence in autopsy series is considered to be in the range of 9% to 10%.[8]

The incidence of clinically apparent metastatic carcinoma to the thyroid gland in life is not known but approximately 180 cases have been reported in the literature.[4–7,10,11,13–31] It is of interest that the frequency of the types of primary carcinomas that metastasize to the thyroid gland varies when comparing autopsy findings with clinically apparent thyroid metastases. There is also a discrepancy in frequency if the autopsy material is analyzed by percentage of primary carcinomas that metastasize to the thyroid gland versus the total number of metastases among the reported autopsy series. When percentage of metastasizing tumors found at autopsy is calculated (see Table 11.1) malignant melanoma tops the list with breast, kidney, and lung primaries trailing far behind.[6] When the absolute percentage of reported autopsy cases in the literature is tabulated, it is apparent that breast and lung primaries are the most common, each accounting for 25%, with melanoma accounting for only approximately 10% and renal, only 8%.[3,4,6,8,20,33,35]

Table 11.1. Site of primary malignancy metastatic to the thyroid gland in 613 cases studied at autopsy

Primary site	Percentage of 613 cases with thyroid metastases
Breast	26.1
Lung	22.1
Melanoma	9.6
Kidney	8.6
Lymphoma and leukemia	5.9
Gastrointestinal	5.6
Nasopharynx/larynx	4.7
Female genital	2.6
Pancreas and liver	1.9
Miscellaneous	12.9

Table 11.2. Site of primary malignancy metastatic to the thyroid gland in 180 clinically diagnosed patients

Primary site	Percentage of 180 cases with thyroid metastases
Kidney	37.3
Breast	14.5
Lung	13.5
Nasopharynx/larynx	7.5
Esophagus/stomach	6.1
Colorectal	3.3
Malignant melanoma	2.8
Cervix	1.6
Miscellaneous (less than 3 cases reported)	13.4

Table 11.2 lists the order of frequency of primary malignancies that metastasize to the thyroid gland as reported in clinical series. Renal cell carcinoma has the highest incidence with breast, lung, nasopharynx, larynx, stomach/esophagus and colorectal occurring in that order.[5–7,10–18,20,21,30,31] Surprisingly, malignant melanoma, which accounts for 10% to 39%[6] of the microscopic metastatic lesions to the thyroid found at autopsy, accounts for less than 3% of the metastatic carcinomas to the thyroid as demonstrated clinically. It is also unclear why renal cell carcinoma, which comprises up to 57%[5] of the clinically evident metastatic malignancies to the thyroid makes up only 8% to 12% of the metastases found in autopsy material.

Among the rare primary sites that fall into the miscellaneous category in Table 11.2 are bladder,[7,18] adrenal,[4] pancreas,[5,18] malignant carcinoid,[27] ovary,[4,27] cervix,[6,7,9,20] testis,[6] angioblastic meningioma,[14] sarcoma,[1,6,18,24] hepatoma,[5] choriocarcinoma,[1,19] fibrous histiocytoma,[29] uveal melanoma,[22] lymphoma/leukemia,[4,6] Hodgkin's disease,[4,6] and Kaposi's sarcoma[28] (in a patient with AIDS.)

Clinical Picture

As would be expected, most patients with carcinoma metastatic to the thyroid gland are in their sixth decade or beyond.[18,20] The clinical picture is similar to that seen in lymphoma of the thyroid gland. The mass may be solitary or multinodular, is usually quite hard and rapidly enlarging; although slower-growing masses have been reported. The mass is usually painless at presentation.[20,31] Dysphagia, dyspnea, stridor, and hoarseness produced by recurrent laryngeal nerve involvement are the most common complaints. When the mass is rapidly enlarging, tracheal compression and occlusion may lead to the patient's rapid demise.[5,6,14,16,18,20,24,27] Because a majority of the patients have metastatic disease elsewhere, systematic symptoms of metastatic carcinoma may be present. Clinical hyperthyroidism has been reported in association with metastatic carcinoma to the thyroid,[6,14] some authors believe that this hyperthyroidism may be coincidental.[6] However, it is also possible that there may be an outpouring of thyroid hormone secondary to tumor invading the thyroid gland. At least seven cases of documented hypothyroidism secondary to near-total replacement of the thyorid gland by tumor have been published. Of the seven cases of hypothyroidism reported, five patients had breast carcinoma and two had rectal carcinoma.[6,19,27]

Laboratory Studies

The results of hematologic and chemical studies vary depending on the overall extent of the metastatic cancer. As mentioned, in rare cases clinical evidence of hyperthyroidism or hypothyroidism may be present. On nuclear scanning the thyroid mass is always "cold".[14,20,31] On Gallium 67 imaging the mass always scans positively; a finding which, although it is nonspecific, strongly suggests the possibility of malignancy and suggests the need for further investigation.[36]

In the case of metastatic carcinoma to the thyroid gland, needle aspiration of the mass has proven to be a most effective diagnostic modality.[14,21,24–27,30,31] Watts reported finding 4 patients with metastatic cancer to the thyroid gland among 70 patients in whom fine needle aspiration of a thyroid nodule was performed. All had a previous history of carcinoma of other organs. The diagnoses included breast cancer, colon cancer, malignant carcinoid and Hodgkin's disease.[27] Smith et al. reviewed the 5426 fine needle aspirations of the thyroid done at the Mayo Clinic between 1980 and 1985, documenting the presence of metastatic cancer in 19 patients, 14 of whom had a prior history of nonthyroidal cancer and 5 of whom had no prior history of cancer. The tumor types identified in this series included breast, lung, esophagus, sarcoma and malignant melanoma.[24] Chacho et al. found 6 metastatic tumors to the thyroid among 549 fine needle aspirations performed at the Albert Einstein Medical Center (Bronx, New York). Three occurred in patients with a prior history of carcinoma in other sites, whereas 3 were found in patients who had not been previously suspected of having nonthyroidal primary cancer.[25] Fine needle aspiration cytology has been reported to be 90% accurate in diagnosing metastatic lesions to the thyroid gland.[24,26] Proponents of fine needle aspiration cite the usefulness of this technique in diagnosing distant spread in known nonthyroidal cancer, diagnosing previously unrecognized carcinoma present elsewhere in the body, and assisting physicians in selecting appropriate surgical or conservative management without adversely affecting patient survival.[14,21,24–27,30,31]

Differential Diagnosis

The differential diagnosis of metastatic carcinoma to the thyroid is similar to that of primary lymphoma of the thyroid (See Chapter 10). Because of its tendency to be stony-hard, grow rapidly, and cause obstruction of the upper respiratory tract, it most closely resembles anaplastic carcinoma of the thyroid, primary lymphoma of the thyroid, and Reidel's struma in its clinical characteristics. Tissue diagnosis by either fine needle aspiration or open biopsy is the most direct way to make the diagnosis. Some authors believe that a subgroup of cases previously diagnosed as anaplastic carcinoma of the thyroid was really metastatic carcinoma to the thyroid from nonthyroidal primaries.[5,6,37]

Pathophysiology

In 1931 Willis speculated that "altered thyroid tissue" (i.e., preexisting abnormalities of the thyroid gland) was more prone to be the site of metastatic disease to the thyroid gland than normal thyroid tissue. In several cases reported in the earlier literature and in six of his own cases, the metastatic disease in the thyroid was noted to be present in areas of the gland exhibiting advanced fibrous or adenomatous changes. He postulated that "structurally altered thyroid tissue may be a chemically more favorable soil than normal tissue for the development of secondary neoplasms."[1] He further theorized that normal thyroid tissue was a poor medium for metastatic tumor growth because of its high degree of vascularity and "high oxygen tension."[1]

More modern studies have failed to corroborate this hypothesis. The current belief is that because the thyroid gland is a highly vascular organ it has a propensity to be the site of blood-borne carcinomas from distant sites. This theory is validated by the fact that the tumors that most commonly metastasize to the thyroid (kidney, breast, lung, and melanoma) are all known to metastasize via the blood-borne route.[4,14]

Although the majority of metastatic lesions discovered at autopsy are found on microscopic examination, approximately 40% are evident on gross examination. It is of interest that in the series of Shimaoka et al., no tumor nodule smaller than 1 cm found at autopsy was clinically palpable in life. Of nodules 1 to 2 cm in diameter only one of 15 was palpable while among nodules greater than 2 cm in diameter, 9 of 16 were palpable in life. Of the 10 palpable masses in this series, 8 were described as solitary nodules, while 2 were described as being multinodular. At autopsy, however, the same ten cases contained solitary nodules in only 4 cases; the remainder were multinodular.[6]

Treatment and Prognosis

In general, the finding of metastatic cancer in the thyroid gland is ominous. However, data from several authors suggests that for certain carcinomas, early recognition and surgical treatment of thyroid metastases may improve chances for survival, or even cure.[5,7,14,16,18,20,31]

When a metastatic lesion is diagnosed in the thyroid gland and there is no clinical evidence of metastatic disease elsewhere, most authors advocate thyroidectomy.[7,14,16,18,20,31] Surgery is also indicated when metastatic disease to the thyroid gland threatens the patency of the airway or other vital functions.

Rapid deterioration is common among patients with metastases to the thyroid from gastrointestinal and lung cancers. When thyroidectomy has been performed in these patients, the mean length of survival from the time of surgery has been reported as being 1.5 to 2 months.[16] On the other hand, the thyroid may occasionally be the only site of metastasis of hypernephroma, in which case surgery may be curative. In contrast to the patients with gastrointestinal and lung cancers referred to above, patients with metastases to the thyroid from renal and breast adenocarcinomas who have undergone thyroidectomies have had mean lengths of survival of 32 and 37 months respectively.[16] There is no controlled study comparing these data with data on patients who have not undergone thyroidectomy for metastatic carcinoma to the thyroid. Chemotherapy and radiation therapy are useful to the same extent that they would be for treating metastatic disease to any other organ of the body.

Overall, despite sporadic reports of long-term survival or cure among patients with metastatic cancer to the thyroid, the expected length of survival from the time of clinical presentation is short, averaging approximately 12 months. Ericsson et al.[14] performed total or subtotal thyroidectomies on 10 patients with metastatic cancer to the thyroid gland. There were five males and five females ranging in age from 47 to 78 years with a mean age of 64. Seven patients had renal cell carcinomas, two had malignant melanomas and 1 had an angioblastic meningioma. The elapsed time between treatment of the primary tumor to the time of thyroid metastasis was 0 to 14 years with a mean of 6.5 years. Three patients lived less than 4 months from the time of thyroidectomy, four patients lived an average of 3.2 years from the time of thyroidectomy and three patients were alive between 1 and 4 years after thyroid surgery. Two patients with renal cell carcinoma and one with melanoma survived for more than 3 years after surgery.

Ivy[18] reported on 30 cases of clinically evident metastatic cancer to the thyroid gland seen at the Mayo Clinic between 1946 and 1982. The primary tumors in this series included 12 renal, 6 breast, 5 lung and one each from bladder, pancreas, esophagus, larynx, nasopharynx, pelvic teratoma and neurofibrosarcoma. All but three of the patients underwent surgery. Either partial lobectomy, subtotal thyroidectomy, or total thyroidectomy with node dissection was performed. Eighteen patients survived one year or less from the time of diagnosis. Nine patients survived for 3 years or more. Three long-term survivors (3 to 7 years) had renal cell carcinoma, three had breast carcinoma, two had lung carcinoma and one had an esophageal primary. The longest survival interval from the time of disagnosis of thyroid metastasis to the time of death was 7 years. The extent of the surgical procedure did not appear to significantly alter prognosis.

It would appear that a surgical approach to metastatic carcinoma to the thyroid should be considered in those patients who fall into the sub-groups that have good survival rates as reported in the above studies; that is, patients with primary malignancies in the kidney, breast, and possibly the lungs. Obviously, surgery must be considered in patients with respiratory compromise. Chemotherapy and radiotherapy in this group of patients has not been adequately studied but metastatic disease to the thyroid from any given primary tumor should respond as well as soft tissue metastases to other parts of the body.

References

1. Willis RA. Metastatic tumors in the thyroid gland. Am J Pathol 1931;7:187–208.
2. Rice CO. Microscopic metastases in the thyroid gland. Am J Pathol 1934;10:407–412
3. Thorpe JD. Metastatic cancer in thyroid gland. Report of 4 cases. West J Surg 1954:62:574–576.
4. Mortensen JD, Woolner LB, Bennet WA. Secondary malignant tumors of the thyroid gland. Cancer 1956;9:306–309.
5. Elliott RHE Jr, Frantz VR. Metastatic carcinoma masquerading as primary thyroid cancer: report of authors' 14 cases. Ann Surg 1960;151:551–565.
6. Shimaoka K, Sokal J, Pickren J. Metastatic neoplasms in the thyroid gland. Cancer 1962;15:557–565.
7. Wychulis AR, Beahrs OH, Woolner LB. Metastatic carcinoma to the thyroid gland. Ann Surg 1964; 160:169–177.
8. Brierre JT, Dickinson LG. Clinically unsuspected thyroid disease. GB 1964;30:94–98.
9. Silverberg SG, Vidone RA. Metastatic tumors in the thyroid. Pacif Med Surg 1966;74:175–180.
10. Sirota DK, Goldfield EB, Eng YF, Unger AH. Metastatic infiltration of the thyroid gland causing hypothyroidism. J. Mt. Sinai Hosp. 1968;35:242–245.
11. Gault EW, Leung TH, Thomas DP. Clear cell renal carcinoma masquerading as thyroid enlargement. J Pathol 1974;113:21–25.
12. Pillay SP, Angorn IB, Baker LW. Tumor metastases to the thyroid gland. S Afr Med J. 1977;51:509–512.
13. Burge T, Lunberg S. Cancer in Malmo 1958-1969. An autopsy study. Acta Pathol Microbiol Scand 1977;Suppl:260.
14. Ericsson M, Biorklund A, Cederquist E, Ingemansson S, Akerman M. Surgical treatment of metastatic disease in the thyroid gland. J Surg Oncol 1981;17:15–23.
15. Treadwell T, Alexander BB, Owen M, McConnell TH, Ashworth CT. Clear cell renal carcinoma masquerading as a thyroid nodule. South Med J 1981; 74:878–879.
16. Czech JM, Lichtor TR, Carney JA, van Heerden JA. Neoplasms metastatic to the thyroid gland. Surg Gynecol Obstet 1982;155:503–505.
17. Lehur PA, Cote RA, Poisson J, Boctor M, Elhilali M, Kandalaft N. Thyroid metastasis of clear-cell renal carcinoma. Can Med Assoc J 1983;128:154–158.
18. Ivy HK. Cancer metastatic to the thyroid: a diagnostic problem. Mayo Clin Proc 1984;59:856–859.
19. Eriksson A, Gezelius C. Metastatic choriocarcinoma during normal pregnancy presenting as thyroid tumor. Arch Gynecol 1984;236:119–122.
20. McCabe DP, Farrar WB, Petkov TM, Finkelmeier W, O'Dwyer P, James A. Clinical and pathologic correlations in disease metastatic to the thyroid gland. Am J Surg 1985;150:519–523.
21. Lasser A, Rothman JG, Calamia VJ. Renal-cell carcinoma metastatic to the thyroid-aspiration cytology and histologic findings. Acta Cytol 1985;29:856– 858.
22. Gherardi G, Scherini P, Ambrosi S. Occult thyroid metastatis from untreated uveal melanoma. Arch Ophthalmol 1985;103:689–691.
23. Lester JW, Carter MP, Berens SV, Long RF, Caplan GE. Colon carcinoma metastatic to the thyroid gland. Clin Nucl Med 1986;11:634–635.
24. Smith SA, Gharib H, Goellner JR. Fine-needle aspiration. Usefulness for diagnosis and management of metastatic carcinoma to the thyroid. Arch Intern Med 1987; 147:311–312.
25. Chacho MS, Greenebaum E, Moussouris HF, Schreiber K, Koss LG. Value of aspiration cytology of the thyroid in metastatic disease. Acta Cytol 1987;31:705–712.
26. Hsu C, Boey J. Diagnostic pitfalls in fine needle aspiration of thyroid nodules a study of 555 cases in Chinese patients. Acta Cytol 1987;31:699–704.
27. Watts NB. Carcinoma metastatic to the thyroid: prevalence and diagnosis by fine-needle aspiration cytology. Am J Med Sci 1987;293:13–17.
28. Krauth PH, Katz JF. Kaposi's sarcoma involving the thyroid in a patient with AIDS. Clin Nucl Med 1987;12:848–849.
29. Ackerman L, Romyn A, Khedkar N, Kaplan E. Malignant fibrous histiocytoma metastatic to the thyroid gland. Clin Nucl Med 1987;12:648–649.
30. Gritsman AY, Popok SM, Ro JY, Dekmezian RH, Weber RS. Renal-cell carcinoma with intranuclear inclusions metastatic to thyroid: a diagnostic problem in aspiration cytology. Diagn Cytopathol 1988;4:125–129.
31. Green LK, Ro JY, MacKay B, Ayala AG, Luna MA. Renal cell carcinoma metastatic to the thyroid. Cancer 1989;63:1810–1815.
32. Bisi H, Fernandes VSO, Asato De Camargo RY, Koch L, Abado AH, DeBrito T. The prevalence of unsuspected thyroid pathology in 300 sequential autopsies, with special reference to the incidental carcinoma. Cancer 1989;64:1888–1893.
33. Abrams HL, Spiro R, Goldstein N. Metastases in carcinoma; analysis of 1000 autopsied cases. Cancer 1950;3:74–85.
34. Hazard JB, Kaufman N. A survey of thyroid glands obtained at autopsy in a so-called goiter area. Am J Clin Pathol 1952;22;860–865.
35. Hull OH. Critical analysis of two hundred twenty one thyroid glands: Study of thyroid glands obtained at necropsy in Colorado. Arch Pathol 1955;59:291–311.
36. Higashi T, Ito K, Nishikawa Y et al. Gallium-67 imaging in the evlauation of thyroid malignancy. Clin Nucl Med 1988;13:792–799.
37. Perloff WH, Schneeberg NG. Problem of thyroid carcinoma. Surgery 1951;29:572–580.

12

External Radiation Treatment for Thyroid Carcinoma

EDWARD MERKER

Introduction

The treatment of thyroid carcinoma is highly controversial, in part because of the often indolent nature of the majority of these tumors, but also because of the absence of adequately controlled prospective studies. There is certainly agreement as to the need for adequate surgery. It is in the area of postoperative management of thyroid carcinoma that views become more controversial. Although many large series demonstrate a small advantage of postoperative I 131 ablation and/or thyroid suppression therapy, because of the long survival in these diseases, there is much debate over the statistics and their implications. It is in the more esoteric arena of external radiotherapy for thyroid carcinoma that there is perhaps the most divergence of opinion. The data from the most extensive of the published studies is presented below. In evaluating these data, careful attention must be paid to such factors as the histology of the tumors treated, extent of the lesion, type and application of therapy field, and dosage-time considerations. Furthermore, a distinction must be made between the use of external radiotherapy for treatment of known persistent disease and its use in prophylaxis of recurrent disease after apparently adequate initial therapy.

In one of the earliest studies of the usefulness of radiotherapy in tne treatment of thyroid carcinoma, Windeyer[1] reported the disappearance or marked regression of "locally inoperable" papillary carcinoma of the thyroid in 10 of 24 patients. Survival rates were analyzed by Frazell and Foote[2] in their report of a 25-year experience. Of 23 patients with inoperable papillary carcinoma of the thyroid, 10 survived 5 or more years after radiotherapy; the longest survival period was 26 years. The problem in evaluating these data is lack of knowledge of the appropriate comparative survival figures for a totally comparable control group of nonirradiated patients with this often indolent disease. In 1966, Sheline et al.[3] reported their 29-year experience. In their analysis of all the patients seen by their section of therapeutic radiology from 1935 to 1964, of 147 patients, 89 had to be excluded fram study because of one or more of the following: there was no convincing evidence of persistent local disease at the time of radiation treatment, the treated lesion was a recurrence of previously radiated disease, no radiation therapy was given to the thyroid area, or extrathyroidal extension involved only the overlying strap muscles. The 58 patients in the study had residual or recurrent extrathyroidal cancer in the surgical field but none had carcinoma demonstrable beyond the cervical region at the time of treatment. Because of tracheal, laryngeal, or esophageal invasion, surgical excision was incomplete in 44 patients, 19 of whom had gross evidence of tumor remaining after surgery was completed. No definitive surgical procedure was performed in the remaining 14 patients "due to obvious involvement of vital structures," a categorical statement not further elaborated on by the authors. The histologic description of these tumors was papillary carcinoma (27 cases), follicular carcinoma (9 cases), anaplastic and giant cell (12 cases), lymphosarcoma (6 cases); there was one case each of fibrosarcoma, angiosarcoma, medullary carcinoma, and Hürthle cell carcinoma. It appeared that these patient groups had, on the average, much more tumor involvement from the beginning than the average thyroid carcinoma patients. Although tracheal invasion was suspected preoperatively in 8 patients, it was present in 35 of the patients who had thyroidectomy performed and was suspected in 12 of the 14 grossly inoperable tumor patients who had only biopsy performed. Curiously, in 4 patients with papillary carcinoma, the tumor appeared as a mass in the tracheal lumen or the hypopharynx. Paresis of one vocal cord was not present preoperatively in 15 patients. Three patients with papillary carcinoma presented with hemoptysis. The specifics of the radiation treatment varied considerably. Radiation doses were calculated in, or just lateral to, the midplane of the neck at the sites of presumed residual cancer. The doses varied from 3000 rad over 15 days to 6000 rad over 50 days. Higher doses of 5000 to 6000 rad over 6 to 7 weeks were used in the patients treated in the later years of the study.

In examining the Sheline study as well as all subsequent studies, the data must be broken down into groups representing the histologic patterns of the different cancers. In the 15 patients with papillary cancer in whom the tumor was grossly evident after surgical treatment, or in whom there was an inoperable recurrence, 9 had tumor that was palpable at the time of radiation therapy. Of these 9 there was a complete disappearance of the lesion in 7 and a decrease in size was noted in the remaining two. There had been cancer within the trachea or hypopharynx in 4 of the 9 patients with palpable tumor. In terms of survival, in the patients with definite persistent or recurrent carcinoma, 8 were alive without local recurrence 1 to 14 years after radiation therapy. Three deaths occurred frcm unrelated causes without local recurrence at 1, 6, and 25 years after therapy. One patient with a local recurrence was living 5 years after treatment and three others died of a local recurrence. The four recurrences occurred from 1 to 18 years after therapy. In the 12 remaining patients with papillary carcinoma there was no gross tumor remaining; however, tumor had been "shaved off" the trachea or thyroid cartilage. In none of these patients was a local recurrence demonstrated after radiotherapy (minimal follow-up time was five years and ten patients were followed-up for 10 to 22 years). One patient did die from distant metastases. These patients were younger than those with grossly apparent residual disease, which raises the question of whether the better statistics were due to treatment at an earlier stage of the disease. The statistics certainly led the authors to believe that patients with persistent microscopically infiltrating papillary carcinoma should be treated with radiation therapy.

Nine patients with follicular carcinoma of the thyroid were treated with external radiation therapy by the Sheline group. Of the 4 with gross residual carcinoma after surgery or inoperable carcinoma, 1 failed to respond to treatment and died 3 years later of tumor growth. The other 3 were living without recurrence 2, 10, and 16 years after treatment. Of the 5 patients with tracheal infiltration but no grossly evident tumor, 2 died of local recurrence 4 and 6 years after radiation, 1 died of an unrelated cause 7 years later, and 2 were living without recurrence 5 and 18 years later. Although radiation therapy was effective in controlling tumor growth in follicular cancer in this study, it was not as effective as it was in patients with papillary cancer. In 12 patients in this study radiation was used to treat anaplastic carcinomas although, at the time, 5 of these were separately described as giant cell carcinomas. One of the patients was alive and well 2 years after radiation. One died 6 years after treatment from metastases but without local recurrence. Ten patients died from local recurrence. All but one died within 2 to 7 months after radiation.

In the Sheline report no serious sequelae of radiation therapy were observed. Tracheostomy was necessitated only when tumor obstructed the airway. It is of interest that at their center (UCLA San Francisco), radioiodine

Table 12.1. Response of papillary thyroid carcinoma to external radiation—microscopic disease

Postoperative status	No treatment		Radiation		Radioiodine	
	No recurrence	Recurrence	No recurrence	Recurrence	No recurrence	Recurrence
No residual	10	2	6*	1†	2	0
Probable residual	3	3	16‡	0	5	1
Residual microscopic	0	1	12§	0	2	1

*1 patient also received radioiodine treatment.
†2,600 rads.
‡7 patients also received radioiodine treatment.
§4 patients also received radioiodine treatment.
Reprinted, by permission, from Simpson, WJ and Carruthers, JS, 1978(4).

therapy was described as being reserved for situations in which the initial lesion and metastases were inoperable and not amenable to external radiation therapy, because they were concerned about giving systemic radiation therapy to younger patients who might live for a long time regardless of the stage of their carcinoma.

Simpson and Carruthers[4] reported on their treatment with external radiotherapy of 137 patients with differentiated thyroid carcinoma from a group of 516 patients with thyroid carcinoma registered at the Princess Margaret Hospital in Toronto from 1958 to 1977. There were 82 patients with papillary carcinoma and 55 patients with follicular carcinoma. The age distribution was older than that found in unselected surgical patients. The authors noted that since their hospital is a referral center for radiation therapy many patients with "favorable" disease are never referred to them for an opinion, whereas patients who either present with advanced disease initially or suffer from recurrences or metastases are often referred for radiation therapy. Many of Simpson and Carruthers' patients had undergone multiple surgical procedures and/or been treated with radioiodine one or more times. Twenty of the patients with papillary carcinoma and 31 of those with follicular carcinoma had infiltrating neck masses, distant metastases at the time of referral, or both. The patients were classified by the degree of completeness of surgical excision. "No residual disease" was defined as removal of all gross tumor, as well as demonstration by histologic examination of an adequate rim of uninvolved tissue at the margin of resection. Patients were said to have probable residual microscopic disease if there was tumor within 2 or 3 mm of the resection margin. Residual microscopic disease described cases in which tumor extended to the resection margin, usually instances in which tumor was removed by sharp dissection from the outer surface of the trachea, larynx, or esophagus. "Gross residual tumor" meant that the surgeon knew that visible tumor was left behind. In this report, the response of microscopic disease to treatment was based on whether local recurrence was observed independently of the occurrence of distant metastases. "Gross disease" included inoperable thyroid masses and nodal involvement but also a few distant metastases, which were the first site of recurrence and had been treated only by external radiotherapy. Reference to Tables 12.1 and 12.2 show that there is a risk of local recurrence in patients with papillary carcinoma with

Table 12.2. Response of papillary thyroid carcinoma to external radiation—gross disease

	Complete regression	Partial regression	No regression
Radiation	3*	8	0
Radioiodine	0	1	3

*1 patient also received radioiodine treatment.
Reprinted, by permission, from Simpson, WJ and Carruthers, JS, 1978(4).

Table 12.3. Response of follicular thyroid carcinoma to external radiation—microscopic disease

Postoperative status	No treatment		Radiation		Radioiodine	
	No recurrence	Recurrence	No recurrence	Recurrence	No recurrence	Recurrence
No residual	3	9	4	0	2	1
Probable residual	1	2	5*	1†	4	0
Residual microscopic	0	0	4*	0	1	0

*2 patients also received radioiodine treatment.
†Marginal recurrence.
Reprinted, by permission, from Simpson, WJ and Carruthers, JS, 1978(4).

grossly complete tumor excision but the risk can be eliminated by radiation in high enough dosage, in this study 4000 rads over 3 to 3.5 weeks. The only recurrence was noted in a patient who received only 2600 rads. The efficacy of external radiotherapy was noted to be better than radioiodine therapy; 2 out of 9 patients who were treated with radioiodine had local recurrences. However, whether the differences were statistically significant in this case is moot. Gross tumor also responded at least partially to external radiotherapy. A reasonable question is whether the response could have been improved with higher doses. This was not determined in this study.

Table 12.3 shows that when only microscopic residual disease was present, external radiotherapy was as effective in preventing local recurrence of follicular carcinoma as it was in preventing papillary carcinoma. In the follicular group with microscopic disease the only local recurrence in the 14 patients treated with external radiotherapy was at the margin just outside the radiation field. This may be compared to the one non-marginal recurrence in the 8 patients with follicular microscopic disease treated with radioiodine therapy. However, gross follicular carcinoma, like papillary carcinoma, responded less favorably. Five out of 14 patients treated in this group had complete regression of disease and 4 more had a partial regression. In comparison, all 7 patients treated with radioiodine responded; 4 responded completely.

The report concludes that microscopic disease can be eliminated by moderate dose external radiotherapy, and that most patients with

Table 12.4. Response of follicular thyroid carcinoma to external radiation—gross disease

	Complete regression	Partial regression	No regression
Radiation	5	4	5
Radioiodine	3	2	1
Radiation and radioiodine	4	3	0

Reprinted, by permission, from Simpson, WJ and Carruthers, JS, 1978(4).

gross disease respond favorably, albeit to higher radiation doses (5000 rads over 4.5 weeks). Results were noted to be improved (Table 12.4) by adding radioiodine treatment in cases in which the tumor took up radioiodine. It is of interest that these authors claimed therapeutic success with more moderate radiotherapy doses than others have described. Reviewing their survival curves (Figs. 12.1 and 12.2) it appears that patients with pure papillary tumors have a better survival than those with mixed papillary-follicular elements. This was thought to simply reflect the smaller number of such patients. The authors stated that patients with mixed tumors have a lower-than-average survival rate for ten years after initial therapy and may later die as a direct result of their thyroid cancer. The patients with follicular carcinoma of the thyroid were noted to have a higher mortality rate than of individuals of the same age and sex in the general population. The average survival rate for more poorly differentiated follicular carcinoma is lower than the rate for well-differentiated tumor. Although it appears

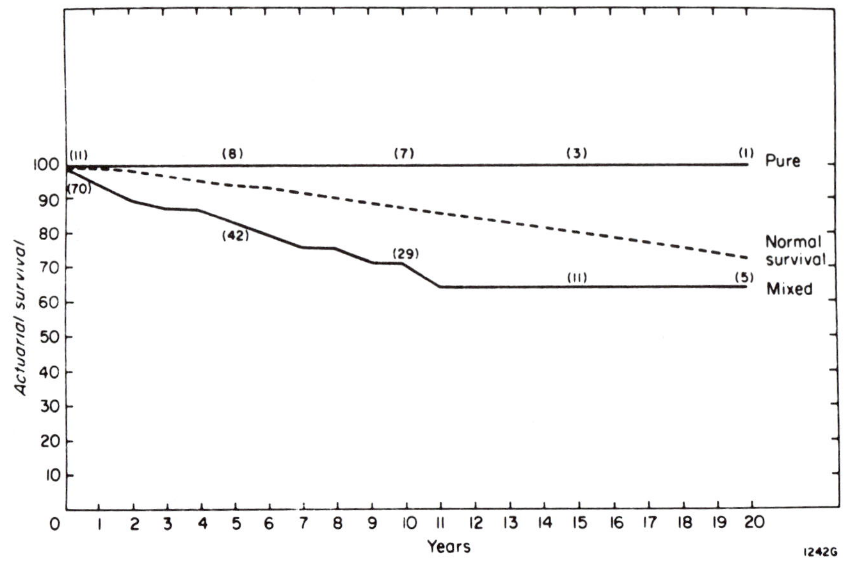

Figure 12.1. Survival of patients with papillary thyroid carcinoma (pure and mixed papillary and follicular) compared with survival of normal patients of same age and sex. Numbers in parentheses indicate the number of patients at risk at 0, 5, 10, 15, and 20 years. Reprinted, by permission, from Simpson WJ, and Carruthers, JS, 1978(4).

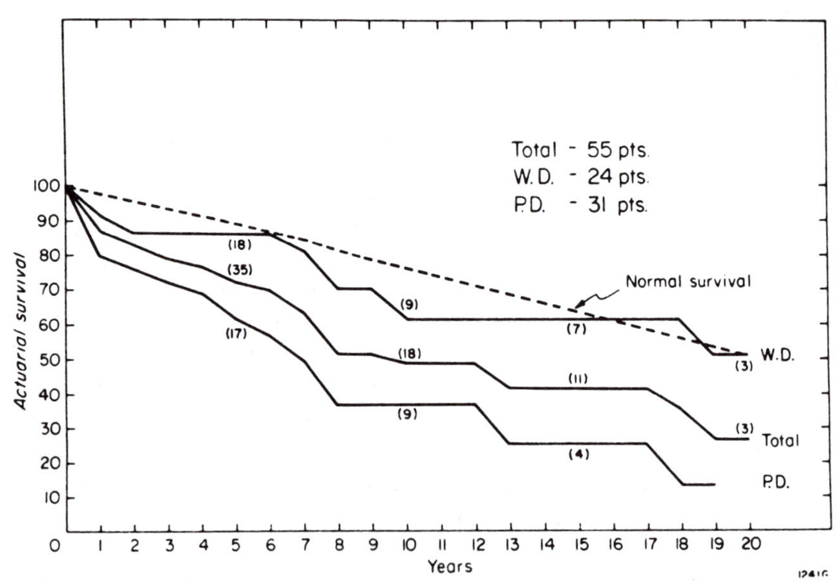

Figure 12.2. Survival of patients with papillary thyroid carcinoma (well differentiated [WD] and poorly differentiated [PD]) compared with survival of normal patients of same age and sex. Numbers in parentheses indicate the number of patients at risk at 0, 5, 10, 15, and 20 years. Reprinted, by permission, from Simpson WJ, and Carruthers, JS, 1978(4).

Table 12.5. Complications of treatment for papillary and follicular thyroid carcinoma

	Complication	No. of patients
Radioiodine (70 patients)	Severe thyroiditis	8
	Acute leukemia	1
Radiation (91 patients)	Severe esophagitis, tracheitis	9
	Lhermitte's syndrome	2
	Tracheal chondritis (with surgery and infection)	1
	Fibrosis of neck tissues	3
	Skin necrosis (overdose)	1
	Brain necrosis (multiple radiation therapy)	1
Surgery (128 patients)	Vocal cord palsy	25
	Hypoparathyroidism	8
	Horner's syndrome	3
	Severe local infection	3
	Tracheal chondritis (with radiation therapy inflammation)	1
	Postoperative thyroid storm	1
	Ear-cough syndrome	1
	Tracheal stoma stenosis	1
	Recurrent Marlex slough (trachea)	1

Reprinted, by permission, from Simpson, WJ and Carruthers, JS, 1978(4).

from the data that patients with papillary cancer have significantly better survival than those with follicular carcinoma, the data are not statistically significant when corrected for age and sex. The authors noted that since two thirds of the deaths in their series were directly due to thyroid cancer, and that only one third of the patients who died of other causes had clinical evidence of cancer at the time of their death; adequate initial treatment is obviously very important. Because papillary carcinomas are more aggessive in older patients, the authors suggest that older patients should be treated more radically than younger patients.

In terms of complications in the Simpson and Carruthers report (Table 12.5), it is noted that in those treated with external radiotherapy, radiation necrosis occurred in two patients: one who received three courses of radiation for uncontrolled brain metastases and one who developed skin necrosis from an accidental overdose of radiation.

The authors discussed the fact that differentiated thyroid carcinomas have traditionally been regarded as radioresistant because they regress very slowly when treated by external radiation. Very little change in tumor size occurs for months after treatment is administered and disappearance or maximum regression is often not apparent for months or even years later.

In 1980 Chung et al.[5] reported 38 patients with residual or recurrent thyroid carcinomas with no uptake of ^{131}I whom they treated with external radiation therapy between 1962 and 1977. These patients had 8 papillary-follicular carcinomas, 15 undifferentiated and 2 medullary carcinomas. Doses of 3500 to 7000 rads were used for local disease control in 23 patients, 8 of whom had successful tumor control. Among these 8 patients, 6 were alive and well 2 to 11 years after treatment. Cobalt 60 or 4-MeV linear accelerator teletherapy was employed in 33 of 35 courses, with a single anterior field directed at the neck and upper mediastinum in 13 of 23 cases. A more complex field arrangement was needed to encompass tumor in 10 cases. Most of the patients received conventional fractionation of 200 rads (2 Gy) a day. There was a variety of time-dosing regimens used in treatment of metastases.

In this series there were 9 follicular and 6 papillary carcinomas. All except one had palpable disease. In all 4 who received more than 1700 rets (6000 rads [60 Gy] in six weeks) local tumor control was achieved. Three of the 4 were alive 46 to 78 months after treatment. One of these patients died of distant metastases despite local tumor control. However, control was not achieved in 4 patients who received less than 1600 rets; they all died 2 to 24 months after therapy (Table 12.6). Fifteen of the 16 patients with anaplastic carcinoma, 11 of whom did not have distant metastases, were treated with local irradiation. They were treated with a spectrum of dosing (Table 12.7). Local tumor control was achieved in 3 of the 5 patients who received more than 1700 rets; one patient remained well at $2\frac{1}{2}$ years, one patient

Table 12.6. Papillary and follicular carcinoma

Patient No.	Sex	Dose rad/fr/day	NSD (rets)	No local recurrence Alive	No local recurrence Dead	Local recurrence Alive	Local recurrence Dead
1	F	5500/11/40	2060	—	16M[a]	—	—
2	M	7000/35/67	1890	46M	—	—	—
3	M	6000/30/57	1715	84M	—	—	—
4	F	5500/25/35	1715	78M	—	—	—
5	F	5200/26/40	1585	—	—	—	9M
6	F	4800/24/33	1520	—	—	—	24M
7	M	4000/14/22	1510	—	—	—	2M[b]
8	F	3500/10/14	1505	—	—	—	2M[c]

[a] Distant metastases.
[b] Intercurrent disease.
[c] Lung, bone metastases.
Reprinted, by permission, from Chung, CT, Sagerman, RH, Ryoo, MC, King, GA, Yu, WS, Dalai, PS, Emmanuel, IG, 1980(5).

Table 12.7. Undifferentiated carcinoma

Patient	Sex	Dose rad/fr/day	NSD rets	No local recurrence Alive	No local recurrence Dead	Local recurrence Alive	Local recurrence Dead
1	F	6000/25/43	1830	—	—	—	6M
2	F	6000/29/40	1780	—	66M	—	—
3	M	6000/30/43	1750	30M	—	—	—
4	F	6000/30/60	1715	54M	—	—	—
5	F	5500/25/35	1715	—	—	—	6M
6	F	5000/24/32	1595	—	—	—	4M
7	M	5000/25/39	1545	—	—	—	4M
8	F	5079/27/50	1525	—	—	—	18M
9	F	4784/23/36	1520	—	—	—	6M
10	F	4023/20/27	1365	—	—	—	1M
11	F	3850/20/25	1319	—	—	—	2M
12	F	3000/10/12	1315	—	—	—	4M
13	M	3495/15/21	1305	—	—	—	7M
14	M	3477/17/23	1250	—	—	—	2M
15	F	920/03/08	560	—	—	—	2D

Reprinted, by permission, from Chung, CT, Sagerman, RH, Ryoo, MC, King, GA, Yu, WS, Dalai, PS, Emmanuel, IG, 1980(5).

remained well at $4\frac{1}{2}$ years, and the third died of distant metastases at $5\frac{1}{2}$ years. Twelve patients had a local recurrence and died within 18 months, 11 in the first 7 months. Metastatic disease was treated in 10 patients with 12 metastatic sites. There were 2 papillary, 5 follicular, 2 medullary, and 1 anaplastic tumors treated (Table 12.8). Palliation was minimally better with higher dose therapy. One patient with papillary carcinoma metastatic to the lung died at 7 months with persistent progressive disease. Four died 1 to 4 years after radiation, but 3 were alive with disease at 3, 6, and 11 years. In one patient with medullary carcinoma, a metastatic focus in the left supraorbital area treated with 6000 rads (60 Gy) remained under control 6 years later. A better survival rate was definitely achieved with higher radiation doses (Table 12.9) in the Chung study, the results of which were consistent with

Table 12.8. Metastatic disease

Patient no.	Sex	Histology	Site treated	Dose rad/fr/day	NSD (rets)	Response	Status
1	F	Medullary	L. Supraorbit	6000/30/41	1765	Local control	Alive—6 yr.
2	M	Follicular	Mediastinum	4800/16/47	1680	Marked regression	2 yrs later
			Hip	2400/06/16	1245	Little relief	Dead—26 M
3	M	Papillary	Lung	4800/16/60	1670	No response	Dead—7 M
4	F	Medullary	Cervical spine	3500/09/11	1585	No change	Alive—11 yr.
5	F	Papillary	Pubic bone	3000/10/14	1290	Some relief	
			Cord compress.	2500/05/07	1375	Stable	Dead—1 yr.
6	F	Undiffer.	Cord compress.	3000/10/14	1290	No response	Dead < 1 M
7	F	Follicular	Ribs	3000/16/16	1270	No response—1 yr. Retreated—O.K.	Alive—3 yr.
8	M	Follicular	Cord compress.	2260/05/14	1150	Stable	Dead—1 yr.
9	F	Follicular	Hip	2000/05/07	1100	Little relief Further I^{131}	Dead—4 yr.
10	F	Follicular	Sternum	2120/08/12	(985)	—	Dead < 1 M

Reprinted, by permission, from Chung, CT, Sagerman, RH, Ryoo, MC, King, GA, Yu, WS, Dalai, PS, Emmanuel, IG, 1980(5).

Table 12.9. Dose–response–survival

	Local				Metastases	
	Undifferentiated		Differentiated			
Dose (NSD:rets)	Controlled/ patients	NED	Controlled/ patients	NED	Controlled/ patients	Alive >2 YR
< 1500	0/6	—	—	—	0/7	2
1500 << 1700	0/4	—	0/4	—	0/4	2
1700 <	3/5	2	4/4	3	1/1	1

NED = no evidence of disease.
Reprinted, by permission, from Chung, CT, Sagerman, RH, Ryoo, MC, King, GA, Yu, WS, Dalai, PS, Emmanuel, IG, 1980(5).

the earlier suggestion of Fuller.[6] It is of interest that in the Chung study anaplastic as well as differentiated carcinoma showed a good local response to external radiotherapy.

In 1981 Mazzaferi and Young[7] stated that external radiation had an adverse effect on outcome in thyroid carcinoma. They reported a retrospective analysis of 576 patients with papillary carcinoma of the thyroid treated in many different hospitals by United States Air Force physicians using highly variable regimens. There were 6 deaths from thyroid cancer and 84 recurrences in this series. Adverse effects on survival were noted in patients who presented at the age of 40 years or older, in patients with tumors larger than 2.5 cm at presentation, and in patients whose tumors demonstrated extracapsular extension. The highest recurrence rates were in those patients with large tumors with local invasion. The group given external radiotherapy and thyroid hormone with (2 patients) or without (16 patients) radioiodine numbered only 18 patients. This group had the highest recurrence rate, 61% (Table 12.10), which was significantly higher than the group treated with radioiodine or thyroid hormone alone. However, the other groups were much larger. The patients treated with external radiotherapy were similar to the rest of the study group in degree of tumor invasion and age at presentation; however, cervical lymph node metastases were noted in more

Table 12.10. Impact of treatment on recurrence and survival

	Recurrence			Deaths from cancer		
	%	No.	p*	%	No.	p†
Thyroidectomy						
"Total"[1]	10.9	34/310	<0.01	0.6	2/310	N.S.
Subtotal	19.2	50/261		1.5	4/261	
Lymph node surgery						
None	12.3	32/255		0.8	2/260	
Simple excision	17.9	31/173	N.S.	1.7	3/173	N.S.
Neck dissection	14.7	21/143		0.7	1/143	
Adjunctive therapy						
None	40.0	12/30	‡	10.0	3/30	
Thyroid hormone	13.1	54/413	<0.001	0.2	1/414	<0.001
^{131}I and thyroid	6.4	7/110		0.9	1/114	
External radiation	61.0	11/18		5.6	1/18	

Note: Denominator in recurrence column contains only patients presumed to have been cured following initial therapy. Denominator in cancer death column contains all patients on whom the observation is made. N.S. = not significant; $p \geq 0.05$.

* Comparing recurrences in each subgroup.

† Comparing deaths in each subgroup.

‡ See text.

Reprinted, by permission, from Mazzaferri, EL and Young, RL, 1981(7).

of those treated with external radiotherapy (78% versus 45%, $p = .02$). The primary lesions were smaller in the group treated with external radiotherapy. Radiation dosage was estimated to be 1000 to 3000 rads in 4 patients, 3000 to 5000 rads in six patients and 5000 to 7000 rads in 5 patients; the authors could not accurately determine radiation dosage in three remaining cases. Applying Simpson's data it is possible that only 5 out of the group of 18 received an adequate radiotherapy dose, hence making the data from Mazzaferi and Young of questionable value. It is also likely that in nonreferral hospitals where radiotherapy is uncommonly administered, as is the case in this report, radiotherapy is given only to those patients thought by their physicians to be at higher risk from their disease. In any case, of the 11 patients treated with external radiation therapy in whom cancer recurred, all had local recurrences and two had distant metastases as well. Two of these patients died, one of thyroid cancer and one of other causes, although this patient still had thyroid cancer. Another patient was living with persistent disease and one was free of disease before being lost to follow-up. The others were living without apparent disease. Recurrent cancer that could not be eliminated was present in 16.7% (3 of 18) of the external radiation group compared to only 2.3% (13 of 558) of those treated with other modalities or no adjunctive therapy, with a p value of .02. The authors stated that the "routine use of external radiation" has an "adverse effect on outcome."[7] Because of the reservations expressed regarding the size of the subgroup and possible inappropriateness of the dosage that were used it is not clear that this study can be interpreted as significant negative evidence against the use of external radiotherapy for thyroid carcinoma.

In 1985 Ampil[8] reported a retrospective series of 20 patients from two institutions in Louisiana, 19 of whom received external radiotherapy. There were 11 papillary carcinomas, 2 follicular carcinomas, 5 anaplastic carcinomas, and 1 Hürthle cell carcinoma in this series. Eleven of 12 patients with possible microscopic residual disease received external radiation treatment, as did all 8 patients with gross residual or recurrent neck disease. Fourteen of the 19 irradiated patients received treatment to the whole neck and upper mediastinum while two patients received local radiotherapy to the lesion only. Another 2 patients had only the whole neck treated while one patient had a temporary interstitial implant in the neck, followed by involved neck field radiotherapy. Cobalt 60 was used to deliver a total dose that varied from 3800 rads in 21 fractions to 6000 rads in 30 fractions. Most patients received more than 4000 rads but less than 6000 rads. There was no comparison group of patients treated with other modalities. Of 12 patients with microscopic residual disease, seven did not get postoperative radiotherapy. Six of these 7 developed a local recurrence in the neck. These 6 were retreated with neck dissection plus external radiotherapy. Five of 6 were alive without disease on follow-up, 2 months to 5 years later—admittedly a short follow-up period. The one nonirradiated patient was alive and free of disease 2 years and 8 months later. Five of the 12 patients with microscopic residual disease had postoperative radiotherapy immediately after thyroid surgery. Of these patients, three were alive and well without disease; one at 20, one at 26 and one at 75 months of follow-up; one lived 6 months without disease and later died of unknown causes; and one patient was lost to follow-up. This represents a 81.8% control rate. In the 8 patients with gross residual disease two were alive without disease, one at 14 and one at 60 months following radiotherapy. One of these two had a follicular carcinoma and the other a Hürthle cell tumor. One of the eight patients was alive with possible residual neck disease, two died with disease present and three were lost to follow-up. Hence there was a 25% control rate in this higher risk group.

In 1985, Simpson and McKinney[9] reported on the results of a Canadian multicenter retrospective chart review of 2214 patients with thyroid carcinoma registered at 13 radiotherapy centers between 1958 and 1978. Each center was asked to abstract charts of 200 patients. If more patients were registered, the number of charts abstracted for each of the study years was to be a fixed proportion of the total number of patients registered during each of the study years. This was thought to provide a uniform selection of types and numbers of thyroid carcinoma permitting comparisons between eras and analysis of long-term recurrence and survival rates. Of 2600 worksheets sent to the centers, 2411 completed forms were returned; of these, 2214 cases were not duplicates and had enough data for analysis. The study group included 608 males from 8 to 95 years of age and 1599 females from 6 to 97 years of age. The data were stored on their PDP-11/70 computer and statistical analyses were performed with their in-house statistics software package.

In this study, certain centers were found to have a much higher proportion of younger patients referred to them. The same institutions had patients referred to them who had a higher proportion of favorable factors such as smaller primaries, lesser frequency of extrathyroidal invasion, and higher frequency of papillary and follicular tumors compared to anaplastic tumors. In this study about one half the patients had papillary carcinoma and one quarter had follicular carcinoma of the thyroid. Table 12.11 shows the statistics for the diameter of the primary tumor and the presence or absence of factors such as extrathyroidal invasion, neck node involvement, and distant metastases. There was a high frequency of extrathyroidal invasion noted in this study, from 25% in patients with papillary carcinoma to 60% in patients with anaplastic carcinomas. Distant metastases as well as neck node involvement was frequent. External radiotherapy was employed in 14% of the papillary carcinomas and 10% of the follicular carcinomas. Combined modality treatment with both external radiotherapy and radioiodine was employed in 6% of the papillary carcinoma patients and 8% of the follicular carcinoma patients. External radiation therapy was used in 31% of the medullary carcinoma cases. Of the anaplastic carcinoma patients, 40% were treated with surgery and postoperative radiotherapy, 40% with external radiotherapy alone (in cases of unresectable disease), and 8% received chemotherapy, usually in combination with radiotherapy. Table 12.12 shows the distribution of tumor histologies.

In terms of follow-up, although most centers had good follow-up, with 94% of patients followed-up to 1980 or later, five centers had only 53% follow-up to January 1980 or later.

Table 12.11. Extent of cancer at time of diagnosis

Variable	Pathological type (and no. of patients); % of patients Papillary (1089)	Follicular (514)	Medullary (91)	Anaplastic (387)
Diameter of primary tumour (cm)				
<1	9	4	2	0.5
1–4	55	45	53	14
>4	18	36	37	68
Not stated	18	15	8	17
Extrathyroidal invasion				
No	60	57	41	11
Yes	26	25	37	60
Not stated	14	18	22	29
Neck node involvement				
No	55	67	35	32
Yes	20	9	37	26
Not stated	25	24	28	42
Distant metastases				
No	84	74	76	54
Yes	5	11	15	25
Not stated	11	15	9	21

Reprinted, by permission, from Simpson, WJ, and McKinney, 1985(9).

Table 12.12. Proportions of pathological types of thyroid cancer by year of registration at 13 Canadian radiotherapy centres*

Year of registration	Pathological type; % of patients Papillary	Follicular	Medullary	Anaplastic	Other	No. of patients
1958–1962	41	26	3	23	7	286
1963–1967	44	23	4	22	7	437
1968–1972	47	24	4	18	7	498
1973–1978	54	22	5	14	5	811

*This report is based on data for 2214 patients; however, since the data were incomplete for some patients, the patient numbers often total less than 2214 in the various analyses.
Reprinted, by permission, from Simpson, WJ, and McKinney, 1985(9).

This resulted in a total follow-up of only 89% of all patients in the study and 80% of those patients currently alive. Local control was defined as the "complete eradication of local and nodal disease, with no recurrence of disease in the thyroid bed or the regional lymph nodes at any time during the entire follow-up period."[9] Initial treatment provided local control in 77% of the papillary carcinoma cases and 70% of the follicular carcinoma cases. Figure 12.3 provides the overall and cause-specific actuarial survival curves of the patients with papillary carcinoma and Fig. 12.4 provides the survival curves for follicular carcinoma. More than half the deaths in the papillary carcinoma group were due to the carcinoma; there was a 10-year survival rate of 82%. Papillary thyroid cancer was a cause of death as long as 20 years after diagnosis. In the follicular carcinoma group the same phenomena prevailed but with lower rates of survival. Figure 12.5 provides the survival curves for medullary thyroid carcinomas. There were only 91 patients in this subgroup, with a 5-year survival of 68%, 10-year survival of 56% and 20-year survival of 31%. Because the thyroid cancer caused

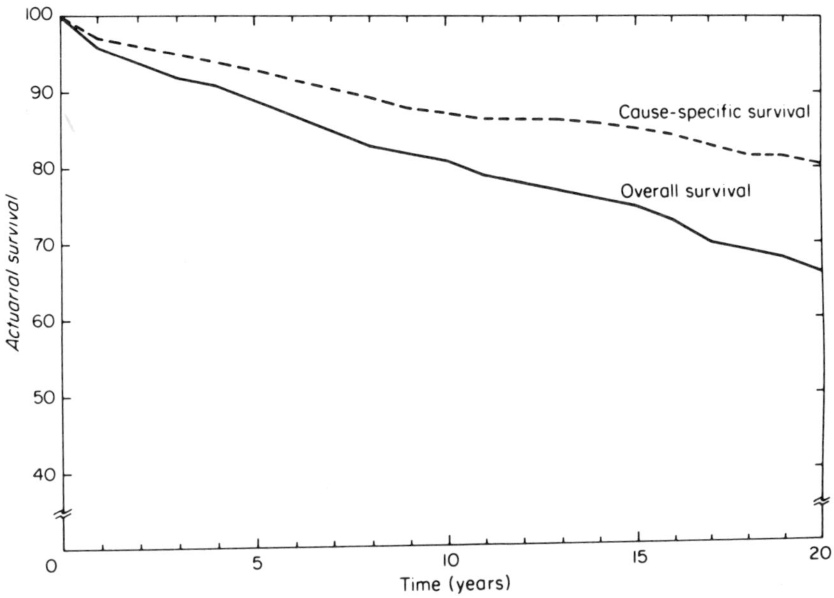

Figure 12.3. Papillary cancers: cause-specific and overall actuarial survival, the specific cause of death being thyroid cancer (1062 patients). Reprinted, by permission, from Simpson, WJ, and McKinney, 1985(9).

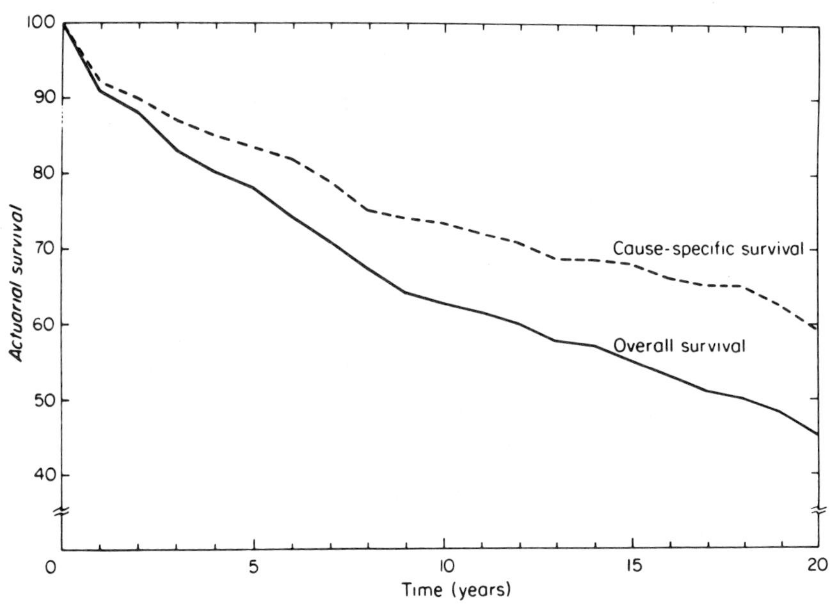

Figure 12.4. Follicular cancers: cause-specific and overall actuarial survival (502 patients). Reprinted, by permission, from Simpson, WJ, and McKinney, 1985(9).

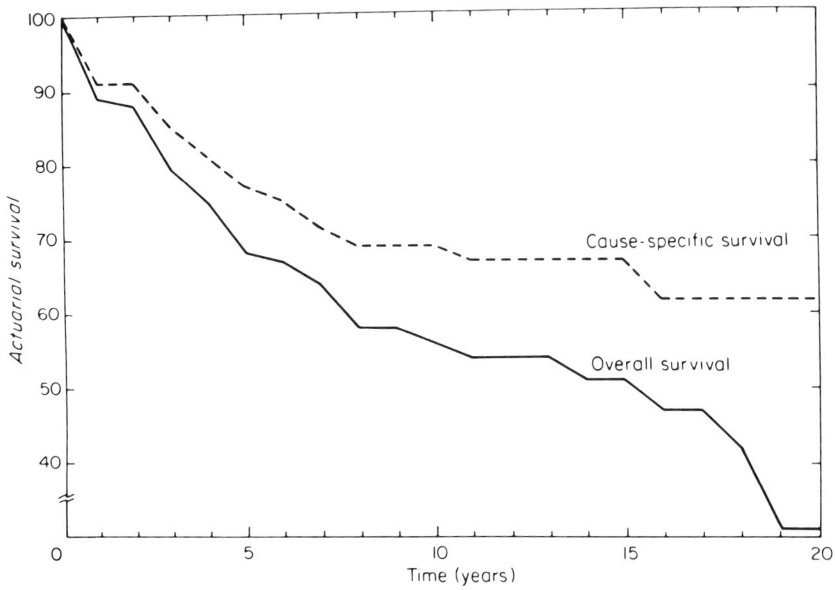

Figure 12.5. Medullary cancers: cause-specific and overall actuarial survival (89 patients). Reprinted, by permission, from Simpson, WJ, and McKinney, 1985(9).

most deaths in the first 15 years the data were interpreted as showing a 60% cure rate of medullary carcinoma by external radiotherapy. In the anaplastic carcinoma subgroup, 377 of 387 patients received some form of treatment. In cases in which surgery was considered possible it was performed. If tumors were unresectable, external radiotherapy was used alone; local control was accomplished in 23% of these cases. Five-year survival was 15% and 10-year survival, 13% (Fig. 12.6). After treatment with radiotherapy alone, survival was better in patients with no distant metastases at the time of diagnosis, with a 5-year survival of 26% and a 20-year survival of 21%. Of the 303 deaths, 89% were from the thyroid carcinoma and 2% from treatment complications. The peculiar finding of a longer-than-expected survival in the anaplastic carcinomas in this survey was thought to be due to mistaken interpretation in the early years of the survey of same medullary carcinomas and lymphomas as anaplastic carcinomas. None of the 116 patients in Simpson's series who had a diagnosis of anaplastic carcinoma confirmed on later review by one pathologist, survived more than 3 years after diagnosis.

The authors of this report analyzed whether survival of the patients with papillary or follicular carcinoma differed over the years included in the survey. When the histologic type of carcinoma and the patient's age at time of diagnosis were included in the analysis, no difference was detected. There was a significant complication rate of therapy noted in this study, particularly in the patients with anaplastic carcinoma and the patients with differentiated carcinoma with more extensive local tumor infiltration. In the 790 patients treated with radiotherapy, there was a significant complication rate of 14% compared to a surgical complication rate of 15%, a radioiodine complication rate of 11%, and a chemotherapy complication rate of 39%. Of the 21 fatal complications among the 2214 patients, 6 were attributed to external radiotherapy as compared to 5 from surgery, 4 from chemotherapy, 2 from radioiodine therapy, and 1 each from combined radiotherapy and radioiodine, combined radiotherapy and chemotherapy, combined radiotherapy, chemotherapy and surgery, and combined radiotherapy and surgery.

In 1985 Tubiana et al.[10] reported their series of 682 patients with differentiated carcinoma

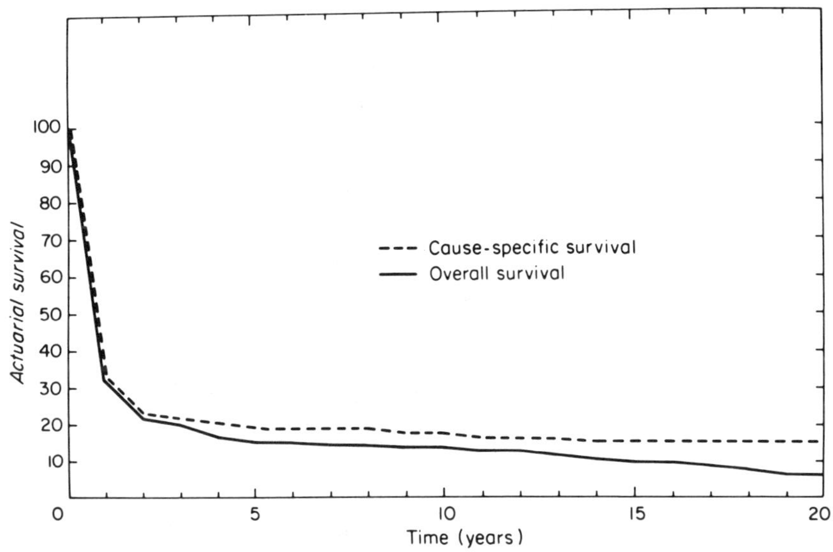

Figure 12.6. Anaplastic cancers: cause-specific and overall actuarial survival (370 patients). Reprinted, by permission, from Simpson, WJ, and McKinney, 1985(9).

of the thyroid. There was a follow-up of 8 to 40 years in this study. Cervical postoperative radiotherapy was given to 203 patients who were suspected of having tumor extension into neighboring tissues, or to patients in whom surgery was incomplete or impossible. From 1945 to 1950 radiotherapy was given by brachytherapy using a radium mold (48 patients), from 1950 to 1960 by conventional 200-kV x-rays (52 patients), and since 1960 by megavoltage (103 patients). Notable in this study was the finding that despite relatively high survival, at 20 years the excess mortality caused by the carcinoma was significant—17% for papillary carcinoma and 15% for follicular carcinoma. It was also noted that about 25% of first relapses occurred after 20 years of complete remission.

In a subsequent paper[11] the same group discussed their results treating 97 of these patients with external radiotherapy after inadequate surgical excision until 1976. They pointed out that there are three major reasons for controversy concerning the role of external radiotherapy in the treatment of thyroid carcinoma. The first is that the slow growth rate of differentiated thyroid carcinoma requires that, in order to adequately evaluate a therapy, follow-up time must be quite long. The second, as mentioned previously, is that not all reported series have adequate controls, and that there is a relative resistance of thyroid carcinoma to radiotherapy, thus requiring the use of doses over 50 Gy. Various centers have differed on the extent of surgery and the dose of radiotherapy required. The third reason for controversy is the failure of many reports to distinguish between prophylactic postoperative radiotherapy, postoperative radiotherapy after incomplete surgery, and radiotherapy for inoperable disease.

This study included 539 patients with differentiated (papillary or follicular) thyroid carcinoma confined to the neck at the time of initial treatment and who could be potentially followed-up for more than 8 years. One hundred eighty of these patients received external radiotherapy. In 66 patients the radiation was given postoperatively for prophylaxis after satisfactory tumor surgery. Another 97 patients were irradiated externally for what the surgeon described as "incomplete surgery." In 17 other patients there was no data concerning adequacy of surgery. In addition, 16 patients not initially radiated were treated for local recurrence of carcinoma with external radiotherapy. There were 23 inoperable patients, 17 of whom were given external radiotherapy.

Table 12.13. Relapse-free survival rate and overall survival rate of patients with differentiated thyroid cancers treated by surgery alone or combined with postoperative radiotherapy by radioiodine or external beam*

	Patients at risk	RFS (%)		Survival (%)	
		5 yr	15 yr	5 yr	15 yr
Surgery alone	275	81	64	94	81
Prophylactic Postop ^{131}I after surgery	61	67	44	93	75
Prophylactic Postop external RT ± ^{131}I	66	70	53	81	62
RT after incomplete surgery	97	58	39	78	57
Inoperable patients	23	55	7	60	14

* Incomplete surgery means macroscopically incomplete.
Postop: postoperative; RFS: relapse-free survival; RT: radiotherapy.
Reprinted, by permission, from Tubiana, M, Haddad, E, Schlumberger, M, et al, 1985(11).

Postoperative radiotherapy to the neck was also given to 35 of 115 patients in this series with medullary carcinoma. Surgery was incomplete in 15 patients with medullary carcinoma who had tracheal, blood vessel, or esophageal involvement. Completeness of surgery was equivocal in 8 other patients. Extensive lymph node involvement with rupture of the capsule was noted in 25 of the 35 patients. Radiotherapy was also administered to eight inoperable patients with medullary carcinoma.

The authors of this report carefully discussed the radiotherapy technique. They point out that a major problem is that the thyroid and draining cervical nodes curve around the vertebrae and the spinal cord, which is sensitive to radiation. They noted that two lymphatic chains must be included in the radiation field. One of these goes from the thyroid to the base of the skull behind the pharynx, the other extends to the mediastinum behind the sternoclavicular joints and the sternum. As with other reports, the technique of therapy varied depending on when the treatment was performed. Radium molds were used from 1943 to 1950. Conventional x-ray with a moderate dose of 25 to 30 Gy over 3 to 4 weeks and two or three fields applied was used until 1955. After 1956, cobalt units were used with an increase in the dosage to an average of 50 Gy in 25 fractions over 5 weeks and a boost of 5 to 10 Gy given to any palpable residual tumor. Usually a direct anterior field with lead blocks to protect the lungs and larynx was used. For radiation to the upper mediastinum, a posterior field was added, which avoided exposing the thoracic spinal cord to a dosage of more than 42 Gy. In more recent years external radiotherapy has been given using megavoltage x-ray and electron beams. For some papillary and follicular carcinomas, radiotherapy was directed only to the thyroid bed and immediately adjacent nodes either unilaterally or bilaterally using an opposing pair of lateral fields. The upper margin of the field was at the level of the hyoid bone and the lower margin directly above the sternal notch. For treatment of anaplastic carcinoma this group radiated the entire anterior half of the neck and the superior 5 cm of the mediastinum.

The group of patients treated prophylactically for papillary or follicular thyroid carcinoma was treated because of surgical findings of extensive nodal involvement, upper mediastinal involvement and neighboring muscle invasion, or after difficult surgery for secondary recurrence. There were also a few in this subgroup who were irradiated after "conservative surgery." Table 12.13 shows the data for total survival and relapse-free survival in the 66 patients who received prophylactic radiation. It is of note that these patients did less well than the subgroup treated with surgery alone. The authors of this report explain this by stating that in this group, radiation was being used for patients with a less favorable prognosis. Results for the 97 patients with incomplete surgery are given in Table 12.13 and Figures 12.7 and 12.8.

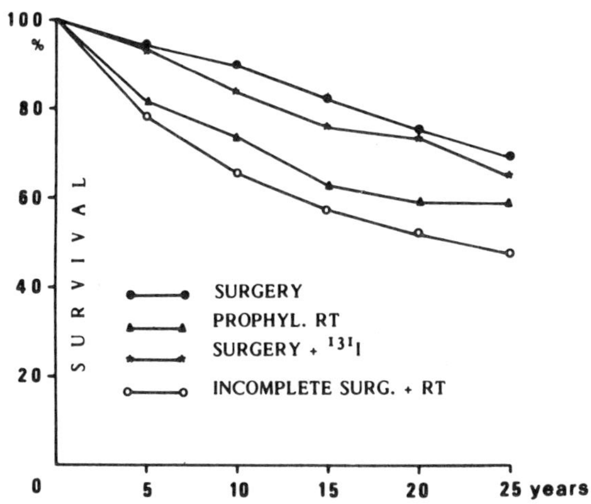

Figure 12.7. Overall survival in various subgroups of patients with differentiated thyroid cancers. Reprinted, by permission from Tubiana, M, Haddad, E, Schlumberger, M, et al., 1985(11).

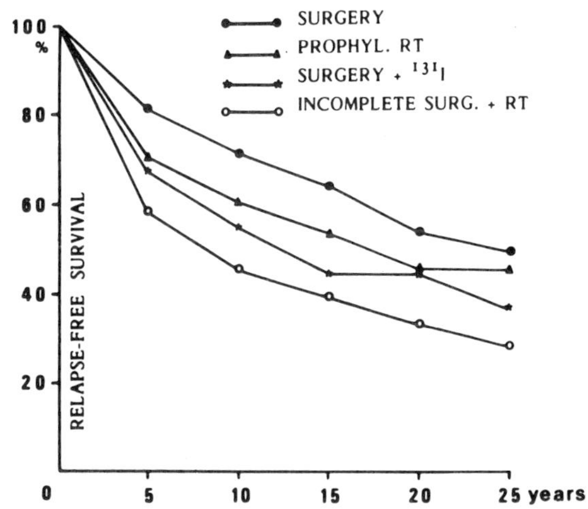

Figure 12.8. Relapse-free survival in various subgroups of patients with differentiated thyroid cancers: patients treated by surgery alone, patients treated by surgery plus 100 mCi of radioactive iodine for ablation of thyroid remnant, prophylactic irradiation after a satisfactory tumor excision, or irradiation after a macroscopically incomplete tumor excision. Reprinted, by permission, from Tubiana, M, Haddad, E, Schlumberger, M, et al., 1985(11).

In the patients treated for local recurrence there were 8 recurrences in the 66 patients who had complete surgery (12%) and 15 recurrences in those radiated after incomplete surgery (15%). No details were provided on the successfulness of surgery for 17 patients two of whom had recurrences. These figures must be compared to the 19% recurrence rate in the 51 of 267 patients treated with "complete surgery" alone, the 29% recurrence rate in 18 of 57 patients treated with dubious completeness of surgery, and the 1 recurrence among the 12 patients for whom surgical completeness was not described. Pooling the above subgroups shows that the local recurrence rate in patients without external radiotherapy and with varying completeness of surgery was 70 of 336 patients (21%), whereas the local recurrence rate in 180 who received external radiotherapy was 25 out of 180 (14%). This difference showed a favorable effect of external radiotherapy and was statistically significant ($p < .05$). It is even more significant that there were only 17 recurrences within the irradiated field ($p = .001$). There were only 5 recurrences within the radiated field noted in the 95 patients (5%) treated with higher doses (average 50 Gy vs. 28 Gy). There were also 5 recurrences outside the irradiated field for a total of 10 recurrences (10.5%). The difference in local recurrence between those treated with surgery alone or surgery followed by high-energy radiotherapy was highly significant ($p = .02$). The difference in recurrence within the irradiated field between the high-energy and conventional x-ray groups was significantly in favor of the former ($p = .04$). Table 12.14 displays the actuarial probabilities of local recurrence and demonstrates the efficacy of sufficient doses of external radiotherapy. The average interval in the irradiated group from initial treatment until local recurrence was 8.5 years. Surgery alone or surgery plus radioiodine resulted in an average delay of 6 years.

Seventeen of 23 inoperable patients with papillary or follicular carcinoma were treated by the Tubiana group with external radiotherapy: at 5 years of follow-up relapse-free survival was 55% and total survival was 60%. At ten years these figures decreased to 22% and 27% respectively.

There were 16 patients described by Tubiana et al. as having received external radiotherapy

Table 12.14. Actuarial probability of local recurrence in patients with differentiated thyroid cancers

	No. of patients at risk	Median follow-up (yr)		Actuarial probability of local recurrence at 5 yr	10 yr	15 yr	
Surgery ± radioiodine	336	16		13%	18%	22%	
Postoperative RT			$p<0.05$				$p<0.05$
Co or high energy	95	20		7%	10%	13%	
200 kV	48	29		5%	11%	18%	
Ra mold	37	33		3%	10%	17%	
Surgery alone	275	16		12%	18%	22%	NS
Surgery + radioiodine	61	17		17%	22%	26%	
Surgery ± radioiodine							
Satisfactory tumor excision	267	16		12%	16%	20%	NS
Dubious tumor excision	57	18		19%	31%	39%	

RT: radiotherapy; Co: cobalt; Ra: radium; NS: not significant.
Reprinted, by permission, from Tubiana, M, Haddad, E, Schlumberger, M, et al, 1985(11).

Table 12.15. Thyroid medullary cancer*

Treatment	Surgical excision: Incomplete	Dubious	Satisfactory	Tumor: Capsul effraction	Extension into walls	Nodes: Involvement	Capsul effraction
Surgery only (n = 57)							
N	3/46	10/46	33/46	10/41	9/43	23/57	16/57
%	6.5	21.7	71.7	24.4	20.9	40.3	28
Surgery + Postop RT (n = 35)							
N	15/32	8/32	9/32	12/26	10/23	29/35	25/35
%	46.9	25	28.1	46.2	43.5	82.8	71.4
χ^2		$p<0.001$		NS	$p=0.06$	$p<0.001$	$p<0.001$

*Characteristics of the patients with medullary carcinomas treated by surgery alone or followed by postoperative RT.
Capsul: capsular; Postop: postoperative; RT: radiotherapy.
Reprinted, by permission, from Tubiana, M, Haddad, E, Schlumberger, M, et al, 1985(11).

for a local recurrence. Eleven of these had incomplete surgery performed prior to treatment of the local recurrence with external radiotherapy. There was no further local recurrence in 9 of these patients. In 2 patients local recurrence was noted 2 and 3 years after external radiotherapy. Of five patients irradiated for inoperable local recurrence, 2 remained relapse-free after a follow-up of more than 20 years, and one patient each had a local relapse 1, 2, and 4 years after external radiotherapy. However, 6 of the 9 patients who had no further local recurrences died; in five patients death was caused by distant metastases.

In the 115 patients with medullary carcinoma of the thyroid reported by Tubiana et al. the relapse-free survival and total survival rates in the 35 patients receiving external radiotherapy was identical to the rates in the 80 patients treated with surgery alone. As shown in Table 12.15, the irradiated patients had a greater degree of disease involvement. In the 8 patients given external radiotherapy for inoperable medullary carcinoma, there was a complete remission in 1 patient, regression of more than 50% of the tumor in 2 patients and less than 50% of the tumor in 5 patients. Two of these patients were living in remission 4 and 6 years after radiotherapy. One was living with a liver metastasis and five had died of their carcinoma, surviving an average of three years after treatment. It was noted that before treatment, the calcitonin level was significantly higher in the patients who were subsequently treated with surgery plus external radiotherapy, implying that they had a greater tumor burden.

No data is presented in the Tubiana et al. report on external radiation for anaplastic carcinoma, but they state that the results were very poor and not improved by combining radiotherapy with chemotherapy.

There were four late complications among patients receiving a dosage of more than 60 Gy. These included a case of tracheal constriction necessitating tracheostomy, two cases of "brachial plexopathy," and a tracheal constriction in a reirradiated patient, again necessitating tracheostomy.

The authors note that the incidence of distant metastases in the patients treated with external radiotherapy documents their poor prognosis. The rate of incidence is similar in those receiving postoperative radioiodine (25%), and those treated with postoperative external radiotherapy with or without radioiodine (29%); by comparison, in the surgery-only group the incidence of distant metastases was 8.7%. This data was interpreted as demonstrating that those given some form of radiation had the greatest tumor bulk. External radiotherapy was noted to be much more effective in local control of thyroid carcinoma than radioactive iodine therapy. The authors attribute this to more even dose distribution from external radiotherapy as compared with the patchy ^{131}I dose distribution.[12] However, since there is no increase in local toxicity when radioiodine is given to patients treated with external radiotherapy, these authors recommend using a combination of these two radiation modalities in patients with poor prognosis in order to sterilize residual disease and more promptly detect local recurrence as well as distant metastatic disease.

In a subsequent report from France by Schlumberger, Tubiana et al.,[13] the authors describe their treatment of a large series of 283 patients followed for up to forty years with lung and bone metastases from papillary and follicular thyroid carcinoma. It should be noted that these patients represented a considerable proportion of the approximately 1200 patients with thyroid cancer reported in the authors' earlier paper. Surgery was performed in 86% of the patients and lymph node dissection in 46% of the patients before metastatic disease was found. Postoperative radiotherapy to the neck was administered to one third of this group and 100 mCi of ^{131}I was given to two fifths of the group. Fourteen percent of the patients were initially treated only with radiation because they had metastatic disease at presentation. All patients in this series were given thyroid medication postoperatively. Follow-up studies included chest radiography and yearly serum thyroxine (T_4) and thyroid-stimulating hormone (TSH) measurements, in addition to clinical examination. When patients had abnormal bone ^{131}I uptake or skeletal symptoms bone x-rays were done. After 1977 serum thyroglobulin was measured yearly with a limit of detectability of 2.5 ng/ml. Total body ^{131}I scanning was performed every year for 2 years and thereafter every 2 or 5 years thereafter. Prior to scanning T_4 was discontinued for 5 weeks. Triiodothyronine (T_3) was then given for 3 weeks and no thyroid medication was given for two weeks prior to scanning. Scanning was performed 72 hours after a dose of 1 to 2 mCi ^{131}I using an Ohio Nuclear 84 FD scanner capable of detecting uptake as low as 1 μCi. Patients with metastases were given 100 mCi of radioactive ^{131}I, and a total body scan was performed 5 days after treatment. T_4 therapy was then restarted. Follow-up scanning was done 3 to 6 months later; again ^{131}I treatment was given to demonstrated metastases. For ablation, 100 mCi was given to patients with abnormal bone or lung x-rays. In patients without detectable metastases after ablation another 100 mCi was administered 3 months after ablative therapy in order to search for metastases. The cumulative dose of ^{131}I in this large group ranged between 54 and 1500 mCi. Patients who had bone metastases visible on x-ray were administered external radiotherapy in a dose of 30 Gy (3000 rads) over 15 days, or 45 Gy over 28 days. It was administered with ^{131}I in the 92 patients whose metastases concentrated radioactive iodine, and by itself in those 18 patients in whom there was no metastatic concentration of ^{131}I. Of the patients with metastases to bone, 44 had surgery performed because of the existence or high risk of orthopedic or neurologic complications. Complete response of bone metastases was defined as absence of ^{131}I uptake and clinical symptomatology for more than 1 year, as well as recalcification of the abnormalities seen on x-ray. Eighty-one patients had bone metastases only and 61 patients had pulmonary metastases in addition to bone metastases. Symptoms were present in 84% of these 142 patients. A single bone metastasis was noted in 29% of patients; 6% of patients had no abnormality on x-ray. The ^{131}I scan revealed metastases in two thirds of the patients with metastases. Of the 79 patients who demonstrated a complete response, 14 had metastatic disease to bone. Only 2 of these were treated with external radiotherapy in addition to ^{131}I. The others were treated with ^{131}I alone. Unfortunately there is no data included in this report concerning incomplete, yet significant responses of bone metastases to external radiotherapy.

Medullary Carcinoma

Data that further substantiates the effectiveness of external radiotherapy in the management of medullary carcinoma of the thyroid is found in a series of studies of 5 patients by Steinfeld[14] and a series of studies of 45 patients by Simpson et al.[15] Steinfeld described 5 patients treated with external radiotherapy after the performance of total thyroidectomy (1 case), hemithyoidectomy (2 cases), and tumor biopsy alone (2 cases). The 2 patients who were treated by tumor biopsy had bulky cervical nodes. One patient treated with a low dose of 2800 rads after total thyroidectomy had locally recurrent disease after one year and underwent repeat treatment with 3000 rads, which provided disease control until the patient's death 4 years later. The four other patients received doses of 4000 to 6000 rads. One patient had locally recurrent disease three years later and one had local control for three years until his death. In the two patients whose only surgical procedure was biopsy, the tumor mass decreased in size. In one case the patient was still alive 6 years later, whereas the other patient died of metastatic disease 1 year later. In the Simpson series of medullary carcinoma patients there were 14 treated with external radiotherapy postoperatively. Eleven had microscopic disease and 3 had no evidence of residual disease. Six of the 20 patients (3%) showed complete tumor regression without recurrence and 9 of the 20 (45%) partially regressed. Three of six patients with complete disease regression died from distant metastatic disease. Because chemotherapy achieved only a partial response in 9 patients with medullary carinoma, Simpson et al. recommended the combination of chemotherapy and radiotherapy in treating unresectable medullary carcinoma.

Anaplastic Carcinoma

Because of the poor response of anaplastic carcinoma of the thyroid to external radiotherapy, 28 patients with anaplastic carcinoma were treated at the Princess Margaret Hospital in Toronto with hyperfractionation radiotherapy as described by Simpson.[16] The results obtained with this technique were compared to a standard fractionation technique of 3500 to 6000 rads administered over 3 to 6 weeks. One group of 14 patients received a large number of small doses of radiotherapy: 11 received 100 rads four times a day for a total of 3600 rads, and 3 received 100 rads only once a day. A second group of 14 patients received doses varying from 1200 rads given in three doses of 400 rads each over 1 to 2 weeks, to as much as 2400 rads given in three 800-rad dose treatments over 3 weeks. Of the 58 patients treated with standard fractionation procedures, 20 had complete tumor regression and 17 partial tumor regression. Among those who had no regression, or only partial regression, there were no patients who survived 5 years. Seven patients with complete regression survived 5 to 20 years. None of the patients treated with the 3 treatment regime had a complete tumor regression, and all died of the thyroid cancer within 9 months. In the group receiving hyperfractionation therapy, 6 patients had a complete regression of tumor, 7 showed a partial regression, and only 1 patient had no response. Of the 11 patients who received 100 rads four times a day, three were alive and free of disease at $6\frac{1}{2}$, 8, and 15 months respectively. The fourth patient died of treatment complications but was free of tumor at 22 months. All 7 who achieved only a partial regression died of treatment complications or tumor, all but one within $9\frac{1}{2}$ months. One patient died 16 months after treatment of complications from the treatment. A modified mantle procedure including the entire neck and the superior half of the mediastinum was recommended by Simpson. Complications of radiation therapy were similar in the groups treated with standard therapy and with hyperfractionation therapy. Although 2 of the 4 deaths from treatment complications were attributed to complications of concomitant Adriamycin therapy, the combined use of external radiation and Adriamycin resulted in complete regression in 4 of 12 patients, and partial regression in 1 patient.

At least five other groups have subsequently reported more favorable results using multimodal therapy for anaplastic thyroid carcinoma. Aldinger et al.[17] reported the experience of MD Anderson Hospital (Houston, Texas) and Tumor Institute in the treatment of 84 patients with anaplastic carcinoma. Prior to 1965, treatment was determined by the extent of disease as initially noted; subsequent results were poor. If at surgery there was thought to be no residual tumor, no further treatment was given. When the tumor was thought to be inoperable, external irradiation either with or without chemotherapy was given. A dose of 6000 rads of external radiotherapy was directed to the neck, bilateral supraclavicular areas, and the mediastinum. After 1965 patients with neck disease were only given combination therapy with surgical removal of as much tumor as possible, 6000 rads external radiation to the above-described areas, and actinomycin D therapy. In the presence of distant metastatic disease, chemotherapy with or without radiotherapy was given. The best results were obtained in those given triple combination therapy. However, of the 84 patients only 6 survived, and only 6 survived 5 years (7.1%). The mean survival was 6.2 months from tissue diagnosis and 11.8 months from the commencement of symptoms. Analysis of the 11 patients who survived at least 12 months revealed that in 8 patients most of the tumor mass was, in fact, differentiated thyroid carcinoma with only small areas of anaplastic transition. Indeed, 89.2% of the 74 cases in which there was sufficient tissue for careful examination revealed evidence of differentiated thyroid carcinoma.

Tennvall et al.[18] reported from Lund on treatment of 13 anaplastic carcinoma patients with combined therapy. Eight patients were treated with external radiation and chemotherapy, and 5 with this combination plus debulking surgery. The field that was radiated included the thyroid and tumor, bilateral cervical nodes up to the mastoid tip, supraclavicular nodes, and upper mediastinal nodes. The dose was 48 Gy administered in 20 fractions over 4 weeks. Chemotherapy included 0.5-gm 5-flurouracil (5-FU) by infusion before radiation fractions 1,3,5,7 and 9 and 0.2-gm Cytoxan intravenously on fractional radiation days 1 to 10. Of the 8 patients treated without surgery, 1 was alive without obvious tumor 59 months after treatment. The others died after 1 to 23 months, with a median of 4 months. Of the 5 patients treated with the addition of debulking surgery, 2 whose surgery was not truly radical died within 4 months. The other three died one at 5 months without tumor; two of these three, one who died at 8 months and one who died at 23 months, suffered from distant metastatic disease, but not from local recurrences. Although using a combination of the three modalities appeared to be move effective, the results were still poor.

Casterline et al.[19] reported a single case of a patient with anaplastic carcinoma from Walter Reed Hospital (Washington, D.C.) treated with triple modality therapy consisting of chemotherapy with Actinomycin-D and external radiation given through two ports with 6000 rads administered over 40 days, with the addition of BCG immunotherapy. This patient was free of disease 48 months after therapy.

Table 12.16. Side effects of radiation treatment of thyroid cancer

Acute Complications (subsides in 2 to 4 weeks after therapy completion)
Skin erythema (moderate): latter part of therapy
More severe skin reaction with dry desquamation (more rarely moist): when high proportion of dose is delivered to superficial tissues
Symptomatic radiation laryngitis: mucous pooling and laryngeal edema
Dysphagia: may require dietary modification and analgesia (hospitalization rarely required)
Superimposed bacterial or fungal infection
Delayed Complications (mild and infrequent)
Mild hypopigmentation or hyperpigmentation for several months following therapy
Skin atrophy with depigmentation, telangiectasia, and loss of subcutaneous fat (only with techniques depositing full dose in skin and subcutaneous tissues)
Edema of subcutaneous and soft tissues (only when extensive prior neck surgery causes impaired lymphatic drainage)
Permanent changes in tracheal, esophageal, or layngeal function: uncommon
Spinal cord injury: not evident until 6 to 36 months later and irreversible (may be avoided with proper dose and volume considerations)

In 1983 Kim and Leeper[20] described their combination of Adriamycin and external radiation therapy in the treatment of 8 patients at Memorial Hospital in New York. Low-dose Adriamycin (10 mg/m^2) was given with 200 rads external radiotherapy 5 times a week for $5\frac{1}{2}$ weeks. Radiation was given in the form of a combination of high energy photon beams and electron beams. Seven out of eight patients who were treated in this fashion achieved a complete tumor regression and, at the time of this report, had survived from 10 months to 3 years.

Werner et al.[21] reported in 1984 from Sweden on 19 patients with anaplastic thyroid carcinoma treated with a combination of preoperative and postoperative hyperfractionated radiotherapy combined with chemotherapy. All of these patients had rapidly growing tumors that were large and bulky, invading tissues adjacent to the thyroid gland. When these tumors were examined by needle biopsy and subsequent histologic examination there was no evidence of any differentiated thyroid carcinoma component. Radiotherapy preoperatively was administered in a dose of 30 Gy in 3 weeks with ^{60}Co or 6-MV x-rays. Two opposing fields were used. Radical thyroidectomy was done 2 to 3 weeks later if possible. Postoperatively, 15-Gy radiation dose was administered with lead shielding used for spinal cord protection. Chemotherapy was given with three drugs combined: bleomycin 5 mg intramuscularly 1 to 2 hours before each radiotherapy fraction, Cytoxan 200 mg intravenously daily, and 5-FU 500 mg intravenously before every other radiotherapy fraction. Additional chemotherapy with Cytoxan and 5-FU was given every other month afterwards for at most 5 courses. Patients with advanced disease had a median survival of 7 months from diagnosis while those with less advanced disease survived an average of 12 months. Those patients who died succumbed to metastatic disease. In this group treatment was well tolerated.

In summary, there is a role for external radiotherapy in thyroid carcinoma of all histologic types. One must balance the rewards against the risks or side effects of external radiotherapy to the thyroid; this has been well summarized by Simpson[22] (Table 12.16). Even with combined modality therapy and hyperfractionation, the results of treating anaplastic carcinoma are poor; this approach requires further careful study. In view of the terrible prognosis, postoperative radiotherapy with approximately 5000 rads to the thyroid or mantle should be given in anaplastic carcinoma. As these tumors rarely concentrate ^{131}I, external radiotherapy should be the treatment of choice in inoperable anaplastic carcinoma of the thyroid. Although the results of external radiotherapy in medullary carcinoma are somewhat questionable, the absence of a better alternative justifies its use in stage III medullary carcinoma, in patients with recurrent tumor postoperatively, and even in nonsurgical candidates with increasing serum calcitonin levels. Radiotherapy may be used effectively for symptomatic relief for isolated metastasis of medullary carcinoma. According to the literature, in all these instances usual doses are approximately 5000 to 6000 rads. More controversial is the indication for the use of external radiotherapy in the treatment of papillary and follicular carcinomas of the thyroid. To maximize survival and lessen morbidity from these tumors postoperatively, radioactive iodine therapy should be the initial approach. In patients over the age of 45 with invasive or possible residual disease, radioactive iodine should be followed by 5000 rads external radiotherapy to the thyroid bed. In patients under the age of 45 with invasive disease, external radiotherapy may be considered but its use is less certainly necessitated. In patients of any age with recurrent papillary or follicular carcinoma in the thyroid bed 5000 rads external radiotherapy to the thyroid bed is appropriate. External radiotherapy treatment of isolated bone lesions in papillary and follicular carcinoma of the thyroid is recommended after radioactive iodine therapy and is mandated in cases in which metastatic lesions do not concentrate iodine. It is to be hoped that further prospective study of combined modality therapy will improve the risk/benefit ratio of the use of external radiotherapy in the treatment of thyroid carcinoma.

References

1. Windeyer B. Cancer of the thyroid and radiotherapy. Br J Radiol 1954;27:537–552.
2. Frazell E, Foote Jr. F. Papillary cancer of the thyroid: A review of 25 years of experience. Cancer 1958; 11:895–922.
3. Sheline GE, Galante M, Lindsay S. Radiation Therapy in the control of persistent thyroid cancer. Am J Radiol 1966;97:923–930.
4. Simpson WJ, Carruthers JS. The role of external radiation in the management of papillary and follicular thyroid cancer. Am J Surg 1978;136:457–460.
5. Chung CT, Sagerman RH, Ryoo MC, King GA, Yu WS, Dalai PS, Emmanuel IG. External irradiation for malignant thyroid tumors. Radiology 1980;136:753–756.
6. Fuller LM. The role and techniques of external irradiation therapy in the treatment of carcinoma of the thyroid. In: Fletcher GH, ed. Textbook of Radiotherapy. 2nd ed. Philadelphia: Lea & Febiger; 1973:311–319.
7. Mazzaferri EL, Young RL. Papillary thyroid carcinoma: a 10 year follow-up report of the impact of therapy in 576 patients. Am J Med 1981;70:511–518.
8. Ampil, FL. Postoperative external irradiation in thyroid carcinoma; a clinical experience of 20 treated patients and literature radiotherapy review. J Surg Oncol 1985;30:83–90.
9. Simpson WJ, McKinney SE. Canadian survey of thyroid cancer. Can Med Assoc J 1985;132:925–931.
10. Tubiana M, Schlumberger M, Rougier P et al. Long-term results and prognostic factors in patients with differentiated thyroid carcinoma. Cancer 1985;55:794–804.
11. Tubiana M, Haddad E, Schlumberger M et al. External radiotherapy in thyroid cancers. Cancer 1985; 55:2062–2071.
12. Scott JS, Halnan KE, Shimmins J, Kostaki P, MacKenzie H. Measurement of dose to thyroid carcinoma metastases from radioiodine therapy. Br J Radiol 1970;43:256–62.
13. Schlumberger M, Tubiana M, De Vathaire F et al. Long-term results of treatment of 283 patients with lung and bone metastases from differentiated thyroid carcinoma. J Clin Endocrinol Metab 1986;63:960–967.
14. Steinfeld AD. The role of radiation therapy in medullary carcinoma of the thyroid. Radiology 1977;123: 745–746.
15. Simpson WJ, Palmer JA, Rosen IB, Mustard RA. Management of medullary carcinoma of the thyroid. Am J Surg 1982;144:420–422.
16. Simpson WJ. Anaplastic thyroid carcinoma: a new approach. Canad J Surg 1980;23:25–27.
17. Aldinger KA, Samaan NA, Ibanez M, Hill, Jr. CS. Anaplastic carcinoma of the thyroid: a review of 84 cases of spindle and giant cell carcinoma of the thyroid. Cancer 1978;41:2267–2275.
18. Tennvall J, Andersson T, Aspegren K et al. Undifferentiated giant and spindle cell carcinoma of the thyroid: report on two combined treatment modalities. Acta Radiol Oncol 1979;18:408–416.
19. Casterline PF, Jaques DA, Blom H, Wartofsky L. Anaplastic giant and spindle-cell carcinoma of the thyroid: a different therapeutic approach. Cancer 1980;45:1689–1692.
20. Kim JH, Leeper, RD. Combination adriamycin and radiation therapy for locally advanced carcinoma of the thyroid gland. Int J Radiat Oncol Biol Phys 1983;9:565–567.
21. Werner B, Abele J, Alveryd MD et al. Multimodal therapy in anaplastic giant cell thyroid carcinoma. World J. Surg 1984;8:64–70.
22. Simon B, Sutcliffe W, Simpson JK, Rosen IB. The place of external radiation therapy for differentiated and undifferentiated thyroid carcinoma. In: Roher HD, Clark OH, eds. Thyroid tumors. Basel: Karger; 1988:147–162.

13

Chemotherapy of Advanced Thyroid Cancer

LI-TEH WU and STEVEN D. AVERBUCH

Principles of Chemotherapy

Biological Basis for Chemotherapy

The biological targets for most chemotherapeutic agents are cellular macromolecules; the drugs usually cause cell death by non-selectively inhibiting DNA, RNA, and/or protein synthesis to disrupt vital cellular function. Selective activity of chemotherapy against malignant cells primarily results from differences in cellular kinetics and lower efficiency of DNA repair in transformed cells as compared with normal cells. Thus, most tumors that are susceptible to chemotherapy tend to be undifferentiated, proliferative tumors that are in rapid cell cycle and that have relatively ineffective DNA repair capacity.[1] Thyroid cancers such as well-differentiated thyroid carcinoma and medullary thyroid carcinoma are slow growing, differentiated tumors that do not exhibit these characteristics and are less susceptible to chemotherapy. Even giant and spindle cell anaplastic carcinoma, which are undifferentiated and characterized by aggressive growth, are usually refractory to chemotherapy. Several hypotheses for the biologic basis of intrinsic resistance of certain tumors to chemotherapy have been suggested[2,3] but none have been substantiated, nor have any been specifically associated with thyroid cancer. General approaches to overcoming tumor resistance in settings where chemotherapy is indicated include the use of combinations of effective agents and the use of dose-intensive regimens.[2,4,5]

Clinical Goals for Chemotherapy

The chemotherapist's approach to the patient with advanced cancer is principally determined by establishing one of three therapeutic goals for that individual: (1) cure, (2) non-curative prolongation of survival, or (3) palliation. The successful achievement of the first two goals requires that the patient's malignancy be responsive (including having the potential for complete remission) to available agents that can be used without causing intolerable toxicity. As discussed above, thyroid cancer is considered to be poorly responsive to cytotoxic chemotherapy. Its use in advanced thyroid cancer has been reserved for palliation of patients with progressive disease that is refractory to other treatment modalities such as surgery, external radiation, and ablative ^{131}I. Largely due to an insufficient number of patients and a lack of well-designed prospective clinical trials, there is very little data from which one can determine the true efficacy of chemotherapy in thyroid cancer. This difficulty is compounded by the fact that many reports of chemotherapy in thyroid cancer do not clearly delineate criteria for tumor response. Furthermore, in the past, many articles did not distinguish histologic subtypes of thyroid cancer or stage of disease, which lead to inconsistent results.[6,7] For example, small cell thyroid cancer was considered anaplastic cancer because of its undifferentiated histology, rapidly progressive course, and failure to be cured by surgery. Today this cell type would be correctly classified as either lymphoma, which is much more sensitive to both radiation and chemotherapy, or medullary thyroid carcinoma, which has a much more indolent course than true anaplastic giant and spindle cell carcinoma.[8,9,10] In this chapter, chemotherapy in thyroid cancer will be reviewed by considering each histologic type separately.

Chemotherapy of Specific Types of Advanced Thyroid Cancer

Well-differentiated Thyroid Cancer

The three histologic subtypes of well-differentiated thyroid cancer—papillary, follicular, and Hürthle cell carcinoma—have an excellent prognosis, with overall cancer mortality of less than 5% at 10 years.[11,12] The primary tumor is usually treated by thyroidectomy. Incompletely resected tumor, local recurrence, or distant metastases are treated with ablative ^{131}I if the tumor concentrates iodine. External radiation may have a limited role in treating tumors that fail to concentrate ^{131}I. For advanced tumors, the major causes of death include respiratory failure from pulmonary metastases, airway obstruction or vascular catastrophe from local tumor invasion, and neurologic complications from brain and spinal cord involvement. In the Mayo Clinic series the mean time to death after initial surgery in patients who died of this disease is 8.5 years, and the mean time to death from the diagnosis of metastasis is 4.2 years.[13] The rarity of advanced well-differentiated thyroid cancer and its relatively indolent natural history has precluded an adequate evaluation of the use of chemotherapy to combat it.

Among single agents, the anthracycline antibiotic doxorubicin is the most extensively studied. Phase II clinical trials of doxorubicin in the early 1970s established this drug as the most active single drug against thyroid cancer.[14,15,16,17] In a summary of the studies conducted at the M.D. Anderson Hospital (Houston, Texas), Gottlieb et al.[18] reported partial responses in 7 patients (32%) and stable disease in 9 patients (41%) out of 22 patients treated with doxorubicin alone. All responding patients had received more than 60 mg/m^2 in each treatment cycle; and the above authors suggested the possibility of a clinical dose response to doxorubicin. In other studies, doxorubicin was responsible for partial remissions in 3 (27%) of 11 patients[16] and in 5 (31%) of 16 patients.[19] In a phase II clinical study the investigational anthracycline analog, aclarubicin, was shown to induce 1 complete remission and 2 partial remissions (complete + partial = 27%) in 11 treated patients[20] and mitoxantrone only produced one brief partial remission among 16 evaluable patients.[21] Other chemotherapeutic agents have not been prospectively studied in advanced well-differentiated thyroid cancer, although scattered anecdotal responses to cisplatin,[22] bleomycin,[23] and semustine[18] have been reported.

Chemotherapeutic agents used in several combinations, most of which include doxorubicin, have been utilized for the treatment of well-differentiated thyroid cancer. The combination of doxorubicin and cisplatin, tested in one arm of a randomized, parallel group study conducted by the Eastern Cooperative Oncology Group (ECOG), induced 2 complete remissions and 1 partial remission (16%) among 19 patients.[19] Using the same combination, only 1 (14%) of 7 patients achieved a partial remission in a Southeastern Cancer Study Group (SECSG) trial.[24] No meaningful responses were observed in 8 patients treated with a combination of doxorubicin, cisplatin, and vindesine as reported by Scherübl et al.[25] Sokal et al. reported 3 (50%) partial remissions in 6 patients treated with doxorubicin, bleomycin, and vincristine,[26] and Hoskin reported 3 (38%) responses in 8 patients treated with the same regimen[22]; however, the same combination with the addition of melphalan accounted for only 1 (20%) partial response in 5 patients in another study.[27]

Locally advanced, unresectable differentiated thyroid cancer is usually refractory to external radiation. In a study of 22 patients, most of whom had received previous treatment with ^{131}I, complete remissions were observed in 20 (91%) following weekly low dose doxorubicin (10 mg/m^2) combined with daily standard external radiation.[28] In these remarkable cases reported by Kim and Leeper, only 5 patients had local recurrences after 2 years. Independent confirmation of their innovative approach has not been published. Nonetheless, since doxorubicin is known to act synergistically with radiation,[2] it is likely that the radiosensitizing property of doxorubicin accounted for this highly positive clinical outcome. Because of the potential for synergistic toxicity in more extensive disease, this combined-modality approach can be utilized only in selective cases of discrete, locally advanced disease.

In summary, although rare complete responses to chemotherapy alone have been reported, there is no evidence that chemotherapy provides any survival benefit or that any combination chemotherapy is more effective than doxorubicin alone used at sufficiently high doses. In view of the indolent course of the disease and the lack of effective chemotherapy, we believe that patients with ^{131}I-refractory metastatic or locally recurrent well-differentiated thyroid cancer should not be treated unless they have symptoms, potentially serious complications, or a rapidly increased tempo of tumor progression. We suggest that outside of investigational trials, doxorubicin be used alone in this setting. In the appropriate patient with locally advanced tumors, the combination of weekly low-dose doxorubicin and daily standard fractionated radiation therapy should be considered.

Anaplastic Thyroid Cancer

Unlike well-differentiated carcinoma, giant and spindle cell anaplastic thyroid carcinoma is one of the most aggressive human malignancies, with a median survival of 4 to 6 months and a 5-year survival of less than 10% in patients treated with surgery alone or with surgery combined with radiation.[29,30,31] The major causes of death include airway obstruction or vascular catastrophe from local tumor progression, or complications of distant metastases.[32] Anaplastic thyroid cancer does not concentrate ^{131}I and its response to external radiation therapy is poor. Patients with stage I disease (disease confined to the thyroid gland) or patients with small foci of anaplastic elements in a well differentiated carcinoma, may have a better outcome following chemotherapy, but patients with a rapidly growing mass with small foci of anaplastic elements do as poorly as patients having pure giant and spindle cell cancer.[33,34]

As for well-differentiated thyroid cancer, doxorubicin is the most active single agent against anaplastic disease. In the studies mentioned previously, Gottlieb et al. reported partial remissions in 4 (29%) of 14 patients[18] and O'Bryan reported partial remissions in 2 (40%) of 5 patients treated with doxorubicin alone.[16] In contrast, only 1 (5%) of 21 patients in the ECOG's randomized trial[19] and none of the 3 patients treated by Schoumacher[35] using doxorubicin alone responded to this agent. Other single agents that, according to anecdotal reports, demonstrate activity include bleomycin,[23] cisplatin[36] and aclarubicin.[20]

In the ECOG randomized study,[19] the combination of doxorubicin and cisplatin produced 3 complete remissions and 3 partial remissions (complete + partial = 33%), but only 1 (14%) of 7 patients had a response to the same combination in the SECSG study.[24] Other doxorubicin-containing combination regimens that also included bleomycin and vincristine were shown to have high activity (60–80%) in two reports of 5 patients each.[26,27] Interpreting these results are difficult because of the small sample size and because, in both studies, the histology of the anaplastic cancers was not specified. One refractory giant cell carcinoma was reported to respond to the combination of 5-fluorouracil, methotrexate, vincristine, thiotepa, and prednisone.[37]

Although the data is scanty and it is possible that thyroid lymphoma may have been diagnosed as anaplastic carcinoma, the occurrence of 3 complete remissions in the ECOG trial leads us to suggest that the combination of doxorubicin and cisplatin should be considered for metastatic disease outside of investigational clinical trials.

Combined modality therapy, employing surgery, radiation, and chemotherapy in various schemas has been used in the hope of achieving improved local control and reduction in distant metastases from anaplastic thyroid carcinoma . Occasionally, there has been a suggestion of improved local control of disease in selected patients. Six patients at the M.D. Anderson Hospital in Houston underwent resection of their thyroid tumor followed immediately by external radiation and actinomycin D, which was continued after treatment with radiation was completed.[34] Three patients (50%) with gross total resection achieved local control and were free of distant metastases for more than 5 years. The other three patients with palpable tumor at the time of radiation had either distant metastatic disease or rapid local recurrence after completion of treatment. Another patient has been disease-free for 4 years after similar combined-modality treatment plus 1 year of methanol extractable residue of BCG (MER).[38] However, when 8 more patients were treated at the same institution using the same approach, none of them achieved long term survival.[33] In another report, 2 of the 3 patients who survived more than one year were treated with chemotherapy that included doxorubicin and radiation after surgery.[39] Durie et al. treated 5 patients with small cell or clear cell undifferentiated thyroid carcinoma with surgery, ^{131}I, and chemotherapy consisting of doxorubicin, phenylalanine mustard, vincristine, and bleomycin for 8 to 10 cycles.[40] Four (80%) of the patients had complete remissions and one patient had a partial remission; yielding an overall response rate of 100%. However, these undifferentiated carcinomas were not typical anaplastic giant or spindle cell carcinoma because they had significant ^{131}I uptake. Two additional patients with spindle cell carcinoma and massive local disease were treated with the same combined modality approach; a partial remission was observed in one patient but the other had no response.[40] In a retrospective analysis of 121 patients with anaplastic thyroid cancer, the mean survival was 7.2 months.[31] Ten of the 12 long-term surviving patients had received radiation and chemotherapy postoperatively, but a univariate analysis failed to show that combined modality therapy had any effect on survival.[31]

The use of hyperfractionated radiation therapy[41] was extended by Kim and Leeper, who combined hyperfractionated radiation therapy and weekly low-dose doxorubicin in 19 patients with anaplastic giant and spindle cell carcinoma who had undergone incomplete resection or biopsy only.[28] The radiation was delivered at a fractional dose of 160 cGy twice a day, three days a week, for a total tumor dose of 5760 cGy in 40 days. The doxorubicin dose was 10 mg/m^2 per week in contrast to the standard dose of 60 mg/m^2 every 3 weeks. Sixteen patients achieved local control, and although only 3 patients had local recurrence, most of them died of distant metastasis. Four patients survived more than 1 year, and the median survival for all 19 patients was 1 year, which is superior to the rates in most published series.

Because surgery and radiation can damage blood supply to residual tumor in the neck and thereby impair delivery of drug to tumor, inductive chemotherapy, administered before surgery or radiation, has the potential for more effective tumor reduction and improved resectability.[2] In addition, tumor shrinkage by inductive chemotherapy has the potential advantage of improving tumor response to radiation by reducing the radioresistant hypoxic fraction. Improved resectability and local control by inductive chemotherapy has been demonstrated in bladder cancer,[42] head and neck cancer,[43] locally advanced breast cancer,[44] and osteosarcoma.[45]

Using inductive chemotherapy with doxorubicin, bleomycin, and cisplatin, Spanos et al.[46] reported that an inoperable giant cell carcinoma of the thyroid was rendered resectable and long-term local control was obtained in a single patient. Tallroth et al. reported 9 cases treated with standard fractionated radiation and concurrent bleomycin, cyclophosphamide, and 5-fluorouracil (BCF).[32] Most of these patients had local recurrence or distant metastases; however, the only long-term survivor was the one patient who underwent surgery at the peak of a remission resulting from combined chemotherapy and radiation therapy. Subsequently, 25 patients were treated with hyperfractionated radiation plus BCF chemotherapy followed by surgery and additional chemotherapy in combination with radiation therapy. Fifteen (75%) of 20 evaluable patients had objective responses to the combined inductive chemotherapy and radiation: 50% of the patients achieved local control.[32] Three patients were disease-free for more than 3 years. Using hyperfractionated radiotherapy, doxorubicin, and debulking surgery in 16 patients, three patients achieved disease-free survival for 10, 30, and 30 months respectively.[47] Although these results are disappointing, they indicate a trend toward higher survival rates and improved local tumor control, thus supporting the use of this combined modality approach.

No randomized study has been conducted to compare different treatment approaches for localized disease in anaplastic thyroid carcinoma. However, from the series reviewed here the following lessons may be learned by examining the few cases in which patients had complete remissions and long-term survival. If feasible, complete resection should be attempted in all cases, followed by adjuvant radiation and using doxorubicin-containing chemotherapy. For unresectable disease, inductive doxorubicin-containing chemotherapy and radiation should be considered followed by surgery if complete resection is feasible. If complete surgical extirpation is achieved, the further use of adjuvant radiation and chemotherapy may be considered. For disease that remains unresectable or that is incompletely resected, the combination of weekly low-dose doxorubicin and hyperfractionated radiation therapy as applied by Kim and Leeper[28] is probably the preferred regimen.

Medullary Thyroid Carcinoma

For the management of medullary thyroid carcinoma (MTC) it is important to determine if the disease is sporadic (80% of patients), or if it is associated with one of several familial endocrine syndromes (20% of patients).[48,49] For all patients with MTC the 10-year survival following surgical resection is approximately 65%. However, patients with familial multiple endocrine neoplasia (MEN)-2b tend to have early metastasis[50] and poor prognosis, while the more common cases of patients with MEN-2a have a much less aggressive course; less than 10% of these patients will die from their thyroid cancer.[49] The median survival for all patients presenting with distant metastases is approximately 3 years.[48] Since MTC is a slow growing tumor and effective chemotherapy has not yet been established, it is appropriate to consider other prognostic factors when deciding if chemotherapy is indicated. For example, tumors that have poor immunocytochemical staining for calcitonin tend to have a more aggressive course.[51,52] Although the serum calcitonin level correlates with the extent of disease, it is not helpful in identifying patients with a poorer prognosis. Instead, high serum carcinoembryonic antigen (CEA), especially a rapidly rising level, is more predictive of a rapid disease course.[53]

Gottlieb et al., reported 3 (50%) partial remissions and resolution of disease-related diarrhea in 6 patients following treatment with doxorubicin.[18] Taken together, additional results reported by others have demonstrated 14 (30%) partial remissions in 46 patients with MTC treated with doxorubicin as a single agent.[19,54–56]

MTC is a tumor of the diffuse neuroendocrine (APUD) system.[57] Therefore a number of single agent and combination chemotherapy treatments that show activity in other "APUD-omas" have been used in advanced MTC. The combination of streptozotocin and doxorubicin, a regimen that shows activity in pancreatic islet cell tumor, did not show activity in a small trial of patients.[58,59] Dacarbazine,[60] 5-fluorouracil,[6] etoposide,[22,61] 5-fluorouracil and dacarbazine,[62] and doxorubicin and cisplatin[63] have all demonstrated limited activity in studies or anecdotal reports.[19,24] The recent report describing the use of the combination of 5-fluorouracil and dacarbazine for MTC is particularly promising as these agents are active against other APUD tumors[62]; however, further experience with this combination is required before its activity can be determined. We have treated a large number of patients with malignant pheochromocytoma and a smaller number of patients with other APUD-omas at the Mount Sinai Medical Center in New York City using a combination of cyclophosphamide, vincristine, and dacarbazine.[64,65] One of two patients with MTC had a partial response for 14 months with complete resolution of pulmonary metastases, improvement of bone pain, and markedly reduced serum calcitonin and CEA. The other patient had stable disease for more than 17 months. Multiinstitutional phase II studies of this combination chemotherapy regimen for patients with metastatic MTC and other neuroendocrine tumors may be warranted.

Biological response modifiers, such as somatostatin analog and alpha interferon, have been shown to be effective with various neuroendocrine tumors, especially pancreatic islet cell and carcinoid tumors in reducing circulating hormones, halting progression, and occasionally reducing tumor size.[66,67] These agents have been shown to prolong survival and ameliorate symptoms due to hormonal excess. It is not clear whether short term administration of the somatostatin or its analog octreotide acetate reduces circulating calcitoninin in patients with MTC.[66,68] Long term subcutaneous injection of octreotide in 18 patients with MTC did reduce serum calcitonin in 8 of them, but CEA levels did not change.[68] Flushing and diarrhea improved in some patients and several of them reportedly had objective tumor response. Continuous subcutomeous delivery of high doses (up to 2.0 mg/day) of Octreotide acetate produced calcitonin and CEA responses in three patients with MTC.[69] Additional clinical studies are required to determine the role for somatostatin analog and, in view of the success of alpha-interferon on islet cell and carcinoid tumors, there may be a rationale for investigating the activity of this agent in patients with metastatic MTC as well.

Thyroid Lymphoma

As discussed in Chapter 10, thyroid lymphomas are rare, accounting for 5% of thyroid cancer, and most thyroid lymphomas are histologically classified as diffuse large cell, non-Hodgkin's lymphoma. Other histologic subtypes occur less frequently; a small number of cases of Hodgkin's disease and plasmacytoma of the thyroid have been reported.[9,70,71] Over 90% of thyroid lymphomas present as localized disease, clinical stage IE or IIE. Cervical lymph nodes are involved in 20% to 48% of patients, and the mediastinum is involved in 30% to 40%. It is important to note that less than half of reported patients have completed recommended diagnostic evaluations for lymphoma staging, including computerized tomography, lymphangiogram, bone marrow (BM) examination, or laparatomy to confirm the clinical stage.[72,73] For this reason, patients have not received consistent treatment approaches within each series, making it difficult to draw any firm conclusion about treatment.

The role of adjuvant chemotherapy following surgery or radiation therapy to reduce local recurrence or to prevent distant relapse depends on the histologic subtype of the lymphoma being treated. For diffuse large cell lymphomas, the addition of combination chemotherapy consisting of cyclophosphamide, vincristine, and prednisolone (CVP) following radiation, results in significant improvement in relapse free and overall 5-year survival.[74–76] For low grade histologies, the number of patients that have been studied preclude formulating definite conclusions.[77,78] In two studies, none of 11 patients relapsed when adjuvant CVP therapy was employed compared to 7 of 18 patients who relapsed when radiation therapy alone was used.[76,79] In contrast, adjuvant CVP therapy failed to affect relapse-free or overall survival in two other studies.[75,80]

More recently developed doxorubicin-containing combination chemotherapy regimens, including cyclophosphamide, doxorubicin, vincristine, and prednisone (CHOP); methotrexate, bleomycin, doxorubicin, cyclophosphamide, vincristine, and dexamethasone (m-BACOD); methotrexate, with leucovorin, doxorubicin, cyclophosphamide, vincristine, prednisone, and bleomycin (MACOP-B); and prednisone, methotrexate, doxorubicin, cylophosphamide, and etoposide combined with mechlorethamine, vincristine, procarbazine, and prednisone (proMACE-MOPP), or with cytarabine, bleomycin, vincristine, methotrexate with leucovorin, and prednisone (proMACE-CytaBOM) as well as other combinations, appear to be more effective than CVP against diffuse large cell lymphomas.[81–83] These regimens have resulted in 60% to 80% complete remissions and 50% long-term

Table 13.1. Chemotherapy for advanced thyroid cancer*

Drug regimens	Number of evaluable patients	Number of responders, (%)	References
Well-Differentiated			
Doxorubicin	49	15 (31)	16,18,19
Aclarubicin	11	3 (27)	20
Mitoxantrone	16	1 (6)	21
Doxorubicin + cisplatin	26	4 (15)	19,24
Doxorubicin + cisplatin + vindesine	8	0 (0)	25
Doxorubicin + bleomycin + vincristine	14	6 (43)	22,26
Doxorubicin + bleomycin + vincristine + melphalan	5	1 (20)	27
Anaplastic			
Doxorubicin	43	7 (16)	16,18,19,35
Doxorubicin + cisplatin	25	7 (28)	19,24,102
Doxorubicin + bleomycin + vincristine	10	7 (70)	26,27

Drugs	Number of evaluable patients	Number of responders (%)	References
Medullary			
Doxorubicin	52	17 (33)	18,19,54–56
Cisplatin	13	1 (8)	22
Doxorubicin + cisplatin	13	3 (23)	19,24,63
Doxorubicin + bleomycin + vincristine	2	2 (100)	22
Streptozotocin	3	0 (0)	57,58,62
Dacarbazine (+/−fluorouracil +/−cyclophosphamide + vincristin)	4	3 (75)	60,62,65
Thyroid lymphoma			
CHOP† +/−bleomycin	8	5 (63)	92,93

1. Table does not include reported responses to chemotherapy as part of a combined modality treatment. For details, see text.
†CHOP = cyclophosphamide, doxorubicin, vincristine, and prednisone.

disease-free survival in advanced nodal large cell lymphoma. In patients with stage I and II large cell lymphoma, these regimens may result in approximately 80% five-year survival.[84,85] Several studies that have combined these chemotherapy regimens with involved field radiotherapy also report relapse-free survival of over 80%.[86–88] Other combined modality studies reported similar results.[89,90] From limited experience in other studies in which chemotherapy was used alone, it is not clear whether the addition of involved field radiation therapy adds significantly to relapse rates or survival.[85,91]

The above discussion refers to the treatment of lymphomas in general, and whereas the same treatment strategies may be applied to thyroid lymphoma, the data available on the chemothermpy of thyroid lymphoma as a seperate entity is limited. The observations of Vigliotti et al,[92] Leedman et al.[93] and Connors et al.[86] have been presented in detail in chapter 10.

Therefore, after adequate staging, thyroid large cell lymphoma can be treated similarly to other stage I and II nodal or extranodal large cell lymphoma utilizing primary combination chemotherapy and involved-field radiation. Although the evidence is not as convincing for low-grade (follicular small cell) lymphoma, it probably should be treated in the same way. Small intrathyroid lymphoma can be treated with radiation alone. For patients with advanced stage III or IV tumors, the use of a current combination chemotherapy regimen as discussed above should be considered.

As discussed in Chapter 10, the prognosis of thyroid plasmacytoma is much better than that of thyroid lymphoma. Thyroid plasmacytoma, which is often associated with chronic lymphocytic thyroiditis, usually presents as a slow-growing thyroid mass. Approximately 33% of these patients have an associated monoclonal gammopathy or urinary Bence Jones protein.[94] Following surgery with or without radiation, 88% of patients respond. Only a few have had local recurrence or systemic dissemination. Therefore, there is usually no role for chemotherapy in the treatment of most patients with thyroid plasmacytoma. For the rare patient that develops multiple myeloma, combination chemotherapy with melphalan and prednisone or other combinations are effective treatment regimens.[95]

Summary and Current Recommendations

For most thyroid cancers, chemotherapy does not completely eradicate tumor, (Table 13.1) nor has it been proven to improve survival in randomized trials. Hence, with the exception of thyroid lymphoma; chemotherapy, alone or in combination with other treatment modalities is mainly a palliative therapy for patients with advanced thyroid cancer. Although the consideration of the major and minor complications associated with chemotherapy treatment is beyond the scope of this chapter, these need to be incorporated into the overall benefit-to-risk consideration that is part of every treatment decision.[2] In general, indications for chemotherapeutic treatment of advanced well-differentiated or medullary thyroid cancer are as follows:

1. Symptoms caused by the tumor, such as pain or the watery diarrhea syndrome associated with MTC.
2. A potentially life or vital function–threatening complication, such as airway obstruction, spinal cord compression from an epidural mass, hepatic dysfunction from metastatic tumor, or pulmonary lymphangitic spread.
3. Rapid tempo of tumor progression.

Anaplastic thyroid carcinoma is such a rapidly fatal disease that all treatment modalities should be used early in the course of disease in order to achieve local control and hopefully prevent metastases. Curative combined-modality treatment should be used for patients with thyroid lymphoma.

References

1. Tannock I. Cell kinetics and chemotherapy: a critical review. Cancer Treat Rep 1978;62:1117–1133.
2. Chabner BA. Clinical strategies for cancer treatment: The role of drugs. In: Chabner BA, Collins JM, eds. Cancer Chemotherapy: Principles & Practices. Philadelphia: J.B. Lippincott Company;1990:1.
3. Goldie JH, Coldman AJ. A mathematic model for relating the drug sensitivity of tumors to the spontaneous mutation rate. Cancer Treat Rep 1979;63:1727–1733.
4. DeVita VT, Schein PS. The use of drugs in combination for the treatment of cancer: rationale and results. N Engl J Med 1973;288:998–1006.
5. Hryniuk WM. Average relative dose intensity and the impact on design on clinical trials. Semin Oncol 1987;14:65–74.
6. Bonadonna G, Beretta G, Tancini G et al. Adriamycin (NSC-123127) Studies at the Istituto Nazionale Tumori, Milan. Cancer Chemotherapy Rep Part 3, 1975;6:231–245.
7. Poster DS, Bruno S, Penta J, Pina K, Catane R. Current status of chemotherapy in the treatment of advanced carcinoma of the thyroid gland. Cancer Clin Trials 1981;4:301–307.
8. Burt AD, Kerr DJ, Brown IL, Boyle P. Lymphoid and epithelial markers in small cell anaplastic thyroid tumours. J Clin Pathol 1985;38:893–896.
9. Compagno J, Oertel JE. Malignant lymphoma and other lymphoproliferative disorder of the thyroid gland. Am J Clin Pathol 1980;74:1–11.
10. Mambo ND, Irwin SM. Anaplastic small cell neoplasms of the thyroid: An immunoperoxidase study. Hum Pathol 1984;15:55–60.
11. Hay ID, Grant CS, Taylor WF, McConahey WM. Ipsilateral lobectomy versus bilateral lobar resection in papillary thyroid carcinoma: A retrospective analysis of surgical outcome using a novel prognostic scoring system. Surgery 1987;102:1088–1095.
12. Mazzaferri EL. Papillary thyroid carcinoma: Factors influencing prognosis and current therapy. Seminars in Oncology 1987;14:315–332.
13. Smith SA, Hay ID, Goellner JR et al. Mortality from papillary thyroid carcinoma. Cancer 1988;62:1381–1388.

14. Gottlieb JA, Hill CS Jr, Ibanez ML, Clark RL. Chemotherapy of thyroid cancer. Cancer, 1972;30:848–853.
15. Gottlieb JA, Hill CS Jr. Chemotherapy of thyroid cancer with Adriamycin. N Engl J Med 1974;290:193–197.
16. O'Bryan RM, Baker LH, Gottlieb JE, Rivkin B et al. Dose response evaluation of Adriamycin in human neoplasia. Cancer 1977;39:1940–1948.
17. Shimaoka K. Adjunctive Management of Thyroid Cancer: Chemotherapy. Journal of Surgical Oncology 1980;15:283–286.
18. Gottlieb JA, Hill CS Jr. Adriamycin (NSC-123127) Therapy in thyroid carcinoma. Cancer Chemother Rep Part 3, 1975;6:283–296.
19. Shimaoka K, Schoenfeld DA, DeWys WD et al. A randomized trial of doxorubicin versus doxorubicin plus cisplatin in patients with advanced thyroid carcinoma. Cancer 1985;56:2155–2160.
20. Samonigg H, Hossfeld DK, Spehn J et al. Aclarubicin in advanced thyroid cancer: A phase II study. Eur J of Cancer Clin Oncol 1988;24:1271–1275.
21. Schlumberger M, Parmentier C. Phase II Evaluation of mitoxantrone in advanced non anaplastic thyroid cancer. Bull Cancer 1989;76:403–406.
22. Hoskin PJ, Harmer C. Chemotherapy for thyroid cancer. Radiotherapy and Oncology 1987;10:187–194.
23. Harada T, Nishikawa Y, Suzuki T, Ito K, Baba S. Bleomycin treatment for cancer of the thyroid. Am J Surg 1971;122:53–57.
24. Williams SD, Birch R, Einhorn LH. Phase II evaluation of doxorubicin plus cisplatin in advanced thyroid cancer: A southeastern cancer study group trial. Cancer Treatment Reports 1986;70:405–407.
25. Scherübl H, Raue F, Ziegler R. Combination chemotherapy of advanced medullary and differentiated thyroid cancer. J Cancer Res Clin Oncol 1990;116:21–23.
26. Sokal M, Harmer CL. Chemotherapy for anaplastic carcinoma of the thyroid. Clinical Oncology 1978;4:3–10.
27. Bukowski RM, Brown L, Weick JK et al. Combination chemotherapy of metastatic thyroid cancer. Am J Clin Oncol 1983;6:579–581.
28. Kim JH, Leeper RD. Treatment of locally advanced thyroid carcinoma with combination doxorubicin and radiation therapy. Cancer 1987;60:2372–2375.
29. Carcangiu ML, Steeper T, Zampi G, Rosai J. Anaplastic thyroid carcinoma. Am J Clin Pathol 1985;83:135–158.
30. Nel CJC, van Heerden JA, Goellner JR et al. Anaplastic carcinoma of the thyroid: A clinicopathologic study of 82 Cases. Mayo Clin Proc 1985;60:51–58.
31. Venkatesh YSS, Ordonez NG, Schultz PN et al. Anaplastic Carcinoma of the Thyroid. Cancer 1990; 66:321–330.
32. Tallroth E, Wallin G, Lundell G et al. Multimodality treatment in anaplastic giant cell thyroid carcinoma. Cancer 1987;60:1428–1431.
33. Aldinger KA, Samaan NA, Ibanez M, Hill CS Jr. Anaplastic carcinoma of the thyroid. Cancer 1978;41:2267–2275.
34. Rogers JD, Lindberg RD, Hill CS Jr, Gehan E. Spindle and giant cell carcinoma of the thyroid: A different therapeutic approach. Cancer 1974;34:1328–1332.
35. Schoumacher P, Metz R, Bey P, Chesneau AM. Anaplastic carcinoma of the thyroid gland. Europ J Cancer 1977;13:381–383.
36. Higby DJ, Wallace HJ, Albert DJ, Holland JF. Diaminodichloroplatinum: A Phase I Study showing responses in testicular and other tumors. Cancer 1974;33:1219–1225.
37. Weisberg A, Luongo V, Bochetto J. Giant cell carcinoma of the thyroid gland: Long survival after combination chemotherapy. Southern Medical Journal 1981;74:638–639.
38. Casterline PF, Jaques DA, Blom H, Wartofsky L. Anaplastic giant and spindle-cell carcinoma of the thyroid. Cancer 1980;45:1689–1692.
39. Spires JR, Schwartz MR, Miller RH. Anaplastic thyroid carcinoma. Arch Otolaryngol Head Neck Surg 1988;114:40–44.
40. Durie BG, Hellman D, Woolfenden JM, O'Mara R, Kartchner M, Salmon SE. High-risk thyroid cancer. Cancer Clin Trials, 1981;4:67–73.
41. Simpson WJ. Anaplastic thyroid carcinoma: a new approach. Canadian J Surgery 1980;23:25–27.
42. Scher HI, Yagoda A, Herr HW et al. Neoadjuvant M-Vac (methotrexate, vinblastine, doxorubicin and cisplatin) for extravesical urinary tract tumors. J Urol 1988;139:475–477.
43. Clark JR, Fallon BG, Dreyfuss AI, Norris CM, Anderson JW, Ervin TJ, Anderson RF, Chaffey JT, Miller D, Frei E. Chemotherapeutic strategies in the multidisciplinary treatment of head and neck cancer. Semin Oncol 1988;15:35–44.
44. Perloff M, Lesnick GJ, Korzun A, Chu F, Holland JF et al. Combination chemotherapy with mastectomy or radiotherapy for stage III breast carcinom: a Cancer and Leukemia Group B study. J Clin Oncol 1988;6:261.
45. Winkler K, Beron G, Delling G, Heise U, Kabish H et al. Noeadjuvant chemotherapy of osteosarcoma: results of a randomized cooperative trial (COSS-82) with salvage chemotherapy based on histological tumor response. J Clin Oncol 1988;6:329.
46. Spanos GA, Wolk D, Desner MR et al. Preoperative chemotherapy for giant cell carcinoma of the thyroid. Cancer 1982;50:2252–2256.
47. Tennvall J, Tallroth E, ef Hassan A et al. Anaplastic thyroid carcinoma. Doxorubicin, hyperfractionated radiotherapy and surgery. Acta Oncol 1990;29:1025–1028.
48. Saad MF, Ordonez NG, Rashid RK et al. Medullary carcinoma of the thyroid. Medicine 1984;63:319–342.
49. Sizemore GW. Medullary carcinoma of the thyroid gland. Seminars in Oncology 1987;14:306–314.
50. Norton JA, Froome LC, Farrell RE, Wells SA. Multiple endocrine neoplasia type IIb. Surgical Clinics of North America 1979;59:109–118.
51. Baylin SB, Mendelsohn G. Medullary thyroid carcinoma: A model for the study of human tumor progres-

sion and cell heterogeneity. In: Owens AH Jr., Coffey DS, Baylin SB, eds. Tumor cell heterogeneity, origins, and implications. New York: Academic Press;1982:12.

52. Saad MF, Ordonez NG, Guido JJ, Samaan NA. The prognostic value of calcitonin immunostaining in medullary carcinoma of the thyroid. J Clin Endocrinology and Metabolism 1984;59:850–856.
53. Saad MF, Fritsche HA, Samaan NA. Diagnostic and prognostic values of carcinoembryonic antigen in medullary carcinoma of the thyroid. J Clin Endocrinology and Metabolism 1984;58:889–894.
54. Husain M, Alsever RN, Lock JP, George WF, Katz FH. Failure of medullary carcinoma of the thyroid to respond to doxorubicin therapy. Hormone Res 1978;9:22–25.
55. Rougier P, Parmentier C, Laplanche A et al. Medullary thyroid carcinoma: Prognostic factors and treatment. Int J Radiation Oncology Biol Phys 1983;9:161–169.
56. Simpson WJ, Palmer JA, Rosen IB, Mustard RA. Management of medullary carcinoma of the thyroid. Am J of Surgery 1982;144:420–421.
57. Pearse AGE, Polak JM. Endocrine tumors of neural crest origin: Neurolymphomas, apudomas and the APUD concept. Med Biol 1974;52:3.
58. Kvols LK, Buck M. Chemotherapy of endocrine malignancies: A review. Sem Oncol 1987;14:343–353.
59. Weiss RB. Failure of streptozotocin in rare hormonally active malignancies. Cancer Treatment Reports 1978;62:847–849.
60. Kessinger A, Foley JF, Lemon HM. Therapy of malignant APUD cell tumors. Cancer 1983;51:790–794.
61. Fiore JJ, Kelsen DP, Cheng E, Dukeman M. Phase II Trial of VP-16 in Apudomas. Proc Amer Assoc Cancer Res 1984;15:174.
62. Petursson SR. Metastic medullary thyroid carcinoma. Cancer 1988;62:1899–1903.
63. Sridhar KS, Holland JF, Brown JC et al. Doxorubicin plus cisplatin in the treatment of apudomas. Cancer 1985;55:2634–2637.
64. Averbuch SD, Steakley CS, Young RC, Gelmann EP, Goldstein DS, Stull R, Keiser HR. Malignant pheochromocytoma: Effective treatment with a combination of cyclophosphamide, vincristine, and dacarbazine. Ann Int Med 1988;109:267.
65. Averbuch S, Wu L, Pertsemlidis D, Drakes T. Cyclophosphamide (C), vincristine (V), and dacarbazine (D) for advanced neuroendocrine carcinomas. Proc Amer Soc Clin Oncol 1990;9:382.
66. Gorden P, Comi RJ, Maton PN, Go VLW. Somatostatin and somatostatin analogue (SMS 201-995) in treatment of hormone-secreting tumors of the pituitary and gastrointestinal tract and non-neoplastic diseases of the gut. Ann Intern Med 1989;110:35–50.
67. Oberg K, Eriksson B. Medical treatment of neuroendocrine gut and pancreatic tumors. Acta Oncol 1989;28:425–431.
68. Modigliani E, Guliana JM, Maroni M et al. Effets de l'administration sous cutanée de la sandostatine (SMS 201.995) en sous cutané dans 18 cas de cancer médullaire du corps thyroïde. Annales d'Endocrinologie 1989;50:483–488.
69. Mahler C, Verhelst J, De Longueville M, Harris A. Long-term treatment of metastatic medullary thyroid carcinoma with the somatostatin analogue octreotide. Clin Endocrinol 1990;33:261–269.
70. Aozasa J, Inoue A, Tajima K, Miyauchi A, Matsuzuka F, Kuma K. Malignant lymphomas of the thyroid gland. Analysis of 79 patients with emphasis on histologic prognostic factors. Cancer 1986;58:L100–104.
71. Tupchong L, Hughes F, Harmer CL. Primary lymphoma of the thyroid: clinical features, prognostic factors, and results of treatment. Int J Radiation Oncology Biol Phys 1986;12:1813–1824.
72. Butler JS, Brady LW, Amendola BE. Lymphoma of the thyroid: Report of five cases and review. Am J Clin Oncol 1990;13(1):64–69.
73. Souhami L, Simpson WJ, Carruthers JS. Malignant lymphoma of the thyroid gland. Int J Radiation Oncology Biol Phys 1980;6:1143–1147.
74. Glatstein E, Donaldson SS, Rosenberg SA, Kaplan HS. Combined modality therapy in malignant lymphomas. Cancer Treatment Reports, 1977;61:1199–1207.
75. Monfardini S, Banfi A, Bonadonna G, Rilke F, Milani F, Valagussa P, Lattuada A. Improved five year survival after combined radiotherapy-chemotherapy for stage I–II non-Hodgkin's lymphoma. Int J Radiation Oncology Biol Phys 1980;6:125–134.
76. Nissen NI, Ersbøll J, Hansen HS, Walbom-Jørgensen S, Pedersen-Bjergaard J, Hansen MM, Rygard J. A randomized study of radiotherapy versus radiotherapy plus chemotherapy in stage I–II non-Hodgkin's lymphomas. Cancer 1983;52:1–7.
77. Gomez GA, Barcos M, Krishnamsetty RM, Panahon AM, Han T, Henderson ES. Treatment of early—stages I and II—nodular, poorly differentiated lymphocytic lymphoma. Am J Clin Oncol 1986;9(1):40–44.
78. Paryani SB, Hoppe RT, Cox RS, Colby TV, Rosenberg SA, Kaplan HS. Analysis of non-Hodgkin's lymphomas with nodular and favorable histologies, Stages I and II. Cancer 1983;52:230–2307.
79. Landberg TG, Håkansson LG, Möller TR, Mattsson WK, Landys KE, Johansson BG, Killander DCF, Molin BF, Westling PF, Lenner PH, Dahl OG. CVP-remission-maintenance in stage I or II non-Hodgkin's lymphomas: Preliminary results of a randomized study. Cancer 1979;44:831–838.
80. Phillips DL. Radiotherapy in the treatment of localised non-Hodgkin's lymphoma. Clin Radiology 1981;32:543–546.
81. DeVita VT, Hubbard SM, Longo DL. The chemotherapy of lymphomas: Looking back, moving forward—The Richard and Hinda Rosenthal Foundation award lecture. Cancer Res 1987;47:5810.
82. Kwak LW, Halpern J, Olshen RA, Horning SJ. Prognostic significance of actual dose intensity in diffuse large-cell lymphoma: Results of a tree-structured survival analysis. J Clin Oncol 1990;8:963–977.

83. Longo DL, DeVita VT Jr, Duffey PL, Wesley MN, Ihde DC, Hubbard SM, Gilliom M, Jaffe ES, Cossman J, Fisher RI, Young RC. Superiority of ProMACE-CytaBOM over ProMACE-MOPP in the treatment of advanced diffuse aggressive lymphoma: Results of a prospective randomized trial. J Clin Oncol 1991;9:25–38.
84. Cabanillas F, Bodey GP, Freireich EJ. Management with chemotherapy only of stage I and II malignant lymphoma of aggressive histologic types. Cancer, 1980;46:2356–2359.
85. Miller TP, Jones SE. Initial chemotherapy for clinically localized lymphomas of unfavorable histology. Blood 1983;62:413–418.
86. Connors JM, Klimo P, Fairey RN, Voss N. Brief chemotherapy and involved field radiation therapy for limited-stage, histologically aggressive lymphoma. Annals of Internal Medicine 1987;107:25–30.
87. Jones SE, Miller TP, Connors JM. Long-term follow-up and analysis for prognostic factors for patients with limited-stage diffuse large-cell lymphoma treated with initial chemotherapy with or without adjuvant radiotherapy. J Clin Oncol 1989;7:1186–1191.
88. Longo DL, Glatstein E, Duffey PL, Ihde DC, Hubbard SM, Fisher RI, Jaffe ES, Gilliom M, Young RC, DeVita VT Jr. Treatment of localized aggressive lymphomas with combination chemotherapy followed by involved-field radiation therapy. J Clin Oncol 1989;7:1295–1302.
89. Mauch P, Leonard R, Skarin A, Rosenthal D, Come S, Chaffey J, Hellman S, Canellos G. Improved Survival Following Combined Radiation Therapy and Chemotherapy for Unfavorable Prognosis Stage I–II Non-Hodgkin's Lymphomas. J Clin Oncol 1985; 3:1301–1308.
90. Prestidge BR, Horning SJ, Hoppe RT. Combined modality therapy for stage I–II large cell lymphoma. Int J Radiation Oncology Biol Phys 1988;15:633–639.
91. Shipp MA, Klatt MM, Yeap B, Jochelson MS, Mauch PM, Rosenthal DS, Skarin AT, Canellos GP. Patterns of relapse in large-cell lymphoma patients with bulk disease: Implications for the use of adjuvant radiation therapy. J Clin Oncol 1989;7:613–618.
92. Vigliotti A, Kong JS, Fuller LM, Velasquez WS. Thyroid lymphomas stages IE and IIE: Comparative results for radiotherapy only, combination chemotherapy only, and multimodality treatment. Int J Radiation Oncology Biol Phys 1986;12:1807–1812.
93. Leedman PJ, Sheridan WP, Downey WF, Fox RM, Martin FIR. Combination chemotherapy as single modality therapy for stage IE and IIE thyroid lymphoma. Medical Journal of Australia 1990;152:40–43.
94. Rubin J, Johnson JT, Killeen R, Barnes L. Extramedullary plasmacytoma of the thyroid associated with a serum monoclonal gammopathy. Arch Otolaryngol Head Neck Surg 1990;116:855–859.
95. Cooper MR, McIntyre OR, Propert KJ et al. Single, sequential, and multiple alkylating agent therapy for multiple myeloma: A CALGB study. J Clin Oncol 1986;4:1331–1339.

Index